THE
PALEO CUPBOARD
COOKBOOK
real food, real flavor

Written and Photographed by
Amy Densmore

VICTORY BELT PUBLISHING INC.

LAS VEGAS

First Published in 2015 by Victory Belt Publishing Inc.

Copyright © 2015 Amy Densmore

ISBN-13: 978-1-628600-84-1

Photography: Amy Densmore
Front Cover Photography by Hayley and Bill Staley
Design: Yordan Terziev and Boryana Yordanova
Personal/Lifestyle Portraits: Patty Brutlag, petulapea.com

Printed in the U.S.A.
RRD 0115

contents

recipes

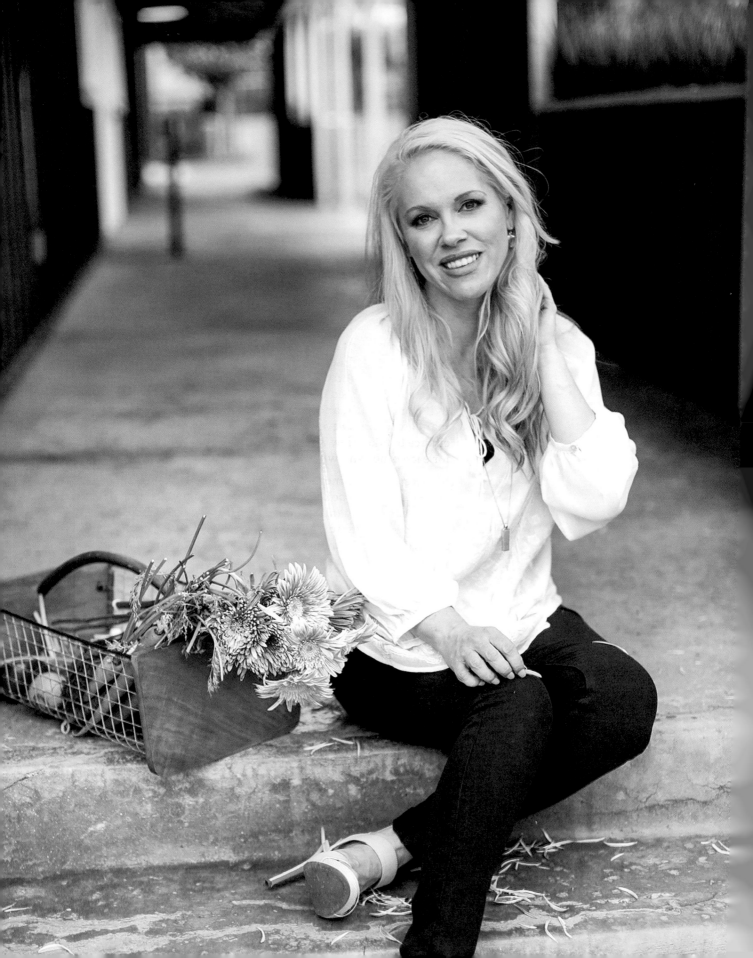

introduction

a LITTLE about ME

Growing up watching my grandmother cook was an experience I will treasure forever. I don't think the word *cook* even does it justice, because she showed me that creating a meal involves so much more than just combining ingredients. She put thought and care into every aspect of it, from thinking up recipes that her family and friends would enjoy to picking out the freshest ingredients she could afford to making sure everyone was sitting, eating, and laughing before she served herself. She put so much love, attention, and care into each meal, and that shone through in everything she made. My mother followed in her footsteps, and no matter where we were living or what ups and downs we were going through, dinner was a mandatory family event. It wasn't fancy or pretentious; it was just a chance to take a few moments out of the day and show appreciation for each other and what we had.

It's because of my mother and grandmother that I have the appreciation for cooking that I do today. I'm not going to pretend that there's some fairy tale going on in my house and there's a fresh-from-the-oven casserole on the table every evening at six p.m. sharp. Sometimes meals are just reheated leftovers or bits and pieces of whatever is in the refrigerator. And every now and then Mommy wishes that instead of making dinner she could just have a glass—or bottle—of wine and go to bed. But there is something so rewarding and therapeutic for me about pausing for a few moments in the kitchen, taking a pile of fresh ingredients, and using my hands to create something that not only tastes amazing but also will nourish me and whomever I might have the pleasure of cooking for. Even though there's usually a kid hanging on my leg, a dog barking, a phone ringing, and all sorts of other chaos going on, I still feel in my element when I am cooking.

WHY PALEO?

When I stumbled upon the Paleo lifestyle, I had started feeling run-down and tired almost every day. I was nauseous a lot of the time after eating and was getting horrible headaches. And at the time, I thought I was doing everything "healthy": I was following a low-fat diet and counting every calorie I put in my body, I led an active lifestyle, and I took a daily multivitamin. With a full-time corporate job and two energetic girls, not feeling well every single day just wasn't an option, and I knew I had to make some big changes. I removed anything from my diet that I thought was not natural for a human to eat. That meant eliminating grains, refined sugars, dairy, and processed foods. I decided I would try it for one month and see how I felt. I figured I could withstand anything for one month.

Within a week I felt amazing. I had so much energy that I was bouncing off the walls, and in less than three weeks I had lost ten pounds. I had been feeling bad for so long that it had become normal for me. I thought stomach pain after a meal was just part of eating and that restless sleep was just something I had to accept. I had forgotten what healthy really felt like. The drastic difference I felt in such a short amount of time made me curious, and after doing some research I discovered that the eating plan I was following was almost identical to the Paleo diet. The more I read, the more I realized that many people had the exact same experience as me, and I decided to adopt Paleo as a lifestyle going forward.

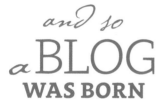

and so a BLOG WAS BORN

I never intended to have a blog. I didn't even know what a blog was. But when friends and family noticed the changes in my health and appearance and wanted to know what I was eating and how to make it, I needed a way for everyone to find my recipes in one central place. So I stumbled along, picked the first domain name I thought of that was available, and started plugging away creating *Paleo Cupboard*.

Very quickly I noticed that other people were visiting my blog, following me on social media, and reaching out to me with their stories. Over time, *Paleo Cupboard* grew to become a big part of my life, and my readers have turned into a wonderful and supportive virtual family. My neighbors may think I am a bit crazy when they pass by my front window and see me standing on my dining room table taking pictures of food, and my kids think it's silly that I have to rush a plate into whichever room has the best lighting before we can all eat, but it is all part of the fun. I'm not going to lie, it takes a lot of time and energy to run a food blog, but hearing stories from those who have found better health and healing through a real-food lifestyle makes every minute spent on it worthwhile.

and Then a COOK-BOOK WAS BORN

Just as running a blog was something I never set out to do, I never in my wildest dreams thought I would be writing a cookbook. And when I was fortunate enough to have the right opportunity presented to me, I instantly went into a state of panic. Not because of the amount of work involved, but because I knew that creating a cookbook that would appeal to everyone was impossible. I have done some slightly scary and weird things in my life, like jumping off a mountain in Austria strapped to a man wearing lederhosen and a parachute, but this situation was far more strange and terrifying. How would I be able to help everyone if I couldn't make a book that appealed to everyone?! Some people want to cook very creative recipes with unique ingredients, while others want recipes that are classic and simple. Some people love to cook and enjoy spending time in the kitchen, while others want to get in and out of the kitchen as quickly as possible. Taking all that into account is enough to almost drive a person crazy, so in the end I decided to stay true to what I know and showcase recipes that I grew up cooking and that my family still enjoys eating to this day. Some may be familiar to you, and some may be more creative and might inspire you to try something new. Some are quick and easy, and others let you spend a little bit more time in the kitchen experimenting.

I am honored to be able to share my stories, tips, thoughts, and recipes with you. I truly believe that good food and humor are the best medicines, and I've tried to fill the pages of this book with as much of both as I could. These are recipes that my family has been cooking for years or that I learned to make on the many journeys and adventures I have had so far in my life. Some I have had to adapt to fit a Paleo diet, and some were already Paleo without my having to change a thing. These recipes are here for you to experiment with and enjoy, and my wish is that they bring you as much health and happiness as they have me and my family.

Since we all have unique tastes that can differ quite a bit, my advice to you is to use the recipes in this book as starting points and make them your own. Think of them as templates to work from, not strict guidelines that you need to follow down to the teaspoon. If your grandmother always added mushrooms to her cottage pie, then add mushrooms. If you just can't get enough garlic, then double the amount. Cooking is more fun when you experiment. At the end of the day, we all need to eat to survive, so whether you have to cook out of necessity or you have a passion for creating amazing food, you still should be eating the best-tasting food possible. My goal for this book is to show that a Paleo diet doesn't have to be boring or restricting, so that instead of worrying about what you can't have, you can see all the wonderful things you can have. So grab your cookware and your spice rack, because you and I are going on a taste bud adventure, and hopefully we'll have some laughs along the way.

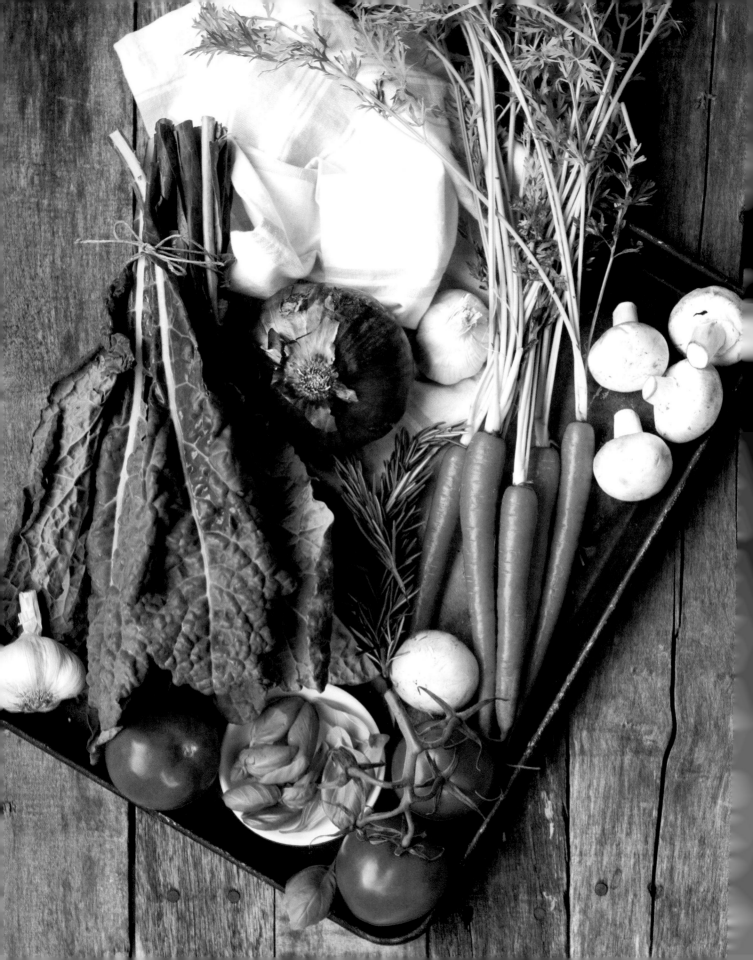

what is paleo?

For many of us, food has become so easily available and accessible that we don't give much thought to what we're putting in our bodies. In a day and age when, in many countries, you can be handed your dinner from a drive-through window, it is easy to forget the significance of food and the role it plays in our lives. What we eat, where our food comes from, how we gather it, how we cook it, and even who we eat it with are all important parts of our overall health and well-being.

The basic premise of the Paleo diet stems from the idea that human DNA has not changed significantly since the Paleolithic era (hence the name *Paleo*), and therefore our bodies are designed to work best on a diet similar to the one our ancestors followed thousands of years ago. While we may not know exactly what the typical diet of ancient humans was, we know that it did not include things like bread, pasta, processed foods, or refined sugars, all of which are foods that have little to no nutritional value. Instead, ancient humans ate a diet based on whole foods found in nature, such as meats, seafood, vegetables, fruits, and nuts, all of which are rich in nutrients.

That said, the point of this lifestyle is not to try to eat exactly what our ancestors ate. It's to make healthy choices and eat foods that our bodies were designed to consume and that will help us function at our very best. A pure hunter-gatherer diet is not very practical in this day and age, unless of course you live in a remote area without any modern technology, in which case you probably aren't reading this book anyway. And while the same exact foods that were available thousands of years ago are not all available today in the exact same form, we can still use the Paleo premise to make good choices with the foods we do have. Most of us who follow a Paleo lifestyle are just trying to eat the most nutrient-dense and minimally processed foods available, while still enjoying what we eat. To keep it simple, it's about eating real food. Make sense so far?

In the following pages, you'll find information about foods that are typically not part of the Paleo diet, foods that are, and some foods that fall into the controversial gray area. Remember that everyone's body is unique, and you need to find which foods work best for you. I also highly recommend the books listed in Resources (page 333) to get a better understanding of the science and nutrition behind the Paleo diet. I am not a trained nutritionist or scientist myself, and these books have been immensely helpful in explaining why so many people have seen such great results on a Paleo diet.

FOODS
TO AVOID

Many of the foods that are avoided on the Paleo diet because they're not whole foods are also those that many people have negative reactions to. This makes sense because the premise of the Paleo diet is that our bodies were never designed to consume those foods in the first place. An easy way to think about it is this: if you eat it and it usually makes you feel bad afterwards, you might not want to keep eating it.

You may read this list and furrow your brow and think things like, "What do you mean, no bread? Are you nuts, lady?!" But stick with me, because very soon we're going to talk about all the great things you do get to eat. So take a deep breath, relax, and read through this overview of the foods you may want to avoid.

Grains

Grains contain proteins called *lectins*, the most famous of which is gluten. For many people, lectins can cause digestive problems and systemic inflammation, which in turn is associated with all sorts of autoimmune problems, from irritable bowel syndrome to food allergies to thyroid problems. In addition, lectins can prevent your body from absorbing many vitamins and minerals. Sounds like a lot of good reasons to avoid them, right?

Including but not limited to:

Wheat (and everything made from it, including bread and pasta)

Barley

Corn

Oats

Rice

Refined Sugars

Refined sugars are pretty much void of nutrients, and consuming too much may cause problems such as insulin resistance, obesity, tooth decay, and digestive problems. And whenever you eat foods with refined sugars, you're not eating more nutrient-dense options, such as proteins and vegetables. Many people on a Paleo diet sweeten foods with raw honey instead—while refined sugars go through a manufacturing process that destroys any natural enzymes and vitamins, raw honey is minimally processed and has antioxidants and antimicrobial properties.

Including but not limited to:

Artificial sweeteners

Brown sugar

Corn syrup

Table sugar

Unclench your jaw; it is going to be all right, I promise. Let's keep going!

Processed Fats and Oils

Natural, minimally processed fats are an important part of a Paleo diet, but highly refined and processed fats and oils—such as vegetable oil, canola oil, sunflower oil, and margarine—should be avoided. These go through a great deal of chemical processing and contain trans fats (often called *partially hydrogenated oils*), which can be especially dangerous because they may lower levels of good cholesterol (HDL) and increase levels of bad cholesterol (LDL), increasing the risk of heart disease.

Including but not limited to:

Canola oil

Cottonseed oil

Margarine

Safflower oil

Soybean oil

Sunflower oil

Vegetable oil

Are there tears streaming down your face yet? Stick with me; it will all be okay.

Processed Foods

Highly processed foods usually contain some refined sugars and/or processed fats, both of which you'll find on this list of foods to avoid. By "processed foods," I'm not referring to things like ground beef or canned tomatoes—even though yes, technically, these have been processed— but rather foods that have been *chemically* processed in some way or have had artificial substances added. Opt for fresh ingredients whenever possible and always check the labels on everything else; even the most innocent-looking items, such as dried fruit, can have some sneaky and unwanted additives.

Including but not limited to:

Soda

Energy drinks

Candy

Packaged snacks and meals

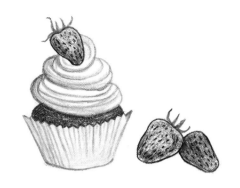

A NOTE ABOUT PALEO TREATS

A few recipes in this book may be considered treats. These include things like waffles, baked goods, and desserts—even though the recipes for these contain Paleo-friendly ingredients, they're less nutrient-dense than other foods.

Many people in the Paleo community have a strong opinion about whether treats can really be Paleo, which can be confusing for people who are new to this lifestyle. Some people think you should never touch a treat, while others make them part of their daily diet. I fall somewhere in the middle of that spectrum and enjoy them in moderation. There are times when I like to make my kids waffles on a Sunday morning or I want to bring a gluten-free dessert to an office event. But just because we slap the word *Paleo* in front of something doesn't mean that we can shove it in our faces with reckless abandon. A cupcake is still a cupcake, whether we call it Paleo or not. I know that I will not hit my health goals if I am eating treats every day, and eating too many means I'm not eating more nutrient-dense foods—I try to focus instead on high-quality proteins, lots of vegetables, and a moderate amount of healthy fats and fruit.

Will eating a treat on occasion totally deter you from your health goals? For most people, probably not. Will eating a treat every day help you reach your health goals? For most people, probably not. But your personal approach to treats needs to tie back to what I mentioned before: you have to eat what is right for your body, lifestyle, and health goals.

FOODS
TO ENJOY

Enough about the stuff we should avoid. Let's talk about the good stuff! The great thing about a Paleo diet is that you get to eat so many amazing and delicious foods. Below is a list of the main foods that are generally enjoyed.

Keep in mind, though, that some people have sensitivities to foods that are in this category, such as eggs, nuts, and nightshades (including eggplant, tomatoes, and peppers). It's important to tailor the diet to work for you, so if you have any food sensitivities, seek the advice of a doctor or nutritionist on how best to adjust the Paleo diet for your needs.

Meat

Meat has had a bad reputation for quite a while, but it contains vital nutrients such as B vitamins, iron, and magnesium, and lean proteins have been shown to support strong bones and muscle development. Proteins found in meat also help keep us feeling fuller longer, which is a nice bonus. Look for grass-fed, pasture-raised meat whenever possible—it's generally free of the chemicals, antibiotics, and growth hormones found in conventional grain-fed meat.

Including but not limited to:

Beef	Lamb
Bison/Buffalo	Pork
Chicken	Turkey
Duck	Veal

Seafood

Most seafood is packed with omega-3 fatty acids, nutrients, and protein, which makes it a great addition to your diet. While you may have heard concerns about mercury levels in fish, for most people, the amounts are so low that the benefits of eating fish far outweigh the risks. (Pregnant women and young children need to be more cautious, though. If you have any concerns, check out the Natural Resources Defense Council's website for a list of fish high in mercury: www.nrdc.org/health/effects/mercury/guide.asp.)

Some kinds of wild-caught fish and seafood are in danger of being overfished, and seeking out sustainably sourced seafood is the best way to protect them and help the environment. The Monterey Bay Aquarium's Seafood Watch (seafoodwatch.org; also available as an app) is a great resource for the most up-to-date news on the best seafood choices.

Including but not limited to:

Clams	Oysters
Crab	Prawns
Fish	Sardines
Lobster	Scallops
Mussels	Shrimp

Eggs

Eggs are a great source of protein, vitamins, and minerals, and although fears about cholesterol gave them a bad reputation for a long time, recent studies have shown that they do not have the negative effect on cholesterol levels that was previously thought.

Just as you consider the quality of the meat you buy, it's important to consider the quality of eggs, too. The food that the hens eat and the chemicals and antibiotics they are exposed to will have an impact on their eggs. Unfortunately, regulations are still fairly loose when it comes to labels like "organic," "free-range," and "cage-free"—they don't always mean that the hens were treated well and fed their natural diet. It's best to look for pastured eggs at your local farmers market, if possible, or at the grocery store—that means the hens were allowed free access to the outdoors and ate their natural diet of grass and bugs.

KINDS OF SWEET POTATOES

Sweet potatoes can be white- or red-skinned, although you'll often find red-skinned sweet potatoes labeled as "yams" in grocery stores. Red-skinned sweet potatoes tend to be softer and creamier when cooked, so they're better for recipes requiring mashed potatoes. White-skinned sweet potatoes are a bit firmer, so they're better for fries and other dishes where you want a more solid bite.

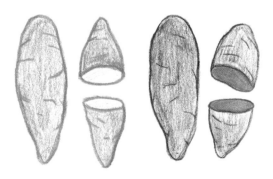

Vegetables and Fruits

Fruits and vegetables are great sources of antioxidants, vitamins, minerals, and fiber. Because of the high amount of natural sugars in fruit, if you're fairly sedentary or looking to lose weight, you may get better results if you eat fruit in moderation. That doesn't mean you have to give up eating fruit entirely; it just means you may not want to chow down on a huge bowl of fruit salad in one sitting.

Organic produce is generally best, since it doesn't have the pesticides that conventionally grown produce may. But if you want to figure out which foods are relatively safe to eat when conventionally grown, the Environmental Working Group (ewg.org) provides lists of foods that are the most and least contaminated by pesticides. These lists are called the "Dirty Dozen" and "Clean Fifteen," even though the count has changed since those names were created. My own rule of thumb, which pretty much follows the EWG lists, is to choose organic whenever the peel or exterior is eaten—apples, kale, strawberries, zucchini—and to choose nonorganic when the peel is removed prior to eating—avocados, bananas, onions.

Including but not limited to:

Apples	Eggplant	Pears
Artichokes	Garlic	Peppers
Arugula	Grapefruit	Pineapples
Asparagus	Grapes	Plums
Avocados	Green onions	Pomegranates
Bananas	Jicama	Radishes
Beets	Kale	Rhubarb
Blackberries	Kiwi	Rutabaga
Blueberries	Leeks	Shallots
Broccoli	Lemons	Spinach
Brussels sprouts	Lettuce	Squash
Cabbage	Limes	Strawberries
Cauliflower	Melons	Sweet potatoes
Celery	Mushrooms	Tangerines
Chard	Nectarines	Tomatoes
Cherries	Onions	Turnips
Collard greens	Oranges	Watermelon
Cucumbers	Peaches	Zucchini

Nuts and Seeds

While nuts and seeds are a good addition to your diet, when eaten in large quantities, they can be hard to digest and can trigger inflammation in some people, so you may want to eat them in moderation. This includes butters and flours made from nuts and seeds, such as almond flour and sunflower seed butter.

Choose nuts and seeds that have not been roasted in oil or covered in salt. And keep in mind that although peanuts have "nuts" in their name, they are a legume, not a nut. (See "Gray-Area Foods" on the next page for more about legumes.)

Including but not limited to:

Almonds	Pistachios
Cashews	Pumpkin seeds (pepitas)
Flax seeds	
Hazelnuts	Sesame seeds
Macadamia nuts	Sunflower seeds
Pecans	Tahini
Pine nuts	Walnuts

Healthy Fats and Oils

As important as it is to avoid unhealthy processed fats (see page 11), healthy, minimally processed fats from natural sources are an essential part of your daily diet. They give you energy, help your body absorb vitamins A, D, E, and K, and also play an important role in brain development and managing inflammation.

Including but not limited to:

Avocado oil	Lard
Coconut oil	Olive oil
Duck fat	Sesame oil
Ghee	Tallow

A NOTE ABOUT FOOD SOURCES AND BUDGETING

As you probably know, the outcome of a recipe partially depends on the quality of the ingredients you use—the fresher the ingredients, the better the dish tastes. Luckily, following the Paleo lifestyle means using quite a lot of fresh ingredients. As I mentioned earlier, using organic produce, grass-fed meats, and wild-caught seafood is ideal, and with good reason. What goes into the food we eat—and with nonorganic produce, grain-fed meat, and farmed seafood, that can include pesticides, grains, hormones, and antibiotics—plays a role in how that food interacts with our bodies.

But while organic and grass-fed are great food choices, for some of us, eating those foods every day is just not practical—they might not fit our budget, they might not be available where we live, or they might be really hard to access. As much as I've rearranged my budget to make healthier foods a priority, sometimes I walk through the organic produce section and my wallet says, "Not this week, honey; just keep on walking."

My advice is to do the best you can with what you have. If you're buying nonorganic produce instead of a bag of chips coated in artificial cheese, you're doing something great for your body and taking a giant leap in the right direction.

GRAY-AREA
FOODS

There are some foods that fall into the gray area when it comes to a Paleo lifestyle: some people embrace them while others believe they should be avoided completely. It's best to eliminate these foods for your first thirty days on Paleo to allow your body to heal in case you're sensitive to them. After that, you can slowly reintroduce them one by one if you want. If you have a negative reaction to any food when you reintroduce it, your body doesn't tolerate it well and you should avoid it in the future. If you have a weaker immune system, are looking to lose weight, or have a chronic illness, you may want to eliminate all these foods entirely from your diet—they may aggravate inflammation and further stress your body.

Alcohol

Most experts say that alcohol made from grains—including beer, whisky, and bourbon—is safe to drink because the distillation process removes gluten. However, not all alcohol is made exactly the same way, and some studies have found gluten in grain-based alcohol. To be on the safe side, many people, particularly those with celiac disease, avoid alcohol altogether. If your primary concern is avoiding gluten but you'd like to have alcohol, reach for tequila, rum, wine, or a gluten-free cider. But keep in mind that alcohol in any form can be hard on your liver and usually contains some form of sugar, so drinking in moderation is a smart choice.

I must confess that I have been known to enjoy an adult beverage on occasion, but as with the other foods on this list, you need to consider your goals and what works best for you.

Dairy

Many people have trouble digesting lactose, the main sugar found in milk and milk-based products, such as yogurt, cheese, and butter. This can cause stomach distress, skin breakouts and rashes, and a number of other issues.

But while ordinary dairy may be hard to digest, many lactose-intolerant people find they can tolerate ghee, which is clarified butter with the milk solids removed. Ghee is becoming more readily available in many stores, but you can also find instructions for making your own on page 320.

If you're one of those who can tolerate dairy well, seek out products from grass-fed animals that are not treated with hormones or antibiotics.

Including but not limited to:

Butter

Cheese

Cottage cheese

Cream

Milk

Yogurt

Legumes

Legumes are notorious for hindering the absorption of nutrients, being difficult to digest, and causing stomach distress and inflammation. They are particularly sneaky because it may take a while for you to begin showing any reactions to them. Some people find green beans, sugar snap peas, and snow peas are easier to digest once cooked, and soaking beans and cooking them over a long period of time can make them easier to digest.

Although it's included here because it's a legume, soy is a special case and really belongs in the "avoid" category. It contains phytoestrogens, compounds that mimic estrogen in the body and could interfere with the body's natural hormones (and that is never a fun thing). And unlike some legumes, soy isn't made more easily digestible by soaking and prolonged cooking, so it's best avoided entirely.

Including but not limited to:

Beans

Lentils

Peanuts

Peas

Soy

(yes, peanuts are a legume, not a nut)

White Potatoes

White potatoes contain lectins (just like grains) and naturally occurring chemicals called saponins, both of which could damage the lining of your intestines over time if consumed regularly. Sweet potatoes don't contain lectins or saponins, so they're often a good substitute. However, people who are more active or require more carbohydrates in their diet often find that white potatoes work well for them.

White Rice

While rice is technically a grain, there is some debate as to whether or not it belongs in a Paleo diet. It's not as nutrient-dense as most Paleo foods and can trigger insulin responses in sensitive individuals, but some more active individuals and athletes have found the extra carbs it provides helpful.

If you choose not to eat white rice, cauliflower rice (pages 200 to 204) is a great substitute.

paleo cheat sheet

Foods to Avoid

Grains

Wheat (and everything made from it, including bread and pasta)

Barley

Corn

Oats

Rice

Refined Sugars

Artificial sweeteners

Brown sugar

Corn syrup

Table sugar

Processed Foods

Candy

Energy drinks

Packaged snacks and meals

Soda

Processed Fats and Oils

Canola oil

Cottonseed oil

Margarine

Safflower oil

Soybean oil

Sunflower oil

Vegetable oil

Foods to Enjoy

Meat

Beef

Bison/Buffalo

Chicken

Duck

Lamb

Pork

Turkey

Veal

Seafood

Clams

Crab

Fish

Lobster

Mussels

Oysters

Prawns

Sardines

Scallops

Shrimp

Eggs

Vegetables and Fruits

Apples

Artichokes

Arugula

Asparagus

Avocados

Bananas

Beets

Blackberries

Blueberries

Broccoli

Brussels sprouts

Cabbage

Cauliflower

Celery

Chard

Cherries

Collard greens

Cucumbers

Eggplant

Garlic

Grapefruit

Grapes

Green onions

Jicama

Kale

Kiwi

Leeks

Lemons

Lettuce

Limes

Melons

Mushrooms

Nectarines

Onions

Oranges

Peaches

Pears

Peppers

Pineapples

Plums

Pomegranates

Radishes

Rhubarb

Rutabaga

Shallots

Spinach

Squash

Strawberries

Sweet potatoes

Tangerines

Tomatoes

Turnips

Watermelon

Zucchini

Nuts and Seeds

Almonds

Cashews

Flax seeds

Hazelnuts

Macadamia nuts

Pecans

Pine nuts

Pistachios

Pumpkin seeds (pepitas)

Sesame seeds

Sunflower seeds

Tahini

Walnuts

Healthy Fats and Oils

Avocado oil

Coconut oil

Duck fat

Ghee

Lard

Olive oil

Sesame oil

Tallow

Gray-Area Foods

Alcohol

Dairy

Butter

Cheese

Cottage cheese

Milk

Yogurt

Legumes

Beans

Lentils

Peanuts

Peas

Soy

White Potatoes

White Rice

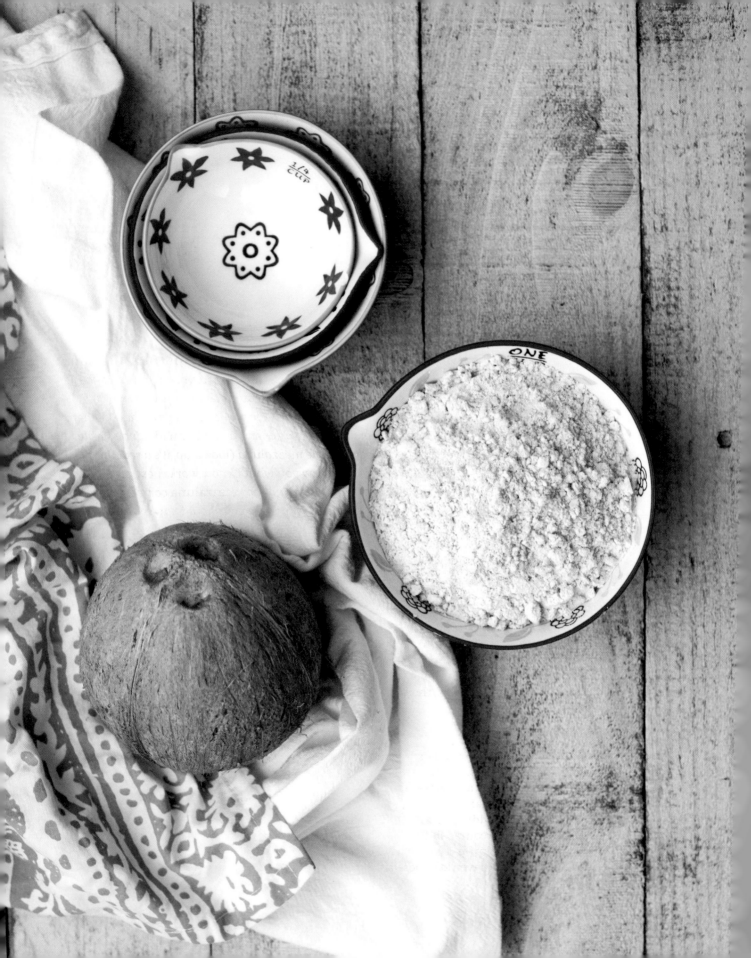

stocking your paleo cupboard and kitchen

EQUIPMENT

Having the right equipment in your kitchen not only makes cooking much easier and faster, it also makes it more likely that your dishes will turn out well. If you are new to cooking, then the best thing you can do for yourself is get the best-quality equipment you can afford. Some people will look at the list of equipment below and think it's outrageous that anyone would have so many things in their kitchen, and others will insist that no kitchen is complete without a marble pastry board and a double mezzaluna (look it up, it's a real thing). But since I am here to show you what I know works best, and there's a good chance I don't even pronounce mezzaluna correctly, these are some of the basic items that I believe you should have handy.

Must-Have Equipment

Baking Mats and Parchment Paper

Baking mats and parchment paper help ensure that your food doesn't stick to your pans or counters. You're on your own when it comes to things sticking to fingers, hair, or small children, though.

Blender or Food Processor

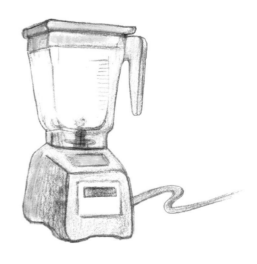

A good blender and/or food processor allows you to make your own milks, flours, batters, and sauces easily and efficiently. I have a higher-end blender that is great for blending and pureeing. A food processor is great for shredding and chopping, but you can usually accomplish the same thing with a good kitchen knife. If you have to pick between one or the other, I would choose a good blender.

Cutting Boards

I keep at least two cutting boards in my kitchen, one for use with meat, poultry, and seafood and the other for everything else. That cuts down on any chance that bacteria from raw meat will contaminate my raw vegetables.

Knives

You don't need a bunch of fancy knives to make it through most recipes, but I recommend having at least one sharp utility knife for most cutting tasks and one quality chef's knife for chopping.

Hand Mixer

A good hand mixer is great for quickly mixing batters and sauces. It will save you a lot of time otherwise spent trying to correctly combine ingredients by hand, and you won't have to keep a huge stand mixer on your counter.

Measuring Cups and Spoons

In addition to measuring spoons, have both wet and dry measuring cups on hand. And yes, there is a difference! While they both hold the same volume, they are designed to help you measure different types of ingredients correctly. (For chopped items like onions or carrots, you can use either kind of measuring cup.)

Dry measuring cups come in a variety of sizes, have long handles, and are flat on top. To measure dry ingredients like flour, dip the cup into the flour, then scrape along the top with the flat edge of a knife to remove any excess. Pouring dry ingredients directly from a bag into the measuring cup can mean you don't get enough of the ingredient.

Wet measuring cups usually come in 1-, 2-, and 4-cup sizes. They're clear, have measurement marks along the side, and have a spout for pouring. They're easier to use for liquids than dry measuring cups because you don't need to fill the cup to get the right amount. When measuring liquids, bend down a bit to look at the measurement marks at eye level, then pour the liquid into the measuring cup until it reaches the appropriate level.

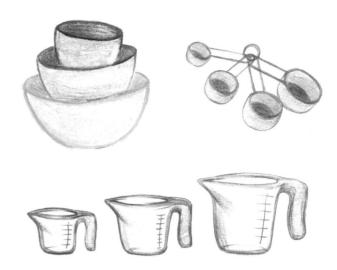

Mixing Bowls

I recommend that you have at least one mixing bowl in each of the basic sizes: small, medium, and large. If you can find a brand with well-fitting lids, such as Cuisinart, your mixing bowls can double as storage bowls for leftovers. Stainless-steel bowls are great for tempering chocolate or warming delicate sauces—instead of investing in a double boiler, you can just place one over a saucepan filled with water.

Microplane Grater

Microplane graters are relatively inexpensive, and they're a huge time-saver when it comes to grating citrus zest and hard foods like garlic, ginger, cinnamon sticks, and nutmeg.

Meat Thermometer

If you are cooking a piece of meat low and slow, a meat thermometer takes the guesswork out of it by letting you know when your food has reached the right internal temperature. If you, like me, are usually doing three things in the kitchen at once, then consider a thermometer with an alarm that alerts you when a set temperature is reached. It prevents you from chatting away with your dinner guests while your poor pork roast gets cooked to a crisp in the oven.

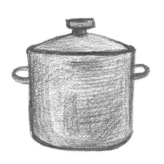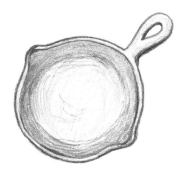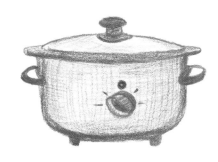

Pots and Pans

The type of pans—cast iron, stainless steel, copper, nonstick, and so on—you use often just comes down to personal preference. I like enameled cast iron because it can go between the stovetop and oven easily and because it conducts heat well. I recommend having at least these kinds and sizes: a large skillet with a lid, a large Dutch oven, two- and six-quart saucepans, a three-quart oven-safe baking dish, two baking sheets 9 by 13 inches or larger, a standard-sized muffin pan, and a pie tin.

No matter what material you use for the rest of your cookware, it's great to have a large cast-iron skillet on hand. When seasoned correctly, a cast-iron skillet is virtually nonstick, can move from the stovetop to oven easily, and will last for decades.

Slow Cooker

A slow cooker is like an assistant in the kitchen. You just hand over the food and when you come back, your meal is cooked and ready. Okay, maybe it's not quite that easy, but on days when you are short on time or just don't feel like doing a lot of cooking, a slow cooker comes in very handy.

Spiral Slicer or Julienne Slicer

Vegetable noodles—zucchini noodles (page 328) and sweet potato noodles (page 327)—are a healthy way to satisfy your pasta cravings, and you can use either a spiral slicer or a julienne slicer to get the perfect noodle shape.

Strainer/Colander

The bigger the better when it comes to a strainer, so you don't have food spilling out all over your sink. Even if you're draining a small amount of food, a large strainer will get the job done.

Wooden Spoons and Rubber Spatulas

You will need larger spoons for stirring, and wooden spoons are great when you're dealing with high temperatures because they won't melt. A rubber spatula is good for scraping bowls and folding egg whites.

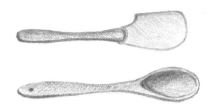

Nice-to-Have Equipment

While the items below are not necessarily a requirement for your kitchen, they are great to have around if you can swing it.

Cheesecloth or Nut Milk Bag

If you plan on making your own coconut milk or nut milks, cheesecloth or a nut milk bag will be a great help. You can strain liquids without having to worry about any tiny pieces slipping through.

Coffee Grinder

Electric blade coffee grinders are relatively inexpensive, and even if you don't drink coffee, they are great to have around if you want to grind your own spices. They can also give coconut flour and nut flours an extra-fine blend before you use them.

Deep-Fry Thermometer

If you don't have a lot of experience gauging how hot your oils and fats are, a deep-fry thermometer is going to help you out.

Fine-Mesh Strainer

I like to keep one small and one large fine-mesh strainer around for straining bacon drippings and making my own lard and ghee. They are very inexpensive, and you will probably use them more often than you think.

Kitchen Tongs

I use tongs all the time, and I have at least three pairs in different sizes. They are great for flipping, frying, transferring food from a plate to a pan (or vice versa), and even giving something a quick stir.

Immersion Blender

While not a requirement, an immersion blender is handy to have around when making mayonnaise, soups, and sauces. Instead of transferring hot liquids to a blender, you can blend everything right in the pot. And with immersion blenders, there's no need to worry about a blender lid flying off and giving you a soup-covered kitchen and face. (It happens.)

Meat Tenderizer/Mallet

Tenderizing your meat is a good way to make cheaper cuts much easier to chew. I can tell you from experience that in a pinch, the flat end can also substitute as a hammer.

Oven Thermometer

I hate to be the one to break it to you, but it's very unlikely that the temperature gauge on your oven is completely accurate. But don't fret, because an oven thermometer will let you know what the real temperature is inside your oven, so you can adjust until you get it to the temperature you really want.

Ramekins

I use small oven-safe ramekins for a few of my dessert recipes in this book. But they serve double duty, because when I am not making desserts (which is most of the time), they are my prep bowls for salt, pepper, and whatever other spices or herbs I happen to be using.

Wire Rack

A wire rack isn't just good for cooling baked goods; it is also helpful in holding breaded items so the coating can adhere before cooking. Look for an oven-safe version if possible so it can serve double duty for both baking and cooling.

INGREDIENTS

There are some ingredients that are particularly common in Paleo recipes; some may be new to you, and others you have probably cooked with before. These are the items I keep stocked in my cupboard and fridge (in addition to a wide variety of spices, which we will get to a little later).

Almond Flour

Almond flour is high in protein and is one of the more common alternatives to wheat flour in many gluten-free and Paleo recipes. Look for finely ground blanched almond flour to give you the best results. Almond flour is not the same as almond meal, which is generally coarse and will result in crumbled baked goods—and nobody likes crumbled baked goods. If your almond flour is not very finely ground, put it in a clean coffee grinder and give it a few bursts. See page 316 for how to make your own almond flour at home.

Almond Milk and Other Nut Milks

Nut milk, particularly almond milk, is a common substitute for dairy milk, and you will see it often in Paleo recipes. If you're using store-bought nut milk, look for one that is unsweetened and has the least amount of additives—but you can also make your own at home (see page 318). If you are allergic to nuts, a seed milk (such as sunflower seed milk) or coconut milk can be substituted in many recipes.

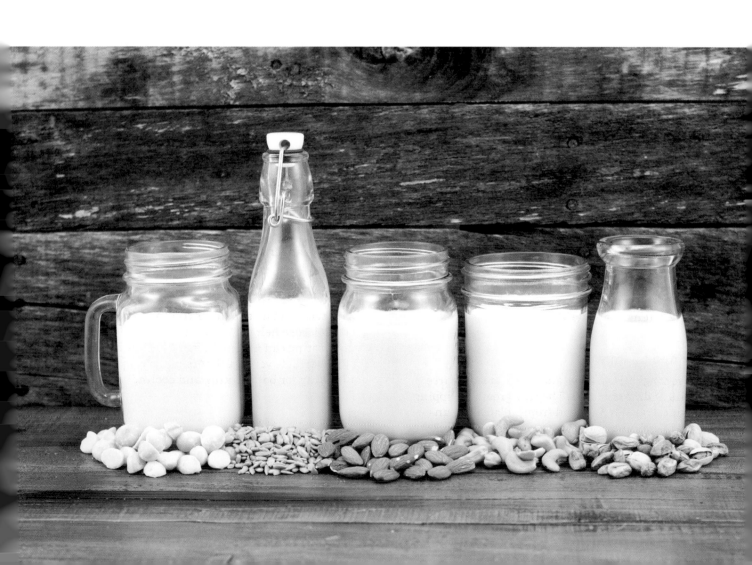

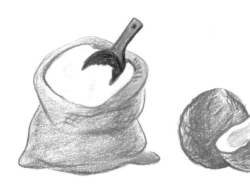

Arrowroot Flour

Arrowroot flour is a great thickening agent that is similar to cornstarch and adds a lighter texture when used in baking. Although they are not the same, you can generally use tapioca flour and arrowroot flour interchangeably in recipes. Arrowroot flour can be found at many natural food stores, or you can order it online.

Baking Powder and Baking Soda

Baking powder and baking soda are both leaveners that are most often used in baked goods. Some people are sensitive to baking powder, but you can easily make your own substitute. Just mix together two parts cream of tartar, one part baking soda, and one part tapioca or arrowroot flour. If you purchase baking powder at the store, make sure it's aluminum-free; the metal may be linked to neurological disorders such as Alzheimer's disease, and it can give your food a metallic taste.

Cacao Powder

Unsweetened cacao powder (not to be confused with cocoa powder) is about the least-processed chocolate you can find. It is made from cold-pressed cocoa beans that are ground into a fine powder, and it is high in antioxidants. It is available at most natural food stores and online.

Coconut Aminos

Coconut aminos are a combination of coconut tree sap and sea salt and are often used as a soy sauce substitute in Paleo recipes. It can be purchased in many natural food stores or online. You can also make your own soy sauce substitute at home (see page 283).

Coconut Cream

Coconut cream (not to be confused with coconut concentrate or coconut butter) is the thicker cream that separates when you leave coconut milk in the refrigerator. It is sometimes sold on its own, but store-bought coconut cream can contain additives, so read the label carefully. You can also get coconut cream from a can of coconut milk or make your own at home (see page 315).

Coconut Flour

Coconut flour is made from dried coconut that is ground until it forms a powder. It is low in carbohydrates and high in fiber, which makes it a great option for gluten-free and Paleo baking (although it's not used in any of the recipes in this book, you will see it in a lot of other Paleo recipes). It is important to note, though, that coconut flour is very absorbent and cannot be used as a one-for-one substitute for other Paleo-friendly flours. See page 313 for how to make your own coconut flour at home.

Coconut Milk

Coconut milk is another common dairy substitute used in Paleo cooking. Look for the canned variety that is full-fat and made from only coconut and water, and check that the cans are BPA-free—or see page 314 for how to make your own.

Fats and Oils

The main fats and oils that I cook with are coconut oil, extra-virgin olive oil, lard, tallow, and ghee. Lard and tallow are good fats for frying and have fairly mellow flavors. You can make your own at home (see pages 322 and 324) or purchase them at some natural food stores and online. Ghee is clarified butter that has had all of the milk solids removed. Most ghee has only trace amounts of lactose, which makes it a good option for people who are lactose-intolerant. Ghee is becoming more readily available in grocery stores, but you can also make it at home yourself (see page 320). I use ghee as a butter substitute, but lard and tallow are also good choices in savory dishes, and coconut oil is great in sweet dishes. (Coconut oil can also be used as a ghee substitute in most dishes; just keep in mind that it may give your food a bit of a coconut flavor.)

Fish Sauce

Fish sauce is used in many Asian recipes and can add a lot of flavor to your dishes. Look for a brand made from only fish, sea salt, and water, such as Red Boat brand.

Gelatin

Gelatin is a good thickening agent and is great for your hair, skin, and nails. Purchase unflavored grass-fed gelatin whenever possible.

Nuts and Seeds

Almonds, cashews, flax seeds, pumpkin seeds, pine nuts, pistachios, and sunflower seeds are all sources of protein. Look for raw nuts and seeds without any roasting or added salt.

Raw Honey

Raw honey is unheated, unpasteurized, and unprocessed, which preserves its natural vitamins and enzymes, and it is the sweetener I use most often for cooking and baking. It has an amazing flavor compared to commercially available honey and is a natural substitute for processed and refined sugars.

Stock

Beef and chicken stock (page 310) and fish stock (page 312) can be purchased at almost any grocery store, or you can easily make your own at home. I find that homemade stock always tastes best, but the store-bought version will work just as well.

Sunflower Seed Flour

Sunflower seed flour is made from ground sunflower seeds and is a great substitute for almond flour if you're allergic to nuts. It can usually be used as a one-for-one replacement for almond flour in most recipes. See page 316 for how to make your own sunflower seed flour at home.

Tapioca Flour

Tapioca flour is made by grinding cassava root into a fine powder. It helps improve the texture of gluten-free baked goods and adds chewiness to recipes. I find that a combination of almond flour and tapioca flour gives me the closest equivalent to wheat flour, so you will often see the two combined in this book. Tapioca flour can be used as a thickener, and just like cornstarch it should be mixed with cold water before being added to a hot sauce or gravy. Tapioca flour can be found at many natural food stores, or you can order it online.

Tomato Products

Canned or jarred sauce, paste, and chopped tomatoes are handy to keep around, especially if tomatoes are out of season.

Vanilla Extract

Look for pure vanilla extract rather than the imitation variety, which often has additives and an unnatural flavor.

Vinegars

I like to have a couple types of vinegar around to help give my recipes a flavor boost when needed. Apple cider vinegar and pure balsamic vinegar are the two I use most often.

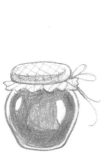
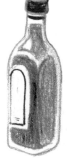
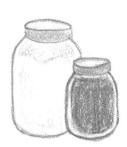
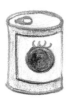

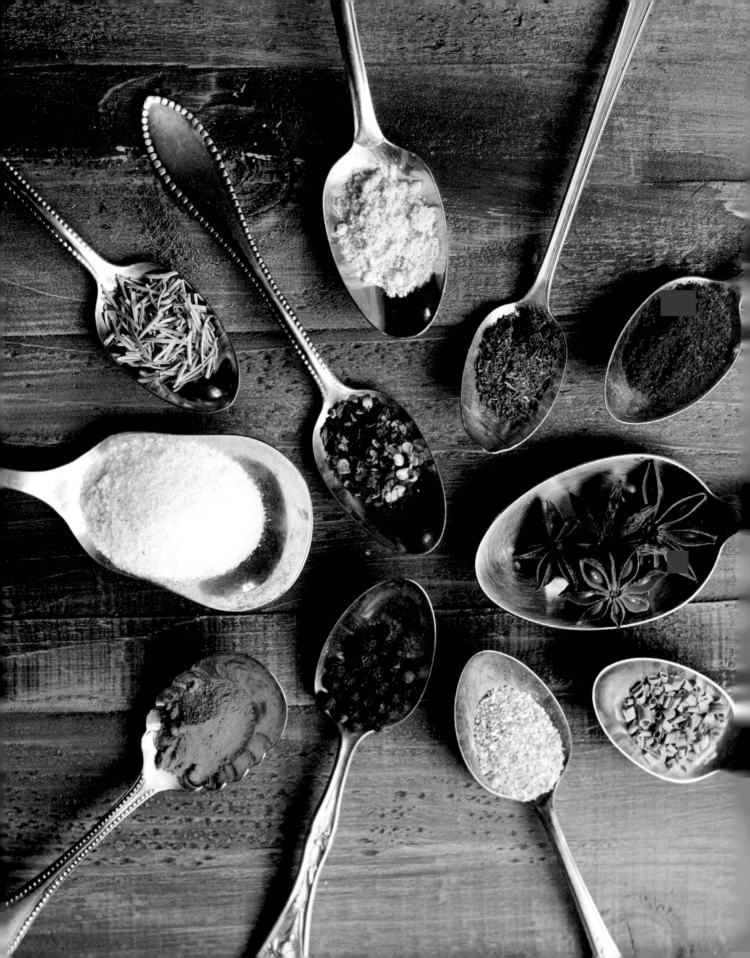

understanding flavor

Understanding flavors and how they combine is critical when preparing food. We all experience the five (maybe six) basic tastes that make up flavors a little differently, and understanding your own preferences and how the different tastes can enhance or balance each another will help you know how to adjust recipes to the way you like them. Once you know how to combine flavors, you can easily build a complex and enjoyable flavor profile. Sounds fancy, right? Actually, it's easier than you think! Here is a breakdown of the basic tastes.

Sweet

Sweetness is probably one of the easiest things to notice in a dish. In the Paleo world, sweet ingredients include fruits, sweet potatoes, butternut squash, carrots, raw honey, maple syrup, vanilla extract, and even some spices like cinnamon, cloves, and nutmeg. Sweet flavors balance out bitter, spicy, and sour flavors while enhancing salty. For example, if you make a tomato-based sauce and it's just a little too bitter, adding a teaspoon of raw honey and a pinch of salt will help to offset the bitterness.

Sour

While sour or acidic flavors may be a little overwhelming on their own, when combined with other flavors they help balance a dish and can add a refreshing zing to a recipe. Most sour flavors come from acidic foods like lime, lemon, or apple cider vinegar. If you have a savory dish that needs a little oomph, try adding a squeeze of fresh lemon juice instead of salt to make the whole recipe come to life. Sour flavors balance out other spicy and sweet flavors in a dish and enhance saltiness.

Salty

Salt is one of the more common and obvious contributors to saltiness in a recipe, but other ingredients, such as coconut aminos or soy sauce substitutes, capers, and fish sauce, provide saltiness as well. I almost always include salty ingredients in my savory dishes, and it's easy to adjust them to your personal liking. As a general rule, the more fat a dish has in it, the more saltiness you need to make the flavors really shine. Salty flavors enhance sweetness and balance bitterness.

Bitter

Bitterness can be an unpleasant experience for some people, but when combined with other flavors it can become highly enjoyable. Dark chocolate, for example, is bitter on its own, but when combined with something sweet, it makes many people jump for joy. Some examples of other bitter foods are spinach, kale, and cacao powder. Adding bitter ingredients to a dish helps balance out salty and sweet flavors.

Umami

Umami is the savory or meaty taste that certain ingredients can add to a dish. Mushrooms, tomatoes, oysters, fish sauce, and caramelized onions are all good examples. You can add umami flavor to a dish to help balance out any bitterness.

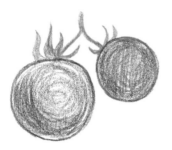

And Then There's Spicy

Although "spicy" is not usually considered its own flavor or taste, I like to call it out because understanding how you experience spiciness and heat is an important part of building flavor profiles. Too much of a spicy element can completely destroy a dish for people who are sensitive to it, while for others, a good amount of heat and spice can add the perfect touch. If you're unsure about how much heat you like or are cooking for someone new, it's best to play it safe and use a very small amount. Examples of ingredients that lean toward the spicier side are radishes, hot peppers, horseradish, hot sauces, crushed red pepper, and mustards. Spicy ingredients help balance out sour and sweet flavors in your dishes.

OTHER THINGS to CONSIDER

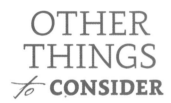

Beyond flavor, there are other aspects of ingredients that contribute to the appeal of a dish. Things like smell, texture, and temperature have a significant impact on your overall experience when eating. For example, the smoky smell of grilled meat plays an important role in the appeal of that food. The way the food feels in your mouth is also key. Smooth and creamy foods can coat your tongue and create a sense of richness, while crispy foods provide a satisfying crunch. Cold foods on a hot day are usually refreshing, while warm foods on a cold day are comforting. These are all things to keep in mind when planning your recipes and tailoring them to suit your mood and taste buds.

ADJUST TO TASTE!

If you're nervous about using new herbs and spices in a dish, try adding small amounts and tasting as you go. The easiest way to figure out if a dish needs more seasoning is to take out a small sample and add a little bit of spices or herbs to it, then taste and compare it to the original. If it tastes better, then add a larger amount of the seasonings to your main dish, tasting as you go. If it tasted better before, then you don't need to adjust your main dish.

Remember, you can always add more, but you can't take it away once you have added it!

One of the easiest ways to make food taste great is to know which spices, herbs, and flavors are compatible with other ingredients. You probably already know how to use salt and pepper, but you may not be as familiar with things like chili powder or coriander. Below is a list of some common spices and dried herbs that you should have around. If you have been cooking for a while, you may already have most of these and know all about them, so feel free to skip ahead—I won't mind. But if spices and herbs are still a mystery to you, then this list should help clear things up a bit. There are many more options available, far too many to list, but think of this as a starting point for understanding the basics of frequently used spices and herbs and which go best with common foods. Once you get the foundation down, you can expand into many other seasonings, but with these basic spices in your cupboard you're going to be able to add amazing flavor to any dish.

let's TALK SEASONINGS

Allspice

Allspice is an aromatic spice that is similar to cloves and cinnamon but more pungent. It is often combined with other spices because it can be overpowering on its own. A little bit goes a long way, so add allspice sparingly if you haven't tried it before.

Tastes great with: apples, baked goods, beef, beets, cabbage, carrots, eggplants, fish, onions, pineapple, pork, soups and stews, spinach, sweet potatoes, and tomatoes.

Works well in combination with: black pepper, cardamom, cinnamon, chili powder, cloves, dry yellow mustard, ginger, nutmeg, rosemary, and thyme.

Basil

Although fresh basil is great when added near the end of the cooking process, dried basil tends to have a slightly sweet flavor and should be added earlier. Using both dried and fresh basil packs an excellent double punch of flavor.

Tastes great with: bell peppers, capers, chiles, chives, cilantro, coconut milk, crab, cucumber, eggplant, honey, lemon juice and zest, lime juice and zest, mussels, onions, oranges, pork, sauces, seafood, soups, stews, and tomatoes.

Works well in combination with: cinnamon, dry yellow mustard, garlic, ginger, marjoram, oregano, parsley, rosemary, and thyme.

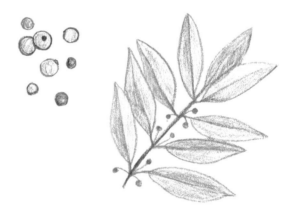

Bay Leaf

Bay leaves are generally sold dried, and they have an aromatic and woodsy taste. They should be added to a dish early on, as it takes a while for the flavor to develop and penetrate the food. You only need one or two bay leaves at the most to flavor your dishes. Any more than that can overpower your recipe and leave it with a bitter flavor. Always make sure to remove the leaves before serving (you don't want one of these guys stuck in your throat).

Tastes great with: apples, beef, cauliflower, chicken, dates, duck, lemon juice and zest, pork, pumpkin, salmon, sauces, sausage, shellfish, soups and stews, and spinach.

Works well in combination with: allspice, black pepper, garlic powder, marjoram, onion powder, oregano, parsley, rosemary, sage, and thyme.

Black Pepper

Black pepper goes with pretty much any savory dish, so always keep it close at hand. While pre-ground black pepper is handy and I use it often, using a pepper grinder to whip up some freshly ground pepper will get you an extra hit of flavor with minimal effort and time. I generally use finely ground black pepper in my recipes and then give my guests the pepper mill at the table so they can add more pepper in whatever size grind they like.

Tastes great with: beef, coconut milk, eggs, fruit, lemon juice and zest, lime juice and zest, pork, seafood, sauces, sausage, soups, stews, and tomatoes.

Works well in combination with: basil, cardamom, cinnamon, cloves, coriander, cumin, garlic, ginger, nutmeg, rosemary, salt, thyme, and turmeric.

Cardamom

Cardamom is a warm, sweet, and pungent spice that is often found in Indian dishes, custards, and some drinks, such as masala chai.

Tastes great with: apples, baked goods, bananas, beef, carrots, chicken, chiles, citrus, coconut milk, fish, honey, hot drinks, lemon juice and zest, lime juice and zest, pears, pork, soups, squash, stews, and sweet potatoes.

Works well in combination with: black pepper, chili powder, cinnamon, cloves, coriander, cumin, curry powder, ginger, and paprika.

Cayenne Pepper

Cayenne pepper is the base of many hot sauces and is frequently used in Cajun and Indian recipes. It adds a lovely bit of sweet heat to food, but use it sparingly if you're sensitive to heat.

Tastes great with: beef, bell peppers, eggplant, fish and seafood, lemon juice and zest, onions, sauces, shellfish, soups, stews, sweet potatoes, and tomatoes.

Works well in combination with: basil, cilantro, cinnamon, coriander, cumin, garlic powder, and paprika.

Chili Powder

Chili powder is a blend of spices that is usually made from dried chiles, cumin, coriander, oregano, and sometimes salt. It's often used to season . . . you guessed it, chili, but it also has many other uses. Chipotle chili powder is delicious in Mexican and southwestern dishes. Don't confuse chili powder with chile powder, which consists purely of dried and ground chiles.

Tastes great with: beef, chicken, eggs, lemon juice and zest, lime juice and zest, pork, soups, stews, and sweet potatoes.

Works well in combination with: allspice, cardamom, cinnamon, coriander, cumin, dry yellow mustard, oregano, and thyme.

Cinnamon

Cinnamon is a sweet, warm spice that comes in stick or ground form. The sticks are good to add to sauces or beverages that need to simmer for a while, and ground cinnamon is great in desserts and sauces. Cinnamon is found in almost every cuisine around the world, in both savory and sweet dishes.

Tastes great with: apples, baked goods, beef, bell peppers, berries, eggplant, honey, maple syrup, nuts, onions, orange juice and zest, pears, pork, sauces, soups, squash, stews, sweet potatoes, and tomatoes.

Works well in combination with: allspice, cardamom, chili powder, cloves, coriander, cumin, ginger, nutmeg, and turmeric.

Cloves

Cloves, like cinnamon, are sold whole or ground. Cloves are sweet and earthy, and a little bit goes a long way. They're commonly used in Asian, African, and Middle Eastern cuisine and are also often used around the holidays and for baking.

Tastes great with: apples, baked goods and desserts, beef, beets, carrots, chicken, ham, honey, lemon juice and zest, orange juice and zest, pork, pumpkin, red cabbage, salad dressings, sweet potatoes, and tomatoes.

Works well in combination with: allspice, bay leaf, cardamom, cinnamon, coriander, cumin, curry powder, garlic, nutmeg, and turmeric.

Coriander

Coriander and cilantro (see page 36) are part of the same plant—coriander is the seed while cilantro is the leaves. Coriander can be bought whole or ground, and it provides a bit of a lemon and pepper flavor. It is often found in Mexican and Indian dishes.

Tastes great with: apples, beef, carrots, chicken, coconut milk, eggs, fish, grapefruit, lemon juice and zest, lime juice and zest, mushrooms, onions, orange juice and zest, pears, pork, sausage, shellfish, soups, stews, and tomatoes.

Works well in combination with: allspice, basil, black pepper, cardamom, cayenne pepper, chili powder, cilantro, cinnamon, cloves, cumin, curry powder, garlic powder, ginger, nutmeg, and turmeric.

Crushed Red Pepper

This tasty spice is usually made from a mixture of dried red chiles that have been crushed . . . hence the name! It can be used to add a smoky flavor to recipes, and it packs a bit of heat. Adding a dash of crushed red pepper will give a kick to many savory dishes.

Tastes great with: avocado, beef, carrots, cilantro, coconut milk, coconut aminos, eggplant, lemon juice and zest, lime juice and zest, mushrooms, onions, orange juice and zest, pork, sauces, sausage, seafood, sesame oil, shallots, soups, stews, tomatoes, and vinegar.

Works well in combination with: basil, bay leaf, cayenne, cinnamon, coriander, cumin, garlic powder, ginger, marjoram, onion powder, oregano, parsley, rosemary, and thyme.

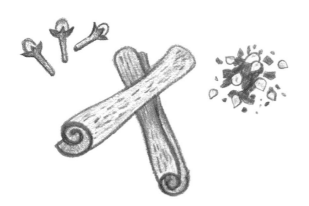

Cumin

Cumin has a smoky and earthy flavor and is often found in Mexican, North African, Middle Eastern, and Indian recipes. While it can be found in whole form, it is more commonly sold already ground.

Tastes great with: beef, bell peppers, carrots, chicken, chiles, eggplant, eggs, fish, honey, lime juice and zest, onions, orange juice and zest, pork, sausage, sauces, soups, squash, stews, sweet potatoes, tahini, and tomatoes.

Works well in combination with: allspice, bay leaf, cardamom, cayenne, chili powder, cinnamon, cloves, coriander, curry powder, dry yellow mustard, garlic powder, ginger, nutmeg, oregano, paprika, and turmeric.

Curry Powder

Curry powder is usually a blend of other spices, such as turmeric, cumin, and chiles. It is most often found in Indian recipes, but a few dashes make a great addition to a mayonnaise-based chicken salad.

Tastes great with: beef, chicken, chiles, cilantro, coconut milk, eggs, fish, lemon juice and zest, lime juice and zest, mayonnaise, mushrooms, onions, sauces, soups, stews, sweet potatoes, tomatoes, and zucchini.

Works well in combination with: cardamom, cayenne, cinnamon, cloves, coriander, cumin, dill, garlic powder, ginger, nutmeg, paprika, and turmeric.

Dry Yellow Mustard

Dry yellow mustard adds a pungent and zesty flavor to sauces and dressings and also works great in most dry rubs and barbecue sauces.

Tastes great with: beef, cabbage, chicken, coconut aminos, curries, eggs, fish, garlic, honey, lemon juice and zest, mayonnaise, onions, and seafood.

Works well in combination with: black pepper, chili powder, coriander, cumin, garlic powder, onion powder, tarragon, thyme, and turmeric.

Garlic Powder

While it's a good idea to always have some fresh garlic on hand, having garlic powder around is handy as well. It's a versatile, must-have spice that works well in combination with almost all other spices and herbs and enhances the flavor of most meats and seafood. Garlic powder should not be confused with garlic salt, which is a mixture of both garlic and salt, or ground or granulated garlic. One fresh clove of garlic equals about ⅛ teaspoon garlic powder or ¼ teaspoon ground garlic.

Tastes great with: asparagus, bacon, beef, broccoli, cabbage, chicken, chiles, chives, cilantro, coconut aminos, eggplant, eggs, fish, leeks, lemon juice and zest, lime juice and zest, mayonnaise, mushrooms, onions, pork, shellfish, shrimp, soups, spinach, stews, tomatoes, vinegar, and zucchini.

Works well in combination with: basil, bay leaf, black pepper, cayenne, coriander, cumin, curry powder, dry yellow mustard, ginger, onion powder, oregano, paprika, parsley, rosemary, sage, tarragon, and thyme.

Ginger

Ginger is a fragrant spice that is used in dishes all over the world. Dried ground ginger is more intense in flavor than fresh ginger and has a different flavor profile, so it does not always work well as a substitute in a recipe that calls for fresh ginger.

Tastes great with: bananas, butternut squash, carrots, honey, nuts, orange juice and zest, pears, pineapple, pumpkin, and sweet potatoes.

Works well in combination with: black pepper, cardamom, cinnamon, cloves, nutmeg, and onion powder.

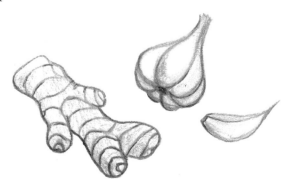

Nutmeg

Nutmeg is a sweet and pungent spice that is frequently used in baked goods but can also add warm notes to savory dishes. It can be found whole or ground, and you can use a Microplane grater to break down the whole version. Nutmeg should be added close to the end of the cooking process to help the dish retain its flavors.

Tastes great with: apple cider, apples, cabbage, carrots, chicken, egg dishes, honey, onions, oranges, pears, pork, and sweet potatoes.

Works well in combination with: black pepper, cardamom, cinnamon, cloves, coriander, cumin, ginger, and thyme.

Onion Powder

Onion powder is onion that has been dehydrated and ground. Like garlic powder, it is a must-have in your spice cupboard. A teaspoon of onion powder equals about ⅓ cup of chopped fresh onion.

Tastes great with: asparagus, bacon, beef, broccoli, cabbage, chicken, chiles, chives, cilantro, coconut aminos, eggs, fish, leeks, lemon juice and zest, lime juice and zest, mayonnaise, mushrooms, onions, pork, shellfish, shrimp, soups, spinach, stews, tomatoes, vinegar, and zucchini.

Works well in combination with: basil, bay leaf, black pepper, cayenne, coriander, cumin, curry powder, dry yellow mustard, garlic powder, ginger, oregano, paprika, parsley, rosemary, sage, tarragon, and thyme.

Oregano

Oregano is aromatic and has a warm, slightly bitter taste. It is a great addition to tomato sauces and stews and is used in many Mexican, Mediterranean, and South American recipes.

Tastes great with: bell peppers, chicken, chiles, eggs, fish, lemon juice and zest, mayonnaise, mushrooms, onions, pork, sauces, soups, squash, stews, tomatoes, and zucchini.

Works well in combination with: basil, black pepper, chili powder, cumin, garlic powder, onion powder, paprika, parsley, rosemary, and thyme.

Paprika

Paprika is not just a garnish for deviled eggs. It adds a sweet note, and of course a vibrant red color, to dishes. It burns easily and can become bitter if overcooked, so treat it gently.

Tastes great with: beef, chicken, chiles, onions, pork, sauces, seafood, soups, stews, and tahini.

Works well in combination with: allspice, black pepper, cardamom, garlic powder, ginger, onion powder, oregano, parsley, rosemary, thyme, and turmeric.

Rosemary

Dried rosemary is usually sold in ground or leaf form. It is probably one of the most pungent of the commonly used herbs, and a little goes a long way. Rosemary has a lemon-pine taste and is often found in French, Italian, and Mediterranean dishes.

Tastes great with: cabbage, chicken, eggs, fish, mushrooms, onions, pork, squash, soups, stews, sweet potatoes, tomatoes, and vinegar.

Works well in combination with: bay leaf, chives, garlic powder, oregano, parsley, sage, and thyme.

Sage

Sage has a strong pine flavor and does well when paired with other strong flavors, such as garlic. I prefer rubbed sage, which is the dried leaves, to the ground variety—sage can be overpowering, and using rubbed sage allows you to keep its flavor more subtle. Rubbed sage is lighter and much less dense than ground sage, so you will need to use twice the amount of rubbed sage to equal that of ground. It goes great in dishes that are rich in fat or oil.

Tastes great with: apples, beef, carrots, chicken, eggs, fish, lemon juice and zest, onions, orange, pineapple, pork, and tomatoes.

Works well in combination with: bay leaf, black pepper, coriander, crushed red pepper, cumin, garlic powder, onion powder, oregano, and rosemary.

Salt

No matter how new you are to cooking, you're probably familiar with salt, but if that's the only seasoning you tend to reach for, then you're really missing out. While using just salt can leave your food a little boring, when combined with other spices, it acts as a great flavor enhancer. Adding salt at the beginning of a recipe helps enhance and build flavors as the food cooks, while adding salt at the end will give you that true salty taste. I like to add a little in the beginning, then sometimes a little more as I cook, and finish it off with one more pinch at the end if needed.

I use finely ground sea salt in my recipes because it has no additives and goes through less processing than most other types of salt. As a general rule, add ½ teaspoon of salt to every quart of liquid and ½ to ¾ teaspoon of salt to every pound of meat. Use less if you're also using any pre-prepared ingredients that may already contain salt, such as broth.

Tastes great with: pretty much everything.

Works well in combination with: see above.

Thyme

Thyme is usually sold in leaf or ground form. It is a fragrant herb that has a woodsy flavor.

Tastes great with: capers, chicken, fish, lemon juice and zest, mayonnaise, mushrooms, onions, pork, sauces, soups, stews, and tomatoes.

Works well in combination with: allspice, bay leaf, chili powder, eggs, garlic powder, nutmeg, oregano, and paprika.

Turmeric

Turmeric is very aromatic and has a pungent, slightly bitter flavor. Bright yellow in color, it's a base for most curry blends. It is often used in Indian and Southeast Asian cooking.

Tastes great with: cabbage, cauliflower, chicken, eggs, fish, spinach, and sweet potatoes.

Works well in combination with: black pepper, cardamom, coriander, cumin, garlic powder, ginger, and paprika.

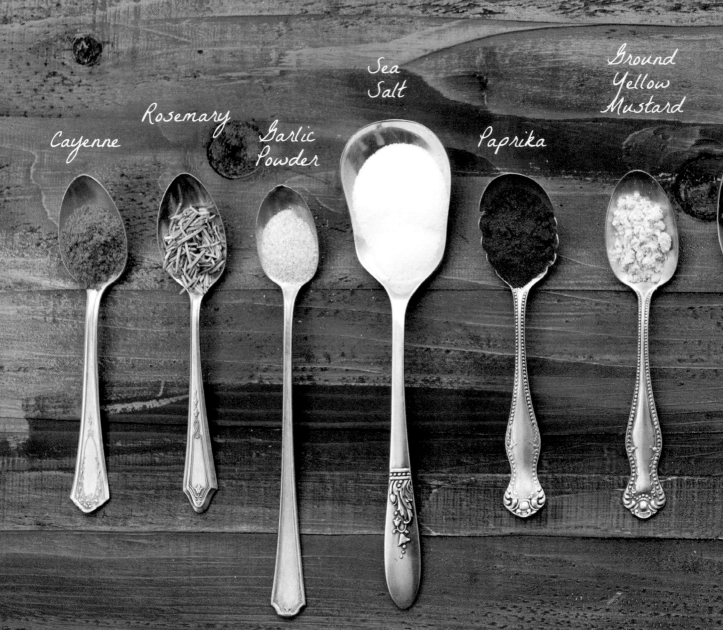

Cayenne

Rosemary

Garlic Powder

Sea Salt

Paprika

Ground Yellow Mustard

STORING DRIED HERBS AND SPICES

Dried herbs and ground spices are best stored in an airtight container away from light and moisture. For the most part, they are at their best when used within one year, although whole spices store well for up to two years. A spice that is older than its suggested shelf life generally won't make you sick, but it will lose its flavor and dishes made with it will lack that fresh, more intense taste. Marking the date you purchased the spices and herbs on the container is a helpful way to know when you need to replace it. You can also rely on your nose to tell if they are still good. If it has a strong and flavorful smell, it is most likely still good. For whole spices, such as peppercorns, crush or grind the spice to help release the aroma before you decide if it's still good.

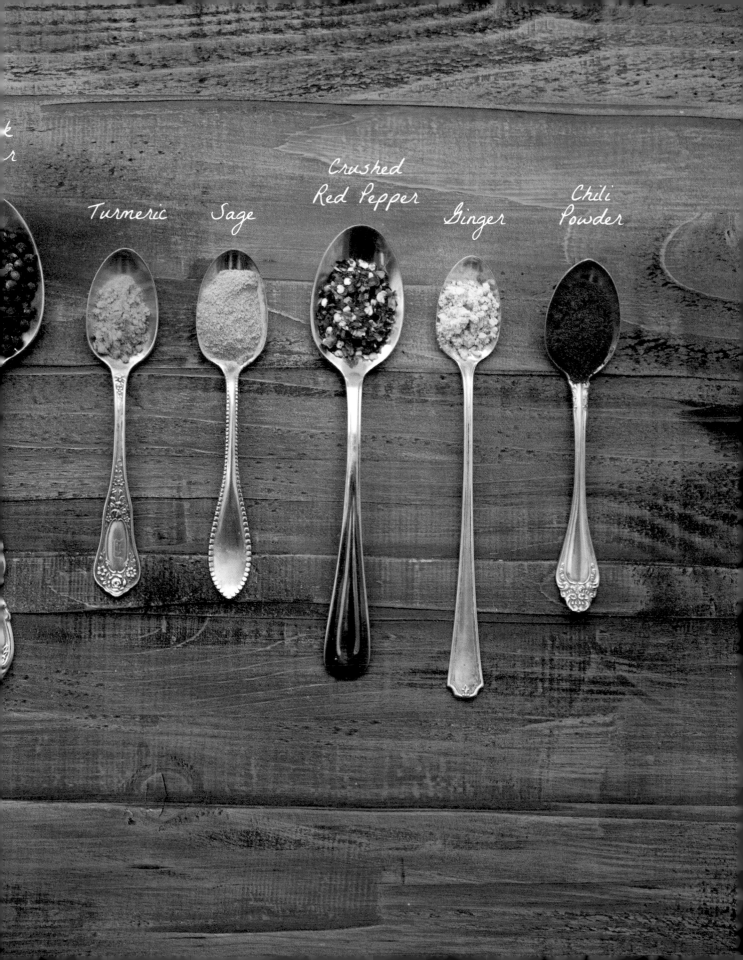

COMMON FRESH
HERBS

Most tender herbs are better fresh than dried—for instance, sprinkling some chopped fresh basil or chives over a dish right before serving results in an amazing flavor. Fresh herbs are usually added close to the end of cooking to help the dish retain their flavor.

There are a couple ways to store fresh herbs. One is to wet a paper towel, wring it out, and wrap the herbs in the paper towel, then place it in a sealed plastic bag and store in the refrigerator. The other method is to trim the base of the stems, place in a glass of water, and place in the refrigerator. Fresh herbs can last one to two weeks if stored properly with one of these methods.

Following are the fresh herbs that I use most often in my cooking and that you'll find throughout the recipes in this book.

Basil

Fresh basil is one of the more popular fresh herbs and is commonly used in sauces and soups. Basil comes in a few varieties, such as sweet basil, which is usually found in Italian recipes, and Thai basil, which is popular in Asian cuisines. In most cases, a recipe is referring to sweet basil unless otherwise indicated. It is a highly aromatic herb that can provide a hint of freshness when added to a dish right before serving, and of course no pesto would be complete without it.

Chives

Although fresh chives may look similar to the grass in your yard, they actually have a light onion flavor and are great sprinkled over savory dishes. It's easiest to cut them with a pair of kitchen shears instead of a knife. I like to call them "nature's edible string" because they are great for tying together foods like lettuce wraps.

Cilantro

Cilantro is an herb that people either love or hate. It has a slight pepper and licorice flavor, and despite being quite delicate, it can deliver a whole lot of flavor when added to a dish right before serving. Although you don't have to use cilantro every time it's suggested, it brings a lot to the flavor party. I frequently use chopped cilantro as a garnish, but if you have picky eaters or guests coming, then serve it on the side so everyone can add as much or as little as they like.

Dill

Dill is a light herb with a pungent flavor. It is great when used in pickling or added to seafood, fish, and egg dishes. Dill is most often added to dishes that require little or no cooking, such as dips and salad dressing. If you do add it to a cooked recipe, add it close to the end of the cooking process so it retains most of its flavor.

Marjoram

Fresh marjoram has a floral and woodsy flavor and is great in sauces and marinades. It is similar to oregano but slightly sweeter and not as pungent; the two can be used interchangeably if necessary.

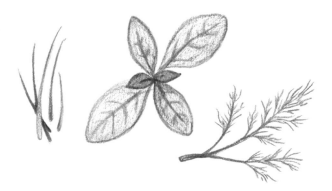

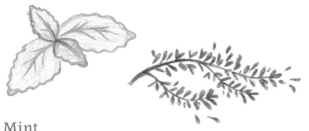

Mint

Mint is a refreshing and cool herb with an intense flavor. The color and smell make it an amazing garnish on many desserts, and muddled mint is light and delicious in many summer drinks. Mojito, anyone?

Oregano

Oregano is a robust herb with a bold flavor that pairs well with meats and vegetables. It is one of the few fresh herbs that can retain almost all of its flavor once dried.

Parsley

Parsley has a mild grassy flavor and comes in both curly and flat-leaf varieties. It can be used as a garnish or added to a dish during cooking to add a hint of bitterness to help balance out the other flavors.

Rosemary

Rosemary is a hearty herb that has hints of pine and lemon. The needles are usually plucked from the woody stem before being used in recipes, unless the whole stem is added to infuse a dish and then removed before serving.

Sage

Fresh sage is a delicate herb with a strong flavor. Look for leaves with a soft, downy coating but no brown spots.

Tarragon

Tarragon has a sweet licorice flavor. Fresh tarragon can stand on its own in many dishes, so you don't need to worry about mixing it with other herbs.

Thyme

Fresh thyme has a lemony and woodsy flavor. Like rosemary, its leaves are usually plucked from the stem before being used, unless the whole sprig is added to infuse a dish and then removed before serving.

DRIED HERBS

Unlike fresh herbs, dried herbs are best added close to the beginning of the cooking process so their flavor has time to develop. More robust herbs like rosemary, thyme, marjoram, bay leaves, and oregano work great when dried and can hold up well in any dish.

You can successfully substitute dried herbs for fresh in many recipes. Dried herbs have a more concentrated flavor than fresh herbs, so my general rule is to use half the amount of dried in any recipe calling for the fresh version. That means if a recipe calls for 1 teaspoon of fresh thyme, you would need only ½ teaspoon of dried thyme leaves. The only time you really should avoid substituting a dried herb is if it's being used as a garnish, in which case the dried form is unlikely to give you the taste you're after.

If you want the best possible flavor, you can use a combination of both fresh and dried herbs. Add your dried herbs toward the beginning and then finish everything off with a sprinkle of fresh herbs right before serving. Voilà!

getting comfortable in the kitchen

If you're new to cooking or just starting out on a real-food lifestyle, the tips below can help make cooking easier and more enjoyable.

Read the Entire Recipe Before Starting

Reading the whole recipe first ensures that you understand the flow of the recipe and what tasks you may be able to do simultaneously—for example, you may be able to start the gravy while the meat is roasting in the oven. It will also let you know if you need to do something before you start, such as chopping an onion or leaving eggs out to reach room temperature, and it will help you know what pans and tools to have ready.

Don't Underestimate the Importance of *Mise en Place*

"Mise en place" is French for "everything in place," and it simply means having all your ingredients and equipment laid out and ready to go before you start. It's an easy way to ensure that your cooking process flows quickly and smoothly. Getting halfway through a recipe and realizing that you can't find your vegetable peeler or that you don't have an important spice is terribly annoying, so have those out and in an easy-to-grab spot before you start.

Prep Ahead of Time

If you have some free time in the morning before a dinner or the night before you plan a nice breakfast, doing some prep work ahead of time can save time later during cooking. Chopping foods that will keep well in the refrigerator for a few hours, like onions or bell peppers, means that you don't have to do it later after a long day. If you have dried ingredients such as flours or spices, you can measure and combine those ahead of time as well, and store in a sealed container until ready to use. Even if you don't have time to prep the food, small things like getting your kitchen equipment laid out and your recipe bookmarked can make a difference.

Cook a Double Batch

Whenever you make soups, stews, sauces, and other basics, double the batch and freeze half. The extras will come in handy on busy days when you are short on time. You'll only need to do this a few times before you have a freezer full of food that you can reheat and serve in minutes.

Don't Be Afraid to Improvise

Once you have read through the whole recipe and you're comfortable in the kitchen, you can wing it—there's no need to follow the recipe letter for letter. Use your senses of taste, touch, and smell, and play with the ingredients. Making mistakes is okay; in fact, it's part of the learning process and will make you a better cook.

Make Cooking Fun

If you're new to Paleo, here's a fact that you may or may not want to hear: there is a good chance you will be spending more time cooking than before. Following a real-food lifestyle means that "fast foods"—including prepared foods from the grocery store, frozen dinners, and a lot of takeout—are no longer a part of your daily routine, and that means you and your kitchen are going to be spending some quality time together. If you absolutely dread cooking or you just want to make it a little more fun, try playing some of your favorite music while you cook. If you live with others, you can invite them to help you out as well—having company while you cook makes it both faster and more fun.

Plan Your Meals

Don't wait until you're headed home from work to think about what you'll make for dinner. Planning your meals ahead of time will help you stay on track with real foods, especially when you are first starting out. Choose recipes that suit your personal tastes and those of your family, and try something new every now and then. You never know what you may wind up loving! One of the best benefits of a real-food diet is that you get to eat a wide variety of foods, so you should never feel deprived or bored, and you never have to sacrifice taste or flavor! Once you have your meals planned for the week, it is easy to create a grocery list with all of the necessary ingredients. The meal plans and shopping lists on pages 42 to 49 can help you get started, but feel free to change it up to suit your tastes!

how to use this book

I wrote The Paleo Cupboard Cookbook *hoping that it would become an essential part of your kitchen and a book that you reach for whenever you want to cook delicious, healthy food. But to get the most out of this book, you will need to do a little bit more than flip through the pages and hope for the best. Here are some of the features you'll find throughout the book and my suggestions for using them for the best results.*

• There's a lot of information before the recipes start about different foods, flavors, and equipment, all of which is designed to help you get the most out of the recipes and the Paleo diet. Take the time to read the introductory material and make sure you understand what will and will not work for you, from the kinds of food you can eat (and like to eat!) to the equipment you might want to pick up before you start cooking.

• Once you start reading the recipes, grab some sticky notes and bookmark ones you'd like to try. I like to use different colors for different categories, such as green for quick dishes, yellow for those I know will be family favorites, and red for something new and interesting that I want to try. That way I can quickly look at the colors and flip to whatever type of recipe I am in the mood for. I recommend you bookmark at least twenty recipes that you want to make, so you'll have items already flagged when you are planning meals and making your grocery lists. And to help make your planning easier, icons on the recipe pages and lists starting on page 336 show you which recipes con be made in forty minutes or less and are nut-free, egg-free, and kid favorites.

• Speaking of meal plans and shopping lists, I have already given you a head start on those! You will find four weeks' worth of meals, along with a shopping list for each week, starting on page 41. You can switch the order of the meals around each week to accommodate how much time you have to cook on that particular day. If the Day 1 meals work best for you on Sunday, cook them on Sunday. If they work better on Thursday, make them on Thursday instead. Don't forget that leftovers make a great breakfast or lunch the next day!

• Many of the recipes in this book have tips for how you can modify them to tweak the flavors. Don't be afraid to experiment! I've also included some of my favorite kitchen tips, from techniques to make-ahead suggestions, and I've sprinkled some of my favorite stories about food, cooking, and life throughout the book. It will be like we're cooking together, except you won't have to deal with me eating all of your food as you try to cook.

• The Basics chapter that starts on page 309 includes recipes for a variety of Paleo staples, such as ghee, lard, tallow, almond and coconut flour, almond and coconut milk, and chicken and beef stock. But if you don't love to spend time in the kitchen, don't freak out! All of these items are available at grocery stores, natural food stores, and online. For a continually updated list of the best places to buy them, see my website at www.PaleoCupboard.com/resources.

BUT WHERE ARE THE MACROS?!

Counting calories and macronutrients—protein, fat, and carbs—is avoided by many people who follow a Paleo lifestyle, which is why you don't see them listed in a lot of Paleo cookbooks. The focus is on putting nutritious food in your body, not on trying to match your food intake to magic numbers that may or may not be right for you. This can be quite a hard idea to accept for people who have lived a long time hearing that they have to plan everything they eat around a number. I know this because I was one of those people, but I can tell you that it is incredibly freeing when you finally realize you don't have to do it anymore. That's not to say that Paleo is a free-for-all and we can shove whatever we want into our mouths, but if you are consciously eating nutrient-dense foods and listening to your body's cues about when you are hungry or full, then you probably don't need to worry about counting calories and macros.

Of course, some people do need or want to count calories and macros for a variety of reasons, and I certainly don't want to discount that. If you fall into that category, there are many online tools and calculators that provide those figures for a wide variety of foods—I've listed a few in the Resources section on page 333.

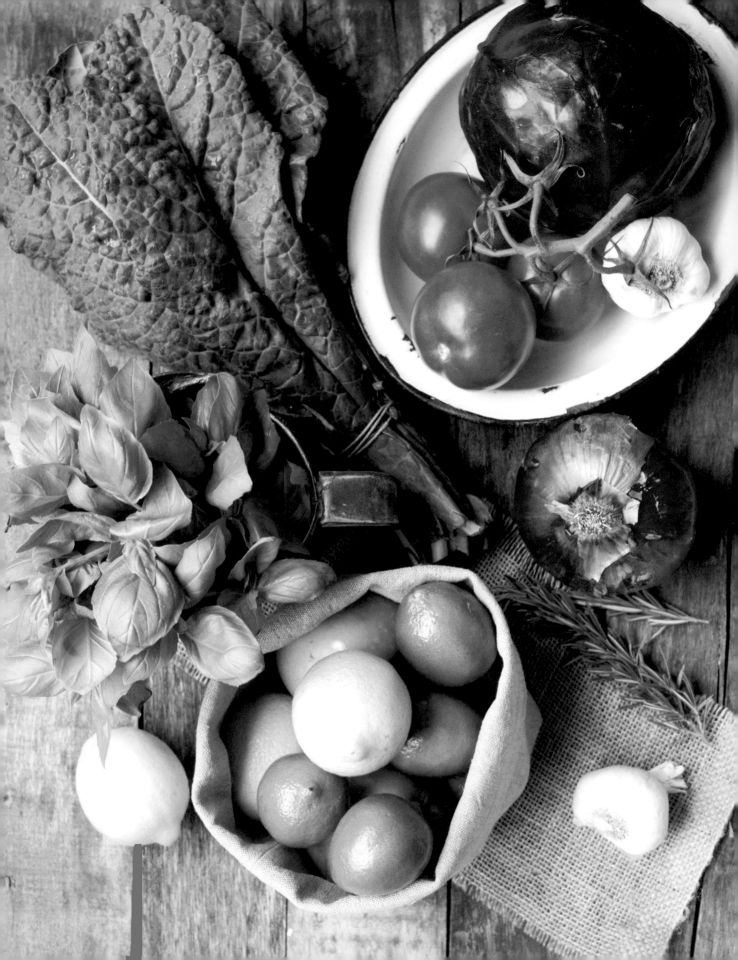

meal plans and shopping lists

Starting out on a Paleo diet can be a little daunting, but having an organized meal plan and grocery list will help you stay on track and make sure you're not stuck wondering, "What in the world am I going to eat today?"

The following meal plans will give you four weeks of Paleo meals. They're designed for a family of four with two adults and two younger kids (like mine), so if you're feeding older kids or four adults, you may want to double the dinner recipes in order to have enough leftovers for lunches (yes, even when I've already called for them to be doubled). You can also supplement your lunches with some of the Paleo snack ideas on page 50.

Remember that you can use breakfast leftovers for lunches as well, and most vegetables, whether raw or cooked, are a great snack or addition to any meal. When I want to add extra vegetables to a dish, I chop some broccoli, carrots, and/ or Brussels sprouts with a little ghee or extra-virgin olive oil, season lightly with salt and pepper, and cook in a 400°F oven for 20 minutes, or until they are just tender. It's an easy and healthy way to make dinners stretch a little more.

Every weekly meal plan has a shopping list to accompany it, organized by categories such as produce, meats, and spices. Each shopping list provides the amount of each ingredient needed for that week's meals, so before you head to the store, you can check your pantry and refrigerator to see if you have enough spices, herbs, condiments, and other basic ingredients. Two things that aren't on the shopping lists? Salt and pepper. Just assume that you'll need to keep plenty of both on hand—I prefer fine sea salt, and although freshly ground black pepper is great, pre-ground often works just as well.

WEEK 1

	Breakfast	Lunch	Dinner	
day 1	Broccoli and Mushroom Frittata / 1 piece/1 cup fruit, your choice [60]	Canned tuna mixed with mayonnaise on a bed of greens with sliced tomatoes and cucumber	Simple Slow Cooker Chicken [130]	Roasted Asparagus with Lemon Sauce [196]
day 2	Turkey slices, tomato, and avocado wrapped in lettuce / 1 piece/1 cup fruit, your choice	Chicken Salad on Apple Slices [114]	Zuppa Toscana [242]	Spicy Smashed Sweet Potatoes [208]
day 3	2 large eggs, cooked any style / Piña Colada Smoothie, no topping (double batch) [304]	Leftover Zuppa Toscana / Leftover Spicy Smashed Sweet Potatoes	Creamy Thai Pasta with Beef Strips [86]	
day 4	Smoked Salmon Deviled Eggs / 1 piece/1 cup fruit, your choice [176]	Asian Sesame Chicken Salad [216]	Cajun Shrimp and Grits [158]	Pan-Roasted Carrots with Gremolata [192]
day 5	2 large eggs, cooked any style / Apple and Sage Sausage Patties / 1 piece/1 cup fruit, your choice [54]	Leftover Cajun Shrimp and Grits / Leftover Pan-Roasted Carrots with Gremolata	Chicken Piccata [112]	Zucchini Noodles [328]
day 6	Sweet Potato Hash with Spicy Hollandaise [76]	Leftover Chicken Piccata / Leftover Zucchini Noodles	Lemon and Thyme Chicken Thighs (double batch) [120]	Brussels Sprouts with Capers and Pancetta [184]
day 7	Blueberry Muffins [56] / Leftover Apple and Sage Sausage Patties	Leftover Lemon and Thyme Chicken Thighs / Leftover Brussels Sprouts with Capers and Pancetta	Pork Vindaloo [140]	Seasoned Cauliflower Rice [200]

Shopping list

FRESH PRODUCE / HERBS

apple, green, 1 small

apples, red, 3 small

asparagus, 1 pound

avocados, 2 large

bananas, 2 medium

bell pepper, red, 1 large

blueberries, ½ cup

broccoli, 1 medium head + 1 small head

broccoli slaw, 1 (18-ounce) bag (or 3 medium carrots + 2 medium bunches broccoli)

Brussels sprouts, 1¾ pounds

carrots, 3 pounds

cauliflower, 1 large head + 1 medium head (about 3½ pounds)

celery, 5 stalks

chives, fresh, 1 bunch (optional)

cilantro, fresh, 1 bunch

cucumber, 1 large

fruit (your choice), 4 pieces/4 cups per person

garlic, 2 heads

ginger, fresh, 1 inch

grapes, red seedless, 1 cup

green onions, 2 (optional)

kale, 1 bunch

lemons, 9 large

lettuce, Bibb or romaine, 1 small head

limes, 3 large

mixed greens, 2 cups per person

mushrooms, white or cremini, 2½ ounces

onions, red, ½ small + 1 medium

onions, white, 2 small

onions, white or yellow, 5 small + 3 medium

parsley, fresh, ¾ bunch + optional ½ bunch

pineapple chunks, 2 cups

sage, fresh, ¼ cup

sweet potatoes, red-skinned, 6 medium (about 2 pounds)

tarragon, fresh, 1 tablespoon

thyme, fresh, 12 sprigs

tomatoes, 2 large

turnips, 4 medium

zucchini, 12 to 16 large (about 6 pounds)

MEATS / SEAFOOD / EGGS

bacon, thick-cut, 17 strips

chicken, 1 whole (5 pounds)

chicken breasts, boneless, skinless, 3½ pounds

chicken thighs, bone-in, skin-on, 12 (4 pounds)

eggs, 25 large + 4 more per person

flank steak, 1 pound

ground Italian sausage, 1 pound

ground pork, 1 pound

pancetta, 4 ounces

pork butt, boneless, 2 pounds

shrimp, large, 1 pound

smoked salmon, 2 ounces

turkey deli meat, sliced, 3 ounces per person

NUTS / SEEDS / BUTTERS

almond butter, ⅓ cup

almonds, sliced, ⅓ cup

cashews, raw, ⅓ cup (optional)

pecans, roasted, ½ cup

pine nuts, raw, ¼ cup

sesame seeds, ¼ cup

SAUCES / CONDIMENTS

apple cider vinegar, ¾ cup

balsamic vinegar, 1 tablespoon

coconut aminos, 2 tablespoons (or homemade soy sauce substitute, page 283)

Dijon mustard, ½ teaspoon

honey, raw, ¾ cup + 2 tablespoons

mayonnaise, ¾ cup + 2 tablespoons per person (or homemade, page 278)

CANNED GOODS

almond milk, 1 cup (or homemade, page 318)

capers, ½ cup + 2 tablespoons

chicken stock, 12¾ cups (102 fluid ounces; or homemade, page 310)

coconut milk, full-fat, 2 (13.5-ounce) cans (or 2 cups homemade, page 314)

tuna, canned in water, 1 (5-ounce) can per person

DRIED SPICES / HERBS

cayenne pepper, ⅛ teaspoon (optional)

chili powder, 1 teaspoon

crushed red pepper, ½ teaspoon + optional 1 teaspoon

dried oregano, ½ teaspoon

dried parsley, ½ teaspoon

dried thyme, 2 teaspoons

dry yellow mustard, ½ teaspoon

garlic powder, 1 tablespoon + ¼ teaspoon

ground cardamom, 1 teaspoon

ground coriander, 1 tablespoon

ground cumin, 2½ teaspoons

ground ginger, 1¼ teaspoons

onion powder, 1 teaspoon

paprika, 2½ teaspoons

turmeric, 1 teaspoon

FATS / OILS

extra-virgin olive oil, ¾ cup + 1 tablespoon

extra-virgin olive oil or ghee, 4 tablespoons (or homemade ghee, page 320)

ghee or coconut oil, ¼ cup (or homemade ghee, page 320)

ghee or palm shortening, ¼ cup (or homemade ghee, page 320)

ghee, lard, or tallow, 1¾ cups + 3 tablespoons (or homemade, pages 320 to 324)

lard or tallow, 1 cup (or homemade, pages 322 and 324)

sesame oil, 2½ teaspoons

FLOURS AND OTHER BAKING INGREDIENTS

almond flour, finely ground and blanched, 2½ cups (or homemade, page 316)

baking powder, ½ teaspoon

pure vanilla extract, 2 teaspoons

tapioca flour or arrowroot flour, ½ cup + 2 tablespoons

_____

_____

_____

_____

_____

_____

WEEK 2

	Breakfast	Lunch	Dinner
day 1	2 large eggs, cooked any style Strawberry Avocado Smoothie (double batch) **306**	Pizza Stuffed Mushrooms **142** Chopped raw vegetables of choice	Orange Chicken (double batch) **118**	Pan-Roasted Carrots with Gremolata **192**
day 2	Turkey slices, tomato, and avocado wrapped in lettuce 1 piece/1 cup fruit, your choice	**Leftover** Orange Chicken	**Leftover** Pan-Roasted Carrots with Gremolata	Taco Soup **236**	Mexican Cauliflower Rice **204**
day 3	2 large eggs, cooked any style 2 slices cooked bacon 1 piece/1 cup fruit, your choice	**Leftover** Taco Soup	**Leftover** Mexican Cauliflower Rice	Mediterranean Fish **178**	Spicy Smashed Sweet Potatoes **208**
day 4	Grab-and-Go Omelets **68** 1 piece/1 cup fruit, your choice	Honey Chipotle Meatballs **88** Chopped raw vegetables of choice	Cajun Chicken Pasta **108** · Zucchini Noodles **328** · Roasted Asparagus with Lemon Sauce **196**
day 5	Grab-and-Go Omelets **Leftover** 1 piece/1 cup fruit, your choice	**Leftover** Cajun Chicken Pasta · **Leftover** Zucchini Noodles · **Leftover** Roasted Asparagus with Lemon Sauce	Spicy Beef and Pepper Stir-Fry (double batch) **98**	Seasoned Cauliflower Rice **200**
day 6	Sweet Crêpes **74** 2 slices cooked bacon	**Leftover** Spicy Beef and Pepper Stir-Fry	**Leftover** Seasoned Cauliflower Rice	Moroccan Chicken (double batch) **122** · Zucchini Noodles **328** · Avocado Basil Cream Sauce **270**
day 7	Breakfast Pizza **58**	**Leftover** Moroccan Chicken	**Leftover** Zucchini Noodles	Slow Cooker Pork Ribs (double batch) **144**	Creamy Coleslaw **188**

Shopping list

FRESH PRODUCE / HERBS

asparagus, 1 pound

avocados, 6 large

baby spinach, 2 cups

basil, fresh, ½ cup + optional 6 leaves

bell peppers, green, 1 small + 4 medium

bell peppers, red, 1 small + 4 medium

cabbage, 1 head (about 1 pound)

carrots, 3 pounds

cauliflower, 2 large heads (about 4 pounds)

cherry tomatoes, 6

cilantro, fresh, ¼ bunch + optional ¼ bunch

fruit (your choice), 4 pieces/4 cups per person

garlic, 2 heads

ginger, fresh, 4 inches

green onions, 7 (optional)

lemons, 9 large

lettuce, Bibb or romaine, 1 small head

limes, 5 large

mushrooms, white, 6 large

mushrooms, white or cremini, 12 (about 1½ pounds)

onion, white, 2 small

onions, red, 1¾ medium + 1 small

onions, white or yellow, 7 small

orange, 1 large

parsley, fresh, 1 small bunch

raw vegetables of choice, 2 cups chopped per person

strawberries, 24

sweet potatoes, red-skinned, 1 pound

tomatoes, 6 large

zucchini, 12 to 16 large (about 6 pounds)

MEATS / SEAFOOD / EGGS

baby back ribs, 6 pounds

bacon, thick-cut, 4 strips + 4 per person

beef sirloin steak, 4 pounds

breakfast sausage, ½ pound

chicken drumsticks and thighs, bone-in, 8 pounds

chicken legs and thighs, bone-in, 8 pounds

chicken thighs, boneless, skinless, 1 pound

eggs, 20 large + 4 per person

ground beef, 2¾ pounds

ground pork, ¾ pound

halibut fillets, 4 (6 ounces each)

pork sausage, ½ pound

prosciutto, 12 slices (6 ounces)

turkey deli meat, sliced, 3 ounces per person

NUTS / SEEDS / BUTTERS

sesame seeds, 4 teaspoons

SAUCES / CONDIMENTS

apple cider vinegar, ¼ cup

barbecue sauce, 2 cups (or homemade, page 272)

coconut aminos, ½ cup (or homemade soy sauce substitute, page 283)

Dijon mustard, ½ teaspoon

honey, raw, 1⅔ cups + 2 tablespoons

mayonnaise, 1 cup (or homemade, page 278)

tomato sauce, 1 (15-ounce) can + 1 cup

CANNED GOODS

almond milk, 1½ cups (or homemade, page 318)

beef stock, 1 cup (8 fluid ounces; or homemade, page 310)

capers, ¼ cup

chicken stock, 2 cups (16 fluid ounces; or homemade, page 310)

coconut milk, full-fat, 4 (13.5-ounce) cans (or 5½ cups homemade, page 314)

green chiles, roasted, 1 (4-ounce) can

Kalamata olives, pitted, ½ cup

olives, sliced black, ¼ cup

pineapple juice, 1 cup

tomato paste, ½ cup (⅔ (6-ounce) can)

DRIED SPICES / HERBS

cayenne pepper, 1 teaspoon + optional ¼ teaspoon

celery seed, ½ teaspoon

chili powder, 1 teaspoon

chipotle powder or chili powder, ¼ teaspoon

crushed red pepper, 2½ teaspoons

dried basil, 1 teaspoon

dried oregano, 1 tablespoon + 1 teaspoon

dried rosemary, 1 teaspoon

dried thyme, 1¼ teaspoons

dry yellow mustard, ¾ teaspoon

garlic powder, 2 teaspoons

ground cumin, 3½ teaspoons

ground ginger, 4 teaspoons

onion powder, ¾ teaspoon

paprika, 3 tablespoons + 2¼ teaspoons

turmeric, 2 teaspoons

FATS / OILS

extra-virgin olive oil, ¾ cup + 3 tablespoons

ghee or coconut oil, 3 tablespoons (or homemade ghee, page 320)

ghee or extra-virgin olive oil, 2 tablespoons (or homemade ghee, page 320)

ghee, lard, or tallow, 1½ cups + 1 tablespoon (or homemade, pages 320 to 324)

sesame oil, 2 tablespoons

FLOURS AND OTHER BAKING INGREDIENTS

almond flour, finely ground and blanched, 2¾ cups + 2 tablespoons (or homemade, page 316)

baking powder, 1½ teaspoons

pure vanilla extract, 1 teaspoon

tapioca flour or arrowroot flour, 1¼ cups + 1 tablespoon

_____

_____

_____

_____

_____

_____

_____

_____

WEEK 3

	Breakfast	Lunch	Dinner
day 1	Smoked Salmon Deviled Eggs **176** 1 piece/1 cup fruit, your choice	**Leftover** **Leftover** Slow Cooker Pork Ribs and Creamy Coleslaw (from Week 2, Day 7)	**238** Thai Coconut Soup **190** Crispy Sweet Potato Wedges
day 2	2 large eggs, cooked any style **304** Piña Colada Smoothie, no topping (double batch)	**Leftover** Thai Coconut Soup **Leftover** Crispy Sweet Potato Wedges	**152** Pork Schnitzel **182** Balsamic Rosemary Mushrooms **207** Slow Cooker Applesauce
day 3	Turkey slices, tomato, and avocado wrapped in lettuce 1 piece/1 cup fruit, your choice	**Leftover** Pork Schnitzel **Leftover** Balsamic Rosemary Mushrooms **Leftover** Slow Cooker Applesauce	**172** Orange and Ginger Glazed Salmon **202** Fried Cauliflower Rice **192** Pan-Roasted Carrots with Gremolata
day 4	2 large eggs, cooked any style **54** Apple and Sage Sausage Patties 1 piece/1 cup fruit, your choice	**Leftover** Orange and Ginger Glazed Salmon **Leftover** Fried Cauliflower Rice **Leftover** Pan-Roasted Carrots with Gremolata	**84** Cottage Pie **218** Brussels Sprouts and Bacon Salad
day 5	**Leftover** Cottage Pie **Leftover** Brussels Sprouts and Bacon Salad	Canned tuna mixed with mayonnaise on a bed of greens with sliced tomatoes and cucumber 1 piece/1 cup fruit, your choice	**168** Grilled Seafood Skewers **198** Roasted Squash and Pesto
day 6	Eggs Baked in Tomato Sauce **66**	BLT Scallops with Herb Mayo **156** Chopped raw vegetables of choice	**102** Swedish Meatballs **328** Zucchini Noodles **189** Mashed Sweet Potatoes
day 7	**72** Lemon Poppyseed Waffles **Leftover** Apple and Sage Sausage Patties	**Leftover** Swedish Meatballs **Leftover** Zucchini Noodles **Leftover** Mashed Sweet Potatoes	Comforting Beef Stew (double batch) **230**

Shopping list

FRESH PRODUCE / HERBS

apple, green, 1 small

apples, 3 pounds

avocado, 1 large

baby arugula, ¼ cup

bananas, 2 medium

basil, fresh, 3 tablespoons (optional)

bell pepper, yellow, 1 medium

bell peppers, green, 1 medium + 1 small

bell peppers, red, 1 medium + 1 small

berries, assorted, 1 cup

blueberries, dried, ½ cup

Brussels sprouts, 1 pound

carrots, 3½ pounds

cauliflower, 1 medium head (about 1½ pounds) + optional 1 large head (about 2 pounds)

celery, 2 stalks

cherry tomatoes, 16 small

chives, fresh, 1 tablespoon (optional)

cilantro, fresh, 1 small bunch

cucumber, 1 large

fruit (your choice), 4 pieces/4 cups per person

garlic, 3 large heads

green onions, 4 (optional)

lemons, 6 large

lettuce, Bibb or romaine, 1 small head

limes, 7 large

mixed greens, 2 cups per person

mushrooms, white, 1½ pounds

mushrooms, white or cremini, 1⅓ pounds

onion, red, ½ small

onion, white, 1 small + optional 1 small

onions, white or yellow, 4 small + 1 medium + 3 large

oranges, 2 large

parsley, fresh, ½ bunch + optional 1 bunch

pineapple chunks, 2 cups

raw vegetables of choice, 2 cups chopped per person

rosemary, fresh, ½ small bunch

sage, fresh, ¼ cup

shallots, 2 small

sweet potatoes, white-skinned, 4 medium (about 1¼ pounds)

sweet potatoes, white or red-skinned, 4 pounds

tomato, Roma, 1 small

tomatoes, 2 large

yellow summer squash, 2 large (about 1 pound)

zucchini, 8 to 10 large (about 4 pounds)

MEATS / SEAFOOD / EGGS

bacon, thick-cut, 9 slices

beef round roast, boneless, 4 pounds

chicken thighs, boneless, skinless, 1 pound

cod fillets, 2 pounds

eggs, 22 large + 4 per person

ground beef, 3½ pounds

ground pork, 1 pound

pork loin chops, boneless, 1½ pounds

salmon fillets, skinless, 1 inch thick, 1½ pounds

sea scallops, large, 6 (about ½ pound)

smoked salmon, 2 ounces

turkey deli meat, sliced, 3 ounces per person

NUTS / SEEDS / BUTTERS

almonds, slivered, ½ cup

poppy seeds, ½ teaspoon

SAUCES / CONDIMENTS

apple cider vinegar, 2 tablespoons

balsamic vinegar, 1 tablespoon

coconut aminos, ¾ cup (or homemade soy sauce substitute, page 283)

Dijon mustard, 2 teaspoons

fish sauce, 1 tablespoon + 2 teaspoons

honey, raw, 1 cup + ½ tablespoon + 2½ teaspoons

mayonnaise, ½ cup + 2 tablespoons per person (or homemade, page 278)

pesto, 3 tablespoons (or homemade, page 280)

pure maple syrup (for serving)

CANNED GOODS

almond milk, ¾ cup (or homemade, page 318)

almond milk or coconut milk, 1 cup (or homemade, pages 318 and 314)

beef stock, 9 cups (72 fluid ounces; or homemade, page 310)

capers, 2 tablespoons

chicken stock, 3½ cups (28 fluid ounces; or homemade, page 310)

chopped tomatoes, 2 (14-ounce) cans

coconut milk, full-fat, 5 (13.5-ounce) cans (or 6⅓ cups homemade, page 314)

diced green chiles, mild, roasted, 1 (4-ounce) can

tomato paste, ¼ cup + 3 tablespoons (⅔ (6-ounce) can)

tuna, canned in water, 1 (5-ounce) can per person

DRIED SPICES / HERBS

bay leaves, 4

celery seed, ⅛ teaspoon

dried oregano, 2⅛ teaspoons

dried parsley, ½ teaspoon

dried rosemary, 2 teaspoons

dried thyme, 3⅛ teaspoons

garlic powder, 1⅛ teaspoon

ground cinnamon, ¼ teaspoon

ground cumin, 1 teaspoon

ground ginger, 1½ teaspoons

onion powder, ½ teaspoon

paprika, 2 tablespoons + 1¼ teaspoons

FATS / OILS

extra-virgin olive oil, ½ cup + 2 tablespoons

ghee or coconut oil, ½ cup, plus more for greasing (or homemade ghee, page 320)

ghee, lard, or tallow, 1¾ cups + 3 tablespoons + optional 2 tablespoons (or homemade, pages 320 to 324)

lard or tallow, 1¼ cup + 2 tablespoons (or homemade, pages 322 and 324)

sesame oil, ½ teaspoon

FLOURS AND OTHER BAKING INGREDIENTS

almond flour, finely ground and blanched, 3½ cups (or homemade, page 316)

baking soda, 1 teaspoon

pure vanilla extract, 1 teaspoon

tapioca flour, ¼ cup + 2 tablespoons

tapioca flour or arrowroot flour, 1½ cups

WEEK 4

	Breakfast	Lunch	Dinner
day 1	2 large eggs, cooked any style Strawberry Avocado Smoothie (double batch) **306**	Comforting Beef Stew (from Week 3, Day 7) **Leftover**	**110** Chicken Curry **200** Seasoned Cauliflower Rice **188** Creamy Coleslaw
day 2	Grab-and-Go Omelets 1 piece/1 cup fruit, your choice **68**	**Leftover** Chicken Curry **Leftover** Seasoned Cauliflower Rice **Leftover** Creamy Coleslaw	Asian Sesame Chicken Salad **216**
day 3	2 large eggs, cooked any style 2 slices cooked bacon 1 piece/1 cup fruit, your choice	**128** Sesame Chicken Wings **218** Brussels Sprouts and Bacon Salad	**164** Cilantro Lime Shrimp **204** Mexican Cauliflower Rice **208** Spicy Smashed Sweet Potatoes
day 4	Grab-and-Go Omelets 1 piece/1 cup fruit, your choice **Leftover**	**Leftover** Cilantro Lime Shrimp **Leftover** Mexican Cauliflower Rice **Leftover** Spicy Smashed Sweet Potatoes	**138** Pork Ragout **189** Mashed Sweet Potatoes **207** Slow Cooker Applesauce
day 5	Turkey slices, tomato, and avocado wrapped in lettuce 1 piece/1 cup fruit, your choice	**Leftover** Pork Ragout **Leftover** Mashed Sweet Potatoes **Leftover** Slow Cooker Applesauce	Cioppino **224**
day 6	Deviled Scotch Eggs 1 piece/1 cup fruit, your choice **64**	**94** Popcorn Chicken-Fried Steak and Gravy **190** Crispy Sweet Potato Wedges	**90** Mongolian Beef (double batch) **206** Sesame Ginger Broccolini (double batch)
day 7	Broccoli and Mushroom Frittata 1 piece/1 cup fruit, your choice **60**	**Leftover** Mongolian Beef **Leftover** Sesame Ginger Broccolini	**92** Pasta Bolognese **328** Zucchini Noodles

Shopping list

FRESH PRODUCE / HERBS

apples, 3 pounds

avocados, 4 large + 2 medium

baby spinach, 1 cup

basil, fresh, ½ small bunch

bell pepper, red, 1 medium

bell peppers, green, 2 medium

blueberries, dried, ½ cup

broccoli slaw, 1 (18-ounce) bag (or 3 medium carrots + 2 medium heads broccoli)

broccoli, 1 small head

broccolini, 2 pounds

Brussels sprouts, 1 pound

cabbage, 1 head (about 1 pound)

carrots, 2 medium + 2 large

cauliflower, 2 large heads (4 pounds)

celery, 2 stalks

chives, fresh, 1 tablespoon (optional)

cilantro, fresh, 2 medium bunches

fruit (your choice), 6 pieces/6 cups per person

garlic, 3 large heads

green onions, 7 (optional)

lemons, 2 large

lettuce, Bibb or romaine, 1 small head

limes, 4 large

mushrooms, white or cremini, 2½ ounces

onion, red, 1 medium

onions, white, 2 small

onions, white or yellow, 4 small + 2 medium + 1 large

parsley, fresh, 1 medium bunch (optional)

shallot, 1 small

strawberries, 24

sweet potatoes, red-skinned, 3 medium (about 1 pound)

sweet potatoes, white-skinned, 4 medium (about 1¼ pounds)

sweet potatoes, white- or red-skinned, 2 pounds

tarragon, fresh, 1 tablespoon

thyme, fresh, 1 teaspoon

tomatoes, 9 large

tomatoes, Roma, 6 large

zucchini, 6 to 8 large (about 3 pounds)

MEATS / SEAFOOD / EGGS

bacon, thick-cut, 11 slices + 2 per person

breakfast sausage, ½ pound

chicken breasts, boneless, skinless, 1 pound

chicken thighs, boneless, skinless, 2 pounds

chicken wings and drumettes, 2 pounds

clams, 1 pound

cube steak, 1¾ pounds

eggs, 23 large + 4 per person

fish fillets (cod, halibut, or mahi mahi), 1½ pounds

flank steak, 4 pounds

ground beef, 1 pound

ground pork, 1 pound

ground pork sausage, 1 pound

mussels, 1 pound

pancetta, 3 ounces

pork shoulder, boneless, 2 pounds

prosciutto, 12 slices (6 ounces)

shrimp, large, 1 pound

shrimp, medium, ½ pound

turkey deli meat, sliced, 3 ounces per person

NUTS / SEEDS / BUTTERS

almonds, sliced, ⅓ cup

almonds, slivered, ½ cup

sesame seeds, ½ cup

SAUCES / CONDIMENTS

apple cider vinegar, ¾ cup + 2 tablespoons + 1 teaspoon

coconut aminos, 2½ cups + 2 tablespoons (or homemade soy sauce substitute, page 283)

Dijon mustard, 2 teaspoons

honey, raw, 2¾ cups

mayonnaise, 1 cup (or homemade, page 278)

tomato sauce, ½ cup

CANNED GOODS

almond milk, 1½ cups (or homemade, page 318)

almond milk or coconut milk, 1 cup + 2 tablespoons (or homemade, pages 318 and 314)

beef stock, 3⅓ cups (27 fluid ounces; or homemade, page 310)

chicken or beef stock, 2 cups (16 fluid ounces; or homemade, page 310)

chicken stock, 1¼ cups (10 fluid ounces; or homemade, page 310)

coconut milk, full-fat, 4 (13.5-ounce) cans (or 3⅔ cups homemade coconut milk, page 314, + ½ cup homemade coconut cream, page 315)

fish or chicken stock, 6 cups (48 fluid ounces; or homemade, page 312 or 310)

pineapple juice, 1 cup

tomato paste, 2 (6-ounce) cans + 1 tablespoon

DRIED SPICES / HERBS

bay leaves, 3

cayenne pepper, ¼ teaspoon

celery seed, ½ teaspoon

chili powder, ½ teaspoon

crushed red pepper, 2½ teaspoons

curry powder, 4 teaspoons

dried basil, 1 tablespoon

dried rosemary, 1 teaspoon

dried thyme, 1 tablespoon

dry yellow mustard, ½ teaspoon

garlic powder, 1¾ teaspoons

ground cinnamon, ¼ teaspoon

ground cumin, 2½ teaspoons

ground ginger, 3 tablespoons

onion powder, 1 teaspoon

paprika, 3 teaspoons

turmeric, ½ teaspoon

FATS / OILS

extra-virgin olive oil, ½ cup + 3 tablespoons

extra-virgin olive oil or ghee, 2 tablespoons (or homemade ghee, page 320)

ghee, lard, or tallow, 2 cups (or homemade, pages 320 to 324)

lard or tallow, 1 cup + 2 tablespoons, plus more for frying (or homemade, pages 322 and 324)

sesame oil, ¼ cup + 2 tablespoons

FLOURS AND OTHER BAKING INGREDIENTS

almond flour, finely ground and blanched, 1½ cups (or homemade, page 316)

tapioca flour, 3⅓ cups

tapioca flour or arrowroot flour, ¾ cup

PALEO
SNACK
IDEAS

Vegetables

Chopped raw vegetables

Dill pickles

Avocado half sprinkled with salt and pepper

Eggplant Dip (page 271), hummus (page 276), pico de gallo (page 282), or guacamole (page 274) with chopped carrots, celery, bell peppers, cherry tomatoes, and/or sliced cucumber

Olives, green or black

Sauerkraut

Simple green salad with olive oil and balsamic vinegar dressing

Nuts and Seeds

Nut or seed butter on celery sticks or apple slices

Small bowl of Granola (page 70), plain or with almond or coconut milk (pages 318 and 314)

Small handful of nuts or seeds

Eggs

Deviled Scotch Eggs (page 64)

Egg salad made with chopped hard-boiled eggs mixed with mayonnaise (page 278) or ripe avocado

Grab-and-Go Omelets (page 68)

Hard-boiled eggs

Scrambled eggs with pico de gallo (page 282)

Smoked Salmon Deviled Eggs (page 176)

Meat / Seafood

Apple and Sage Sausage Patties (page 54)

Bacon

Chicken Salad on Apple Slices (page 114)

Cooked shrimp

Sardines

Smoked oysters

Smoked salmon (great on cucumber slices)

Tuna, plain or mixed with mayonnaise (page 278) or ripe avocado

Turkey, tomato, and avocado wrapped in lettuce

Fruit

Slow Cooker Applesauce (page 207)

Cantaloupe wrapped in prosciutto

Coconut Milk Yogurt (page 62) with fresh berries

Fresh fruit

Piña Colada Smoothie (page 304)

Strawberry Avocado Smoothie (page 306)

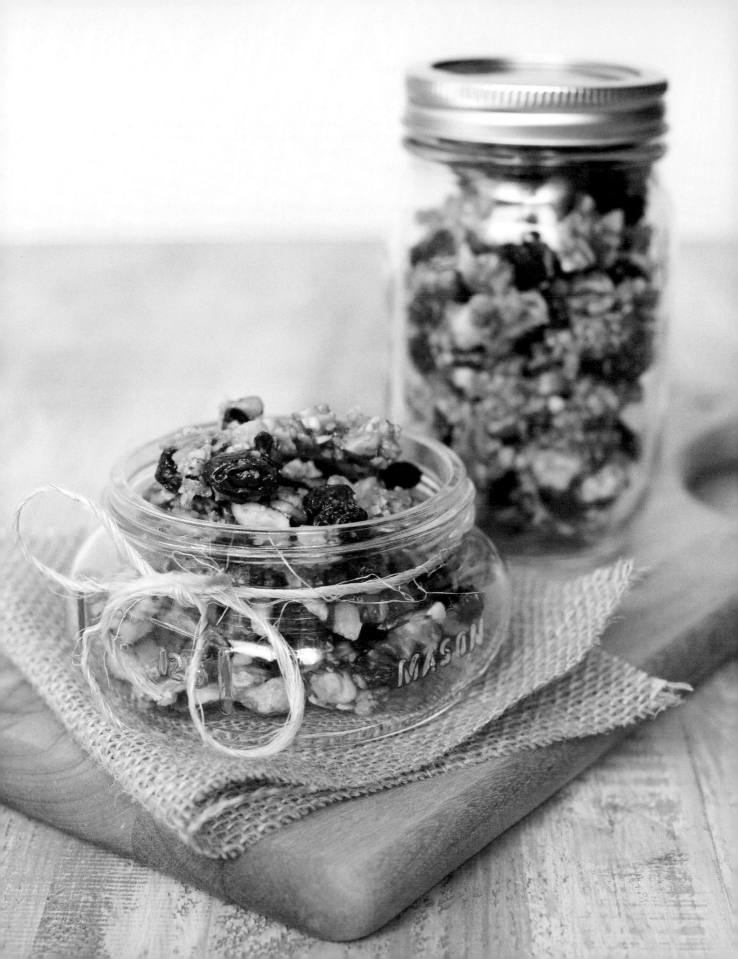

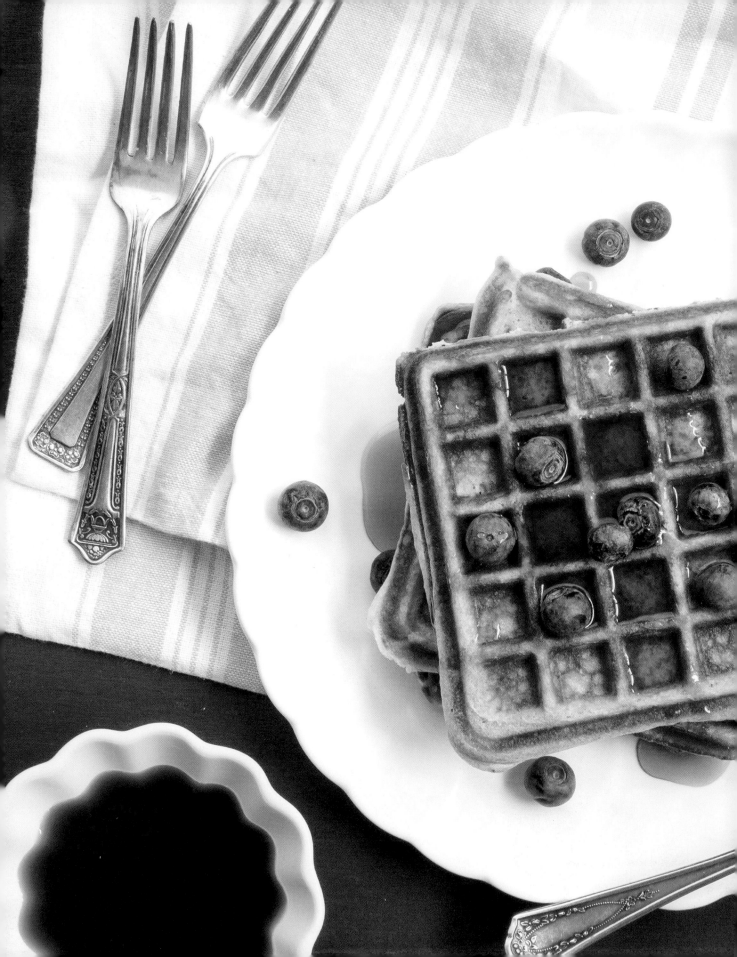

breakfast

APPLE *and* SAGE SAUSAGE PATTIES

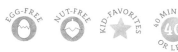

EGG-FREE NUT-FREE KID-FAVORITES 40 MINUTES OR LESS

Making your own breakfast patties at home is an easy way to ensure that your sausage doesn't contain any unhealthy mystery ingredients. The sweet and tart flavors of green apples combined with aromatic sage make these a nice alternative to traditional breakfast sausage. Substituting ground chicken thighs for the pork also works well for this recipe.

Prep Time: 10 minutes   Cook Time: 30 minutes   Yield: 10 patties (4 to 5 servings)

3 tablespoons ghee (page 320), lard (page 322), or tallow (page 324), divided

1 small onion, finely chopped (about ½ cup)

1 small green apple, such as Granny Smith, peeled, cored, and finely chopped (about ½ cup)

1 pound ground pork

¼ cup fresh sage, sliced into thin strips

½ teaspoon fine sea salt

½ teaspoon ground black pepper

½ teaspoon dried parsley

1. Melt 1 tablespoon of the ghee in a large skillet over medium heat. Add the chopped onion and apples and cook for about 4 to 5 minutes, until the apples and onion begin to soften. Transfer the apples and onion to a large mixing bowl and let cool for 5 minutes. Set the skillet aside.

2. Add the ground pork, sage, salt, pepper, and parsley to the apples and onion and mix with your hands until well combined. Form the mixture into 10 patties about 1 inch thick.

3. Return the skillet to the stove and melt the remaining 2 tablespoons of ghee over medium heat. Working in batches so you don't overcrowd the pan, cook the sausage patties for 5 minutes on each side, or until browned and cooked through. Serve right away or store in a sealed container in the refrigerator for up to 3 days.

KITCHEN TIP

These sausages are freezer-friendly! After shaping the patties, lay them out evenly on a baking sheet lined with parchment paper. Freeze for 1 to 2 hours, until hardened, then transfer to a sealed container and store in your freezer. The night before you want to cook them, place them in the refrigerator to defrost overnight.
For a quick and easy lunch, pack leftover cooked sausage with some chopped vegetables and a piece of fruit.

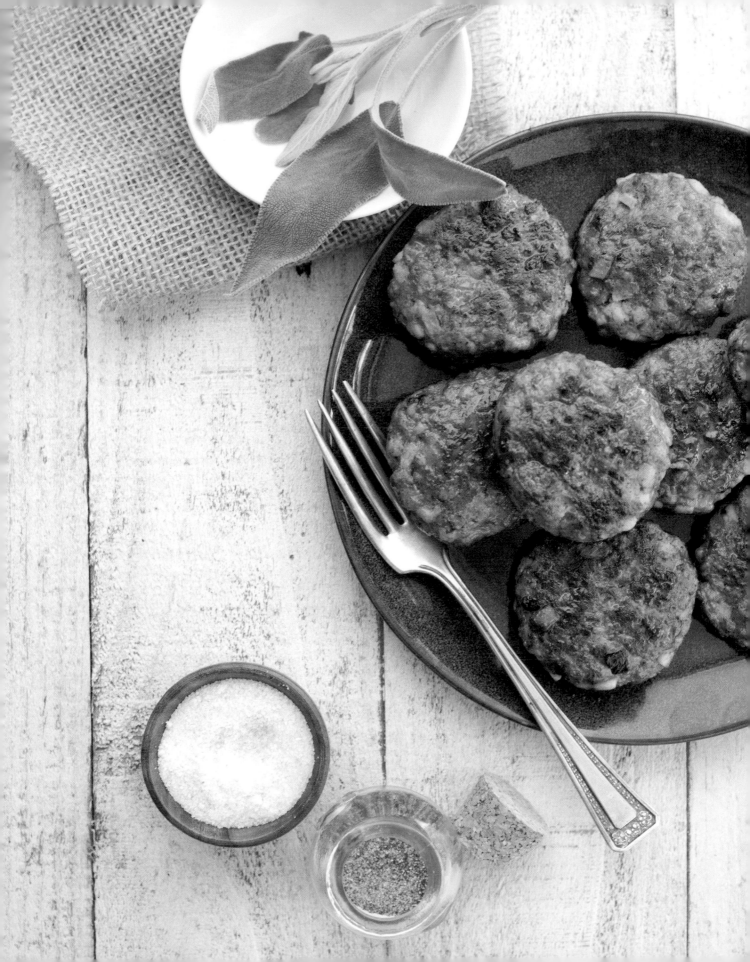

BLUEBERRY
MUFFINS

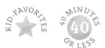

While I don't eat baked treats very often, I am a sucker for a good blueberry muffin. If you're using frozen blueberries, add them to the batter without thawing; otherwise, they will turn your muffins purple. These muffins are easy to pack and make a nice occasional treat for lunch. If you have younger kids, make sure to peel off the liners before packing their muffins. My kids have eaten many a liner in their day. I like to think of it as extra fiber.

Prep Time: 10 minutes   Cook Time: 25 minutes   Yield: 6 muffins

1 cup almond flour (page 316)

¼ cup plus 2 tablespoons tapioca flour or arrowroot flour

½ teaspoon baking powder

¼ teaspoon fine sea salt

¼ cup raw honey

¼ cup ghee (page 320) or coconut oil

2 teaspoons pure vanilla extract

1 large egg, room temperature

½ cup blueberries

1. Place an oven rack in the middle position and preheat the oven to 350°F. Line 6 cups of a muffin pan with baking liners.

2. Combine the almond flour, tapioca flour, baking powder, and salt in a medium-sized mixing bowl and stir to combine.

3. Place the honey, ghee, and vanilla in a separate medium-sized mixing bowl and beat with a hand mixer on medium speed for about 30 seconds, or until well combined. Add the egg and beat for another 30 seconds.

4. Reduce the mixer speed to low and gradually add the dry ingredients, mixing until fully combined. Gently fold in the blueberries, then spoon the batter into the lined cups of the muffin pan.

5. Place the muffins in the oven and bake for 22 to 25 minutes, until a toothpick inserted into the middle of a muffin comes out clean. Remove from the oven and let cool for at least 15 minutes before serving.

TRY THIS!
For a bright citrus flavor, whisk 1 teaspoon of fresh lemon zest and 1 teaspoon of freshly squeezed lemon juice into the wet ingredients before adding the dry ingredients.

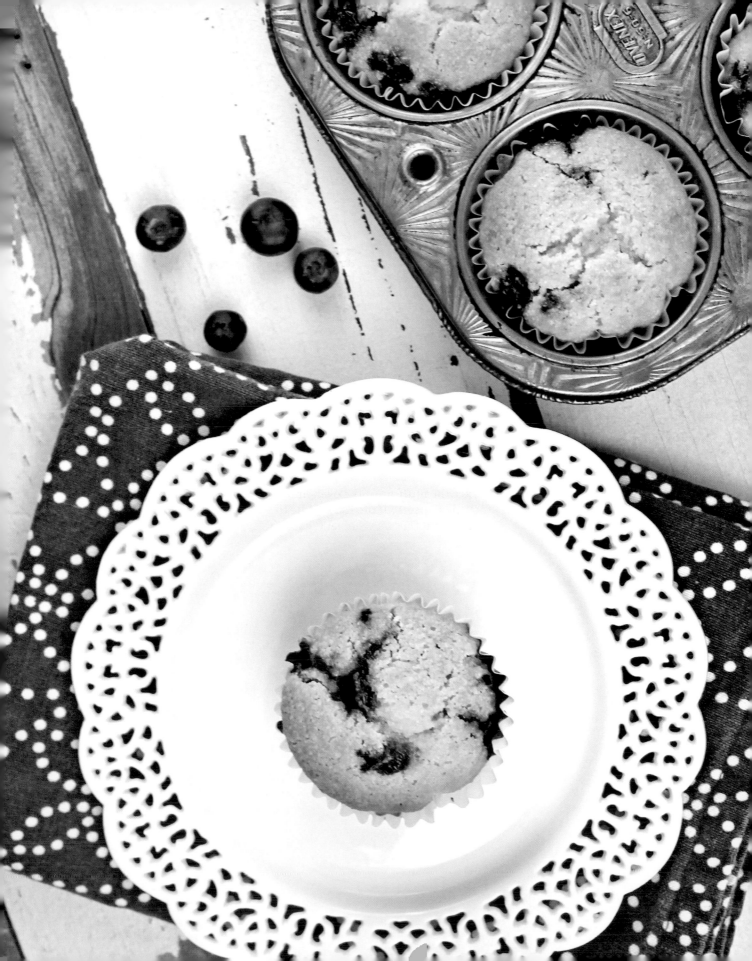

BREAKFAST
PIZZA

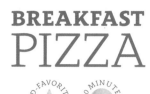

Pizza purists may turn their noses up at me for calling this pizza, but they can snub all they want; the rest of us will be over here chowing down. The tomatoes release a bit of liquid while baking, and that combined with a bit of runny egg yolk makes a delicious creamy sauce. Don't feel like you can only eat this for breakfast—it's good any time of day!

Prep Time: 10 minutes   **Cook Time:** 25 minutes   **Yield:** One 9-by-13-inch pizza (4 to 6 servings)

FOR THE CRUST

2 cups almond flour (page 316)

1 cup tapioca flour

3 large eggs

½ cup almond milk (page 318)

1½ teaspoons baking powder

1 teaspoon fine sea salt

½ teaspoon garlic powder

½ teaspoon dried basil

½ teaspoon ground black pepper

FOR THE TOPPINGS

1 large tomato (about ½ pound), thinly sliced

1 cup fresh baby spinach

½ cup thinly sliced red onion (about 1 small)

4 strips thick-cut bacon, cooked and crumbled

6 large eggs

1. Place an oven rack in the middle position and preheat the oven to 425°F. Line a 9-by-13-inch baking sheet with parchment paper or a baking mat.

2. Place all the crust ingredients in a food processor or blender and blend for 30 seconds, or until you have a thick but smooth batter. Use a rubber spatula to spread the batter in a thin layer on the prepared baking sheet, leaving about an inch between the batter and the edge of the pan on all sides. Bake for 10 to 12 minutes, until the dough is light golden brown.

3. Remove the crust from the oven and add the toppings in layers, starting with the sliced tomatoes, then the spinach, onion, and bacon. Crack an egg into a small bowl or measuring cup and then slide it onto the top of the pizza toppings. Continue with the rest of the eggs, leaving a bit of space around each egg.

4. Return the pan to the oven and bake for another 10 to 12 minutes, until the egg whites are cooked through and the yolks are cooked to your liking. Remove from the oven, sprinkle with a little ground pepper if desired, slice, and serve.

TRY THIS!

You don't have to stick to the toppings listed here! Try mixing and matching whatever toppings you like, such as sliced mushrooms, cooked sausage, or chopped broccoli, or add fresh toppings, such as sliced avocado or a sprinkle of chopped cilantro, right before serving.

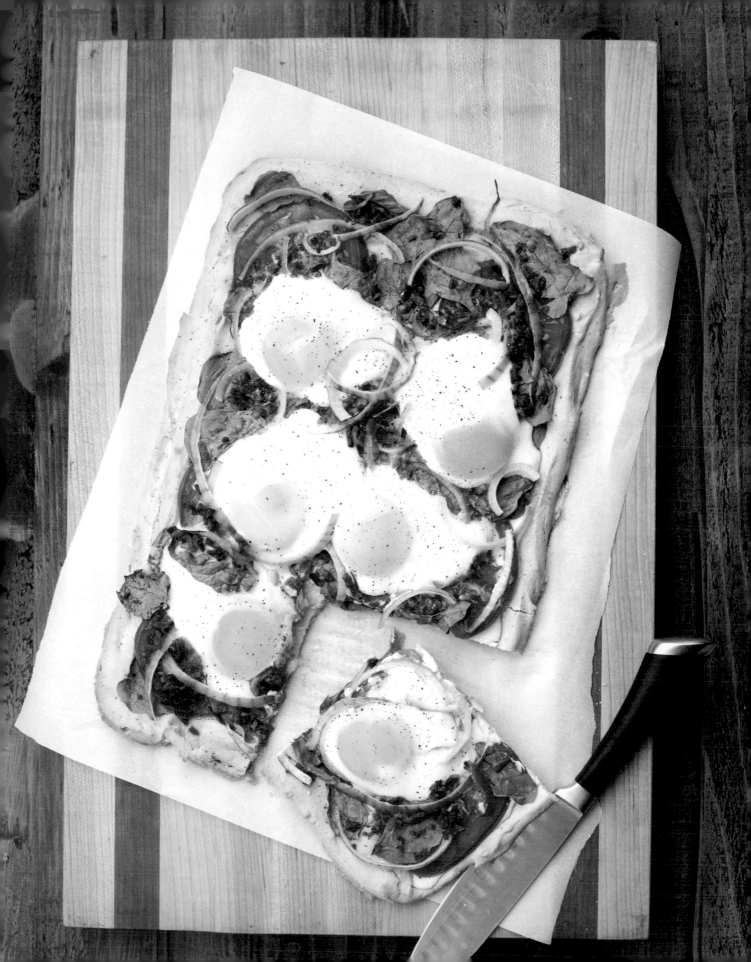

BROCCOLI *and* MUSHROOM FRITTATA

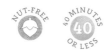

NUT-FREE · 40 MINUTES OR LESS · 40

The great thing about a frittata is that it's basically the same thing as an omelet, but without all the flipping and bother that making an omelet entails. All you need to do is pour the eggs and whatever other ingredients you like into a pan, and the oven does the rest for you. Frittatas are good served warm or cold, and a leftover slice is perfect for a packed lunch. This is a great base recipe for a frittata, but you can get as crazy as you like with the ingredients—just follow your taste buds.

Prep Time: 7 minutes   Cook Time: 23 minutes   Yield: 4 to 6 servings

8 large eggs

½ teaspoon fine sea salt

¼ teaspoon ground black pepper

5 slices thick-cut bacon

½ cup chopped onion

¾ cup chopped broccoli

1 clove garlic, minced

¾ cup sliced white or cremini mushrooms

1 tablespoon chopped fresh tarragon

1 tablespoon chopped fresh parsley, for garnish (optional)

1. In a medium-sized bowl, whisk together the eggs, salt, and pepper until well combined, then set aside.

2. In a medium-sized oven-safe skillet over medium-high heat, cook the bacon until crispy, then transfer it to a paper towel–lined plate and crumble once cooled.

3. Reduce the heat to medium and pour out most of the bacon drippings from the pan, leaving enough to coat the bottom of the pan. Add the chopped onion to the pan and sauté for 4 minutes, or until just softened. Add the broccoli, garlic, and mushrooms and sauté for another 2 minutes. Turn off the heat and add the chopped tarragon.

4. Preheat the oven to broil on high.

5. Give the egg mixture one more whisk and then pour it into the pan and stir to combine. Cook for 5 to 7 minutes without stirring, until the egg mixture begins to set on top.

6. Transfer the skillet to the oven (remember the handle might be hot) and broil for 2 to 3 minutes, until the top of the frittata is light golden brown and fluffy. Remove the skillet from the oven, sprinkle with parsley, if desired, then slice to serve.

TRY THIS!

For a spicier note, add ¼ teaspoon of crushed red pepper at the same time as the chopped garlic and substitute ¼ cup chopped fresh chives for the fresh parsley.

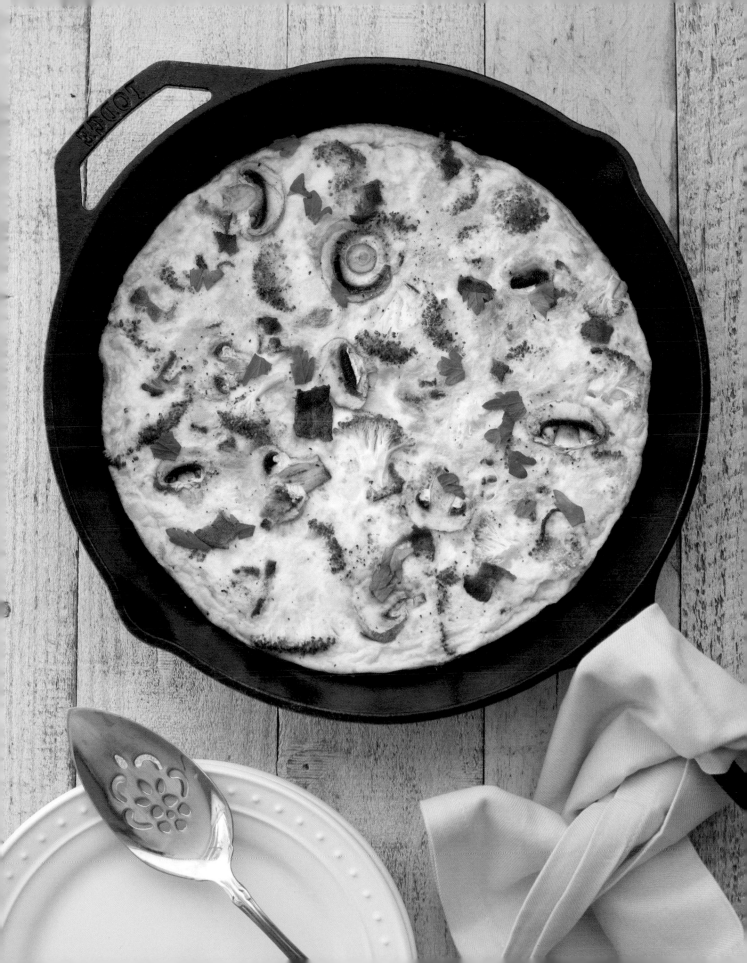

COCONUT MILK YOGURT

EGG-FREE · NUT-FREE · KID-FAVORITES

When I was a young child, my grandmother would say "Always check for teddy bears" before she opened the oven door, peeked inside, and then preheated the oven. It wasn't until I was an adult that I found out that my mother used to like to hide her teddy bears in the oven. Many times my grandmother had unknowingly preheated the oven with the poor stuffed animal still inside, and soon the smell of burnt hair filled the kitchen. To this day, I still peek in the oven before turning it on, which is a good thing because every now and then I find my batch of yogurt from the day before.

Prep Time: 5 minutes, plus 10 to 24 hours to culture   Yield: 2 cups (about 4 servings)

2 capsules probiotics (about 1 teaspoon probiotic powder)

Cream from 2 (13.5-ounce) cans full-fat coconut milk (see page 315) or 2 cups homemade coconut cream (page 315)

2 tablespoons raw honey

1 teaspoon pure vanilla extract

1. Open the probiotic capsules and empty them into a large bowl. You'll have about 1 teaspoon probiotic powder. Add the coconut cream, honey, and vanilla extract and blend on low with a hand mixer for 30 seconds, or until smooth and fully combined.

2. **To use a yogurt maker:** Scoop the yogurt mixture into jars and place the jars in the yogurt machine. Cook the yogurt according to the machine instructions (usually between 10 and 20 hours).

   To use the oven: Place the yogurt mixture in clean jars with tight-fitting lids (mason jars work well) and wrap the jars in kitchen towels. Place an oven rack in the top third of the oven and place the wrapped jars on the rack. Turn the oven light on and keep the door shut. You do not actually need to turn the oven on; it only needs to reach about 110°F inside the oven to culture the coconut milk, and the light and towels provide enough warmth. Leave the jars in the oven for at least 10 hours and up to 24 hours. The longer you leave them in the oven, the tangier the yogurt will be.

3. Store in the refrigerator until chilled. The yogurt will keep for up to a week in the refrigerator in sealed containers. It's normal for it to separate slightly after sitting. Just give it a good stir before eating.

TRY THIS!

To make strawberry yogurt, place 2 cups fresh sliced strawberries, 1 teaspoon raw honey, and 1 teaspoon freshly squeezed lemon juice in a small saucepan over medium heat. Mash the berries until they break down and form a sauce, about 5 minutes. Let cool to room temperature, then stir into the cultured yogurt. Enjoy right away or store in the refrigerator until ready to eat.

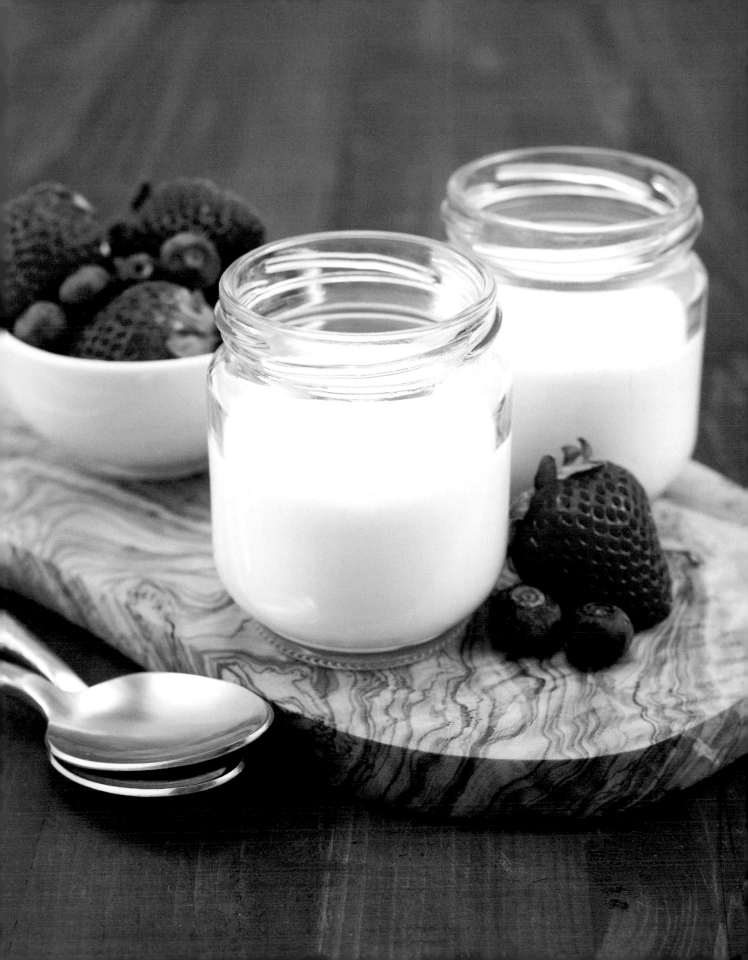

DEVILED
SCOTCH
EGGS

 NUT-FREE

The idea for this recipe came to me one day when I was thinking about how much I like Scotch eggs and deviled eggs, and suddenly it became very obvious to me that the two needed to unite and become one. A creamy ripe avocado makes a great dressing for the egg yolks, but mayonnaise (page 278) works just as well.

Prep Time: 10 minutes   Cook Time: 45 minutes   Yield: 5 servings

5 large eggs

1 pound ground pork sausage

1 teaspoon chopped fresh thyme

¼ teaspoon fine sea salt

¼ teaspoon ground black pepper

1 large ripe avocado, halved, pitted, and peeled, or ¼ cup plus 2 tablespoons mayonnaise (page 278)

1 tablespoon chopped fresh chives, for garnish (optional)

½ teaspoon paprika, for garnish (optional)

1. Preheat the oven to 375°F.

2. To hard-boil the eggs, place the eggs in a small saucepan and cover with water. Place over high heat and bring just to a boil. Turn off the heat, cover the pan, and allow to sit for 12 minutes undisturbed. Remove the eggs from the hot water with a slotted spoon and transfer to a bowl filled with ice water. Leave the eggs to cool in the ice water for 5 minutes, then peel and set aside.

3. In a large mixing bowl, mix the sausage, thyme, salt, and pepper by hand until well combined. Separate the sausage mixture into 5 equal portions. Flatten one portion of sausage in the palm of your hand, place a peeled hard-boiled egg in the center, and form the sausage around it. Make sure that the sausage is completely sealed around each egg. Continue with the rest of the eggs and sausage.

4. Place each egg in the cup of a muffin pan or on an unlined baking sheet and bake for 25 minutes, or until the sausage is golden brown and cooked through.

5. Remove the eggs from the oven and slice each in half. Gently scoop the yolk out with a spoon and transfer it to a small mixing bowl. Add the ripe avocado and mash until well blended.

6. Scoop an even amount of the yolk and avocado mixture back into each egg. Sprinkle with the chopped chives and paprika, if desired, and serve.

TRY THIS!
For extra kick, swap the paprika for chili powder or add a few dashes of hot sauce to the avocado mixture.

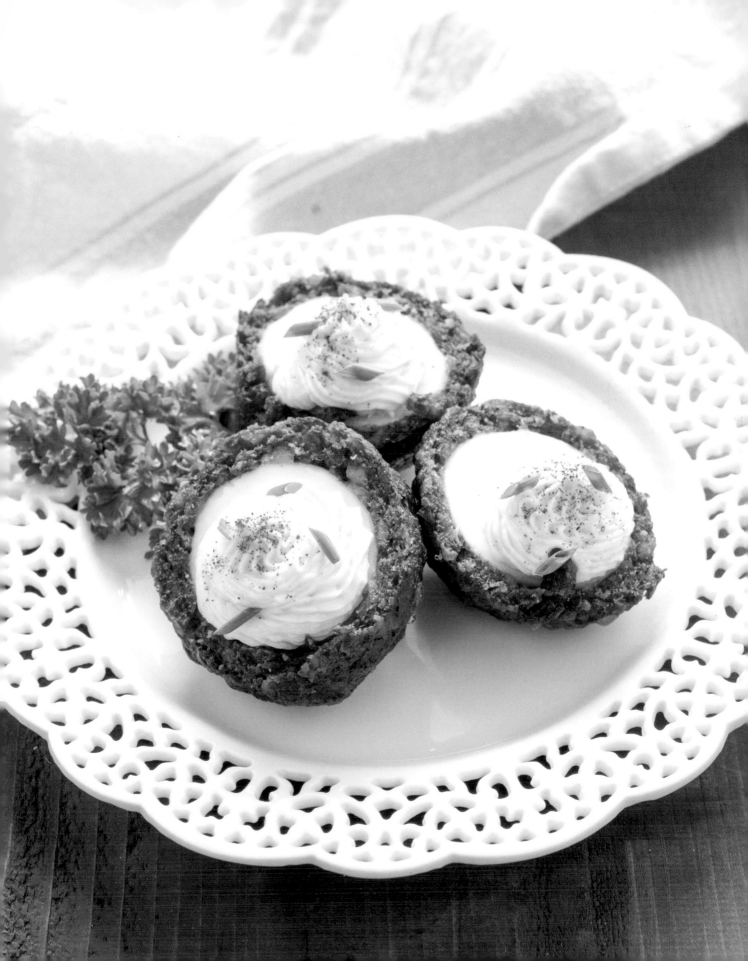

EGGS
BAKED in
TOMATO
SAUCE

It's amazing how something as simple as eggs baked in tomato sauce can impress people, but lucky for us it totally does! Nobody has to know how easy this dish is to make; all they have to do is sit back, enjoy, and praise your cooking wizardry. This recipe is inspired by the flavors of shakshouka, a spicy Middle Eastern egg dish, and huevos rancheros, and I like to serve it with some fresh sliced avocado and tortillas (page 210).

Prep Time: 15 minutes   Cook Time: 25 minutes   Yield: 4 to 6 servings

1 tablespoon ghee (page 320), lard (page 322), or tallow (page 324)

1 medium onion, chopped (about ¾ cup)

1 small red bell pepper, chopped (about ⅓ cup)

1 small green bell pepper, chopped (about ⅓ cup)

2 cloves garlic, minced

2 (14-ounce) cans chopped tomatoes, with juice

1 (4-ounce) can mild diced green chiles, drained

1 teaspoon paprika

1 teaspoon ground cumin

½ teaspoon fine sea salt

¼ teaspoon ground black pepper

6 large eggs

¼ cup chopped fresh parsley or cilantro, for garnish

1. Preheat the oven to 375°F.

2. Melt the ghee in a large oven-safe skillet over medium-high heat, then add the onion, bell peppers, and garlic and sauté for 5 minutes, or until the onions are softened. Add the tomatoes, green chiles, paprika, cumin, salt, and pepper and stir to combine. Bring just to a boil, then reduce the heat to low and simmer for 10 minutes.

3. Using the back of a large spoon, make 6 shallow indentations in the tomato sauce. Crack an egg into a small bowl and gently pour it into an indent in the sauce, then repeat with the remaining eggs. Transfer the pan to the oven and cook for 10 minutes, or until the egg whites are set and the yolks are cooked to your liking.

4. Remove the pan from the oven, sprinkle with parsley, and serve.

KITCHEN TIP

Store any leftover chopped onion and bell pepper in the freezer. For an easy and tasty breakfast, just grab some, heat it up in a pan until soft, add some whisked eggs and a pinch of salt and pepper, and cook until the eggs are cooked through.

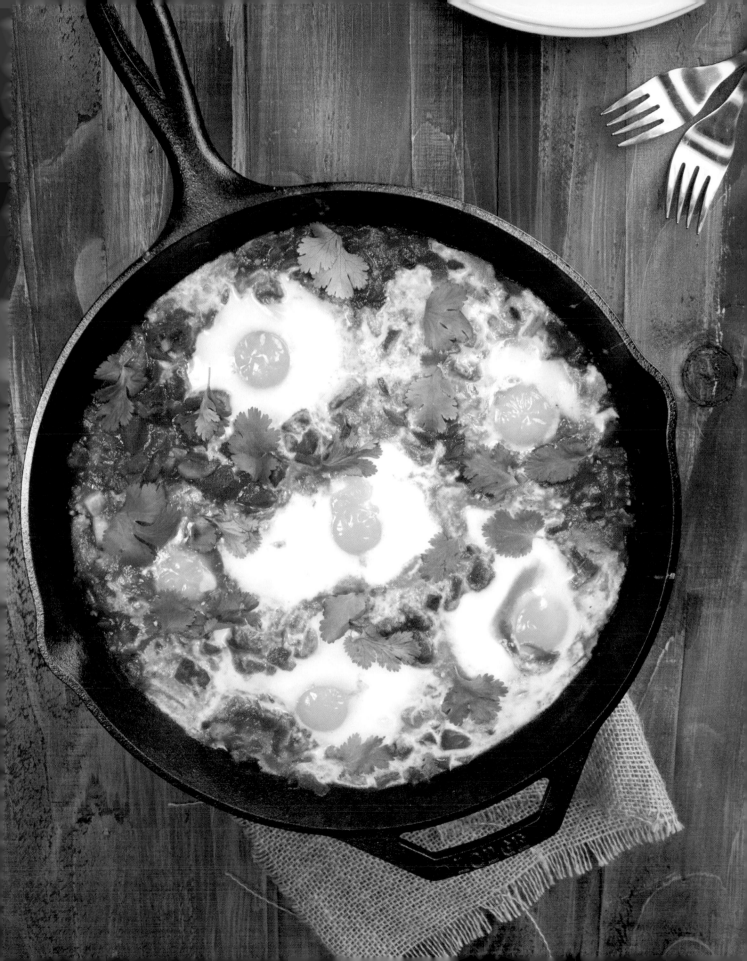

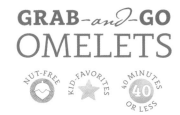

GRAB-and-GO OMELETS

NUT-FREE · KID-FAVORITES · 40 MINUTES OR LESS

If you're as busy as I am, you probably have days when you feel you should get an award just for showering and keeping a houseplant alive. And even though breakfast is one of my three favorite meals of the day, some mornings I just don't want to be bothered with cooking. Having a go-to recipe that you can make ahead of time is a great solution, and this one allows you to get as creative as you want with your ingredients and seasonings. These mini omelets don't need to be restricted to breakfast. Pack them for lunch and eat them cold; they're just as delicious and totally portable.

Prep Time: 10 minutes   **Cook Time:** 15 minutes   **Yield:** 12 mini omelets (about 4 servings)

12 slices prosciutto (about 6 ounces)

8 large eggs

1 small onion, finely chopped (about ½ cup)

1 cup chopped baby spinach

1 medium green bell pepper, finely chopped (about ½ cup)

1 medium red bell pepper, finely chopped (about ½ cup)

½ pound breakfast sausage, cooked and crumbled

¼ teaspoon ground black pepper

1. Place an oven rack in the middle position of the oven and preheat the oven to 375°F. Lightly grease the inside of a 12-cup muffin pan.

2. Place one slice of prosciutto inside each muffin cup. Make sure the prosciutto covers the bottom and sides of the cup so the egg will not seep through.

3. In a medium-sized mixing bowl, whisk the eggs, then add the onion, spinach, bell peppers, sausage, and pepper and stir until all ingredients are mixed.

4. Pour about ¼ cup of the mixture into each muffin cup. Bake for 15 minutes, then remove from the oven and let cool for 5 to 10 minutes. Run a small knife around the outside of each muffin to help separate it from the muffin pan, then remove. Eat right away or store in the refrigerator in a sealed container for up to 3 days.

TRY THIS!

Just as with a frittata, you can get as wild as you like with the ingredients in this recipe. Use chopped tomato, shallots, fresh basil, and cooked sausage for an Italian twist, or some finely chopped jalapeño, dashes of cumin, crumbled bacon, and a couple tablespoons of chopped green chiles for a Mexican flair.

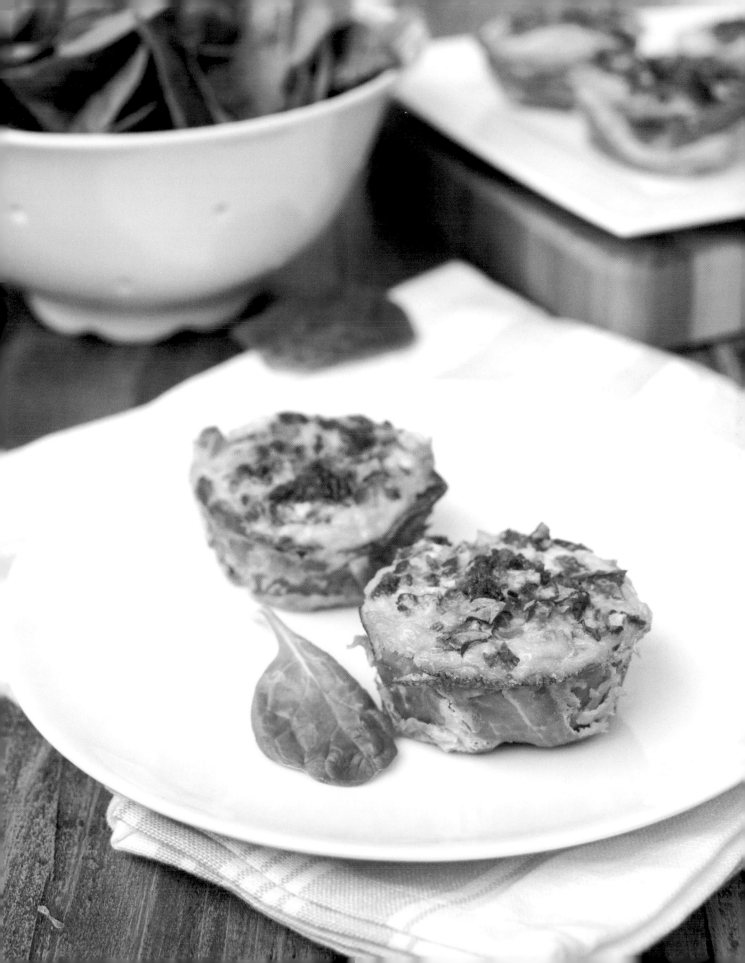

GRANOLA

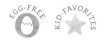

Granola was not something I thought to eat before I turned to a real-food lifestyle, mainly because it was always hidden away in grocery stores, but now I've found that it's a great healthy replacement for a bowl of cereal or as a crunchy, salty, and sweet snack. Pour some almond or coconut milk over it and you have a yummy cereal, or pack a small handful in your lunch for a quick snack. You can mix and match the seeds and nuts to suit your tastes; just keep the volumes roughly the same.

Prep Time: 10 minutes, plus 20 minutes to cool   **Cook Time:** 25 minutes   **Yield:** About 5 cups (6 servings)

1 cup raw almonds

1 cup raw cashews

¼ cup raw shelled pumpkin seeds (pepitas)

¼ cup raw shelled sunflower seeds

½ cup unsweetened coconut flakes

½ cup raw honey

¼ cup ghee (page 320) or coconut oil

1 teaspoon pure vanilla extract

1 cup raisins

1 teaspoon fine sea salt

1. Preheat the oven to 275°F. Line a 9-by-13-inch baking sheet with parchment paper or a baking mat.

2. Place the almonds, cashews, pumpkin seeds, sunflower seeds, and coconut flakes in a food processor or blender and pulse a few times to break into small chunks.

3. In a medium-sized saucepan over medium-high heat, melt the honey, ghee, and vanilla extract. Stir to combine, then add the nut mixture and stir until fully coated.

4. Spread the granola mixture evenly on the prepared baking sheet and cook for about 20 to 25 minutes, until lightly browned, stirring once or twice.

5. Remove the granola from the oven, add the raisins, and sprinkle with the salt. Press down on the top of the granola to create a flat surface.

6. Let cool for at least 20 minutes, or until hardened, then break into chunks. Store in an airtight container on the counter for up to a week.

TRY THIS!
If you want to switch up the flavors of this granola, adding a pancake-like maple taste, try substituting pure maple syrup for the honey and add a few dashes of cinnamon at the same time as the salt.

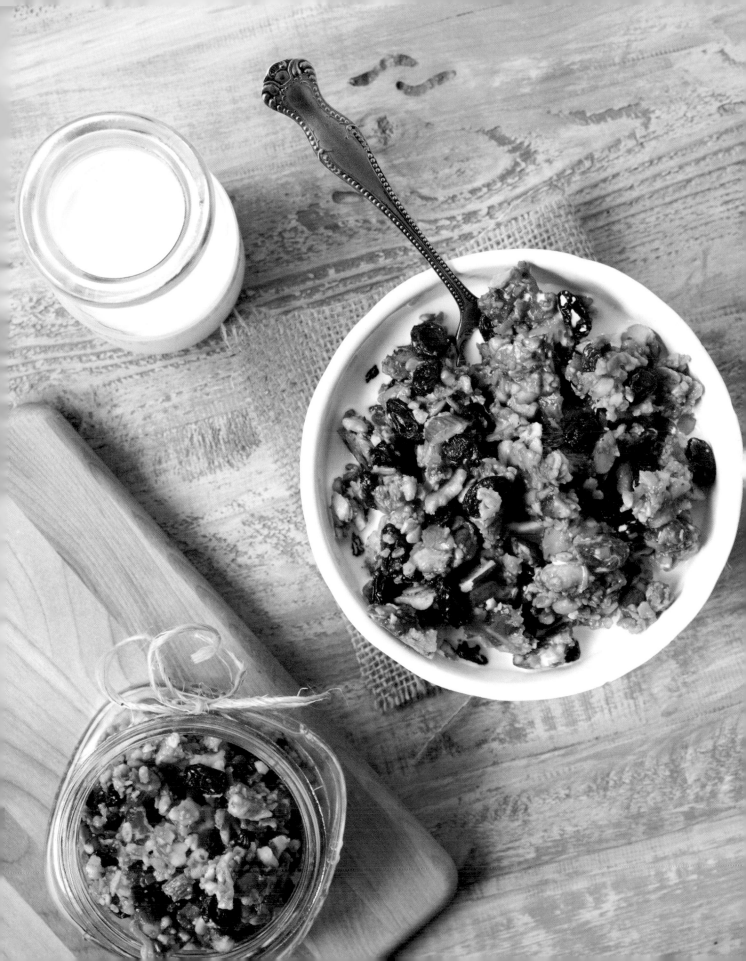

LEMON
POPPYSEED
WAFFLES

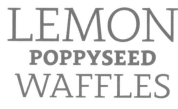

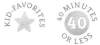

For the first few years of her life, my youngest daughter would much rather have been tearing apart the house than eating, so oftentimes getting food into her involved chasing her with a plate and trying to shove bites into her mouth. But one thing that did get her to sit down was waffles, and who can blame her? The smell of waffles and warm maple syrup wafting through the house on a Sunday morning is enough to bring even the wildest of children and morning-hating adults to the table. If you make them, they will come.

I prefer to use a regular, thinner waffle iron instead of a Belgian waffle iron for this recipe because the waffles come out crispier, but either one will work. You can omit the lemon juice, zest, and poppy seeds and still have a great basic waffle recipe.

Prep Time: 10 minutes **Cook Time:** 15 minutes **Yield:** 8 to 10 waffles

2 cups almond flour (page 316)

1 cup tapioca flour

1 teaspoon baking soda

½ teaspoon fine sea salt

½ teaspoon poppy seeds

2 large eggs, separated

½ cup ghee (page 320) or coconut oil, warmed, plus more for greasing the waffle iron

1 cup coconut milk (page 314)

2 tablespoons raw honey, warmed if solid

1 tablespoon freshly squeezed lemon juice

1 teaspoon finely grated lemon zest

1 teaspoon pure vanilla extract

1 cup fresh berries, for serving

Pure maple syrup, for serving

1. Preheat the waffle iron.

2. Combine the almond flour, tapioca flour, baking soda, salt, and poppy seeds in a large mixing bowl.

3. In a separate large mixing bowl, whisk together the egg yolks, ghee, coconut milk, honey, lemon juice, lemon zest, and vanilla extract. Slowly pour the dry ingredients into the wet ingredients, whisking to combine.

4. In a separate medium-sized mixing bowl, beat the egg whites with a hand mixer on high speed just until soft peaks form, about 2 to 3 minutes. Gently fold the egg whites into the batter until just combined, being careful not to overmix.

5. Grease the waffle iron and pour in enough batter to fill the bottom. Close the lid and cook according to the manufacturer's instructions, or until lightly browned and cooked through. Repeat until no batter remains.

6. Serve with maple syrup and fresh berries.

KITCHEN TIP

When baking with grain-free flours like almond and tapioca flour, separate the egg yolks and egg whites and whip the whites until soft peaks form, then fold the whites into the batter right before transferring it to your baking pan. This will make your baked goods less dense and more cakelike.

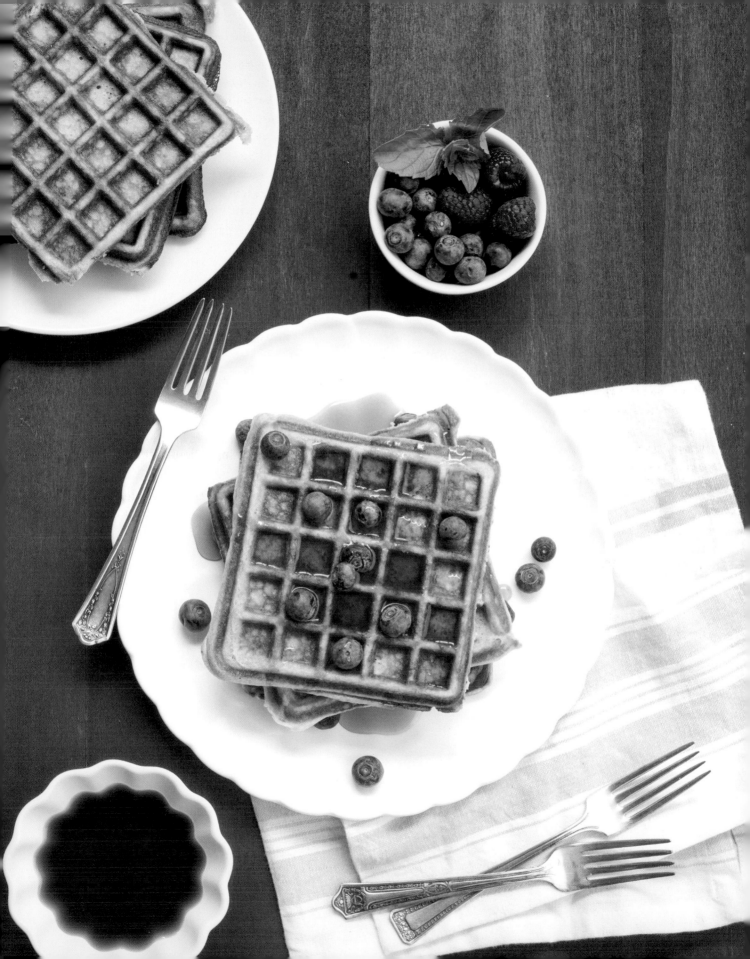

SWEET CRÊPES

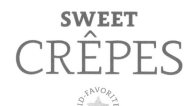

Getting the pan to the right temperature is one of the most important parts of cooking crêpes. If the temperature is too high, the batter will cook before you have finished swirling it around the pan. If it's not high enough, you will wind up with a mushy, misshapen crêpe. The batter should lightly sizzle when it hits the pan, while still allowing a minute or two of cooking time. The first crêpe in the pan is always the test crêpe, or, as I like to call it, my pre-breakfast snack.

Prep Time: 8 minutes   **Cook Time:** 35 minutes   **Yield:** 8 crêpes

¾ cup almond flour (page 316)

¼ cup tapioca flour

1 cup almond milk (page 318)

2 large eggs

2 teaspoons raw honey

1 teaspoon pure vanilla extract

½ teaspoon fine sea salt

3 tablespoons ghee (page 320) or coconut oil, divided

TOPPING IDEAS

Fresh fruit

Almond butter

Pure maple syrup

1. Place the almond flour, tapioca flour, almond milk, eggs, honey, vanilla extract, and salt in a large mixing bowl. Using a hand mixer, blend on medium speed for about 1 minute, or until well combined. The batter should be thin.

2. Heat an 8-inch skillet over medium heat for about 2 minutes. Melt 1 teaspoon of the ghee in the skillet and swirl to coat the bottom. Pour ⅓ cup of batter into the center of the skillet and swirl again until you've coated the bottom of the pan and created a thin circle. Cook for 2 minutes, or until the bottom of the crêpe is set, then gently flip the crêpe over and cook for another 1 to 2 minutes, until the top is very lightly browned and slightly crispy around the edges.

3. Remove the crêpe from the pan, set it on a wire rack to cool, and repeat until all of the batter is gone. Serve with your favorite toppings.

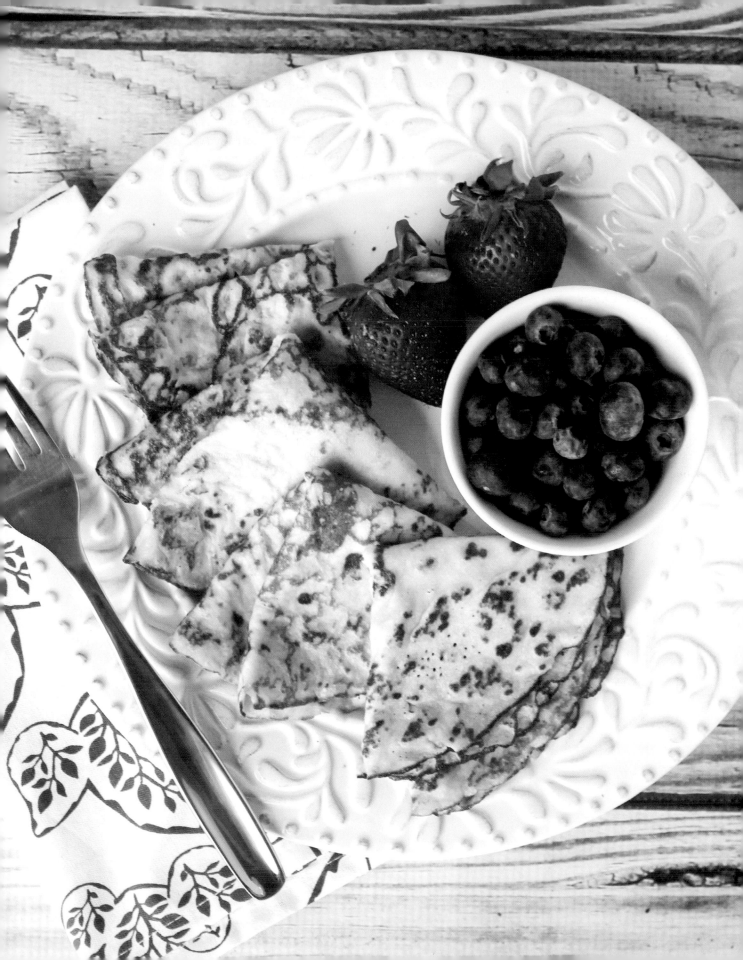

SWEET POTATO HASH
with SPICY HOLLANDAISE

NUT-FREE · 40 MINUTES OR LESS

This is one of my favorite indulgent breakfasts, mostly because I have a deep love of hollandaise. Add in crispy bacon and sweet potato, creamy avocado, and a sprinkle of fresh chives, and I practically swoon. I hope you enjoy this dish as much as I do!

If you use palm shortening instead of ghee, try to look for brands from smaller, family-owned farms, which are more likely to use sustainable production practices.

Prep Time: 10 minutes   **Cook Time:** 30 minutes   **Yield:** 4 servings

8 slices thick-cut bacon

3 medium sweet potatoes (about 1 pound), cut into ½-inch cubes

1 small onion, chopped (about ½ cup)

2 tablespoons raw honey

½ teaspoon dried thyme

½ teaspoon fine sea salt

½ teaspoon ground black pepper

FOR THE SPICY HOLLANDAISE

2 large egg yolks

2 tablespoons freshly squeezed lemon juice

¼ cup ghee (page 320) or palm shortening, melted and hot

½ teaspoon chili powder

Pinch of fine sea salt

8 large eggs

1 large ripe avocado, sliced, for serving

3 tablespoons chopped fresh chives, for garnish (optional)

TRY THIS!
Omit the chili powder for a basic hollandaise sauce that goes great over cooked asparagus, broccoli, beets, artichokes, pork, steak . . . pretty much everything.

1. In a large skillet over medium-high heat, cook the bacon until crisp. Transfer the cooked bacon to a paper towel–lined plate and crumble into large pieces.

2. Make the hash: Drain most of the bacon fat from the pan, reserving 1 tablespoon in a small bowl and leaving enough in the pan to coat the entire bottom of the skillet (about ¼ cup). Add the sweet potatoes and onion to the pan and cook for about 10 minutes, or until the potatoes are browned, stirring occasionally. Add the honey and toss to coat the potatoes, then cook for an additional 2 minutes, or until the potatoes are crispy. Add the thyme, salt, and pepper and stir. Taste and add additional salt and pepper if desired. Reduce the heat to the lowest setting possible to keep the potatoes warm.

3. Make the hollandaise: Place the egg yolks and lemon juice in a blender or food processor. Turn the blender on to medium speed and very slowly pour in the hot melted ghee, drop by drop. Take your time so that the ghee can emulsify with the eggs and lemon juice and form a creamy sauce. Add the chili powder and salt and blend for another 5 seconds, or until fully combined. Set the blender aside.

4. Cook the eggs: Melt the reserved tablespoon of bacon fat in a separate large skillet over medium-high heat. Gently crack each egg into the pan, allowing a bit of space between eggs, working in batches if needed. You can also crack each egg into a small bowl first and then gently pour it into the pan. Cook the eggs until the whites are set and the yolks are cooked to your preferred doneness (usually between 4 and 7 minutes).

5. To serve, place the sweet potato hash on a large serving platter or in individual serving bowls. Add the crumbled bacon, eggs, and sliced avocado, and drizzle the hollandaise sauce over the top. Sprinkle with the chopped chives, if desired, and serve.

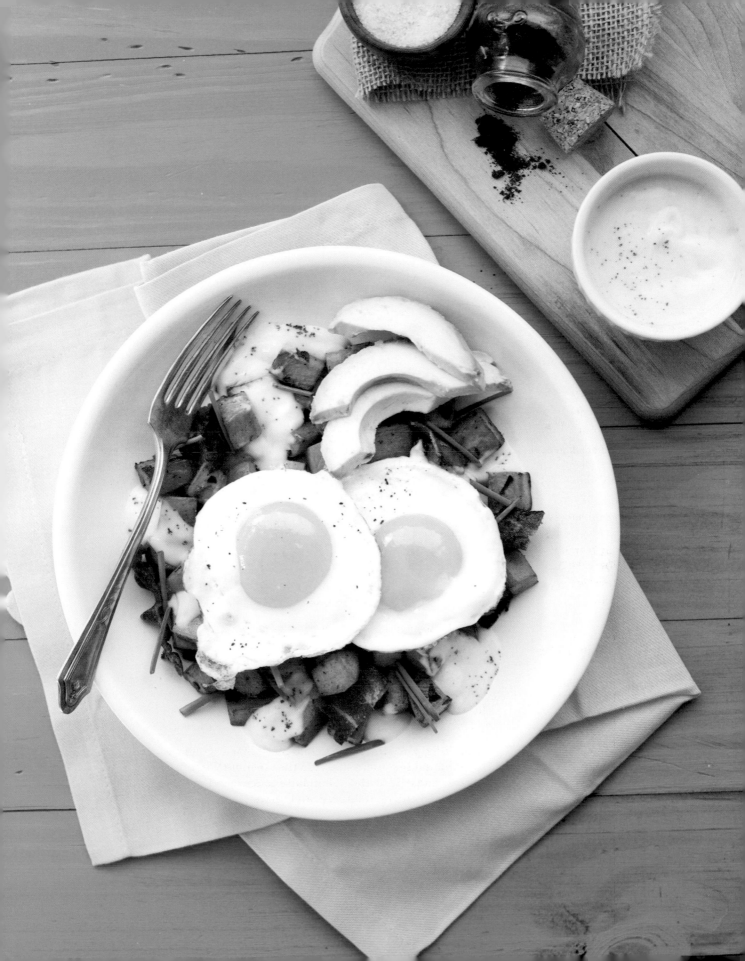

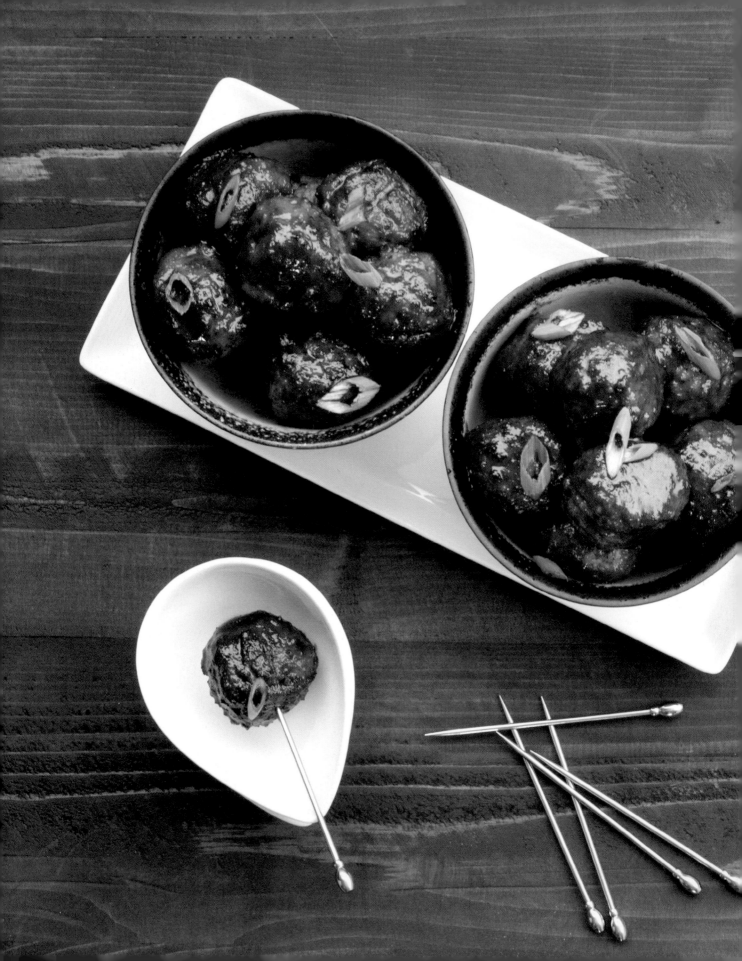

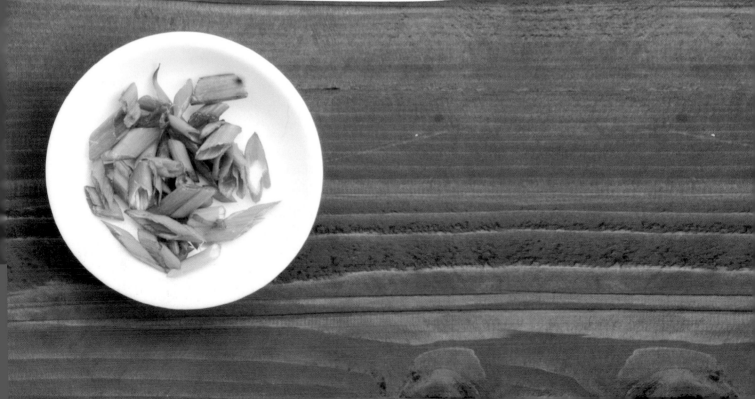

beef

BARBACOA

This recipe needs just a minimal amount of prep and then the slow cooker does the rest of the work, leaving you with moist and flavorful meat. Serve this with your favorite sides, such as Mexican Cauliflower Rice (page 204), tortillas (page 210), guacamole (page 274), and pico de gallo (page 282), and your favorite toppings, such as chopped onion, cilantro, ripe avocado slices, and lime wedges.

Prep Time: 15 minutes   Cook Time: 6 to 8 hours   Yield: 6 servings

4 pounds boneless chuck roast, trimmed of fat and cut into 6 pieces

1 teaspoon fine sea salt

1 teaspoon ground black pepper

2 tablespoons ghee (page 320), lard (page 322), or tallow (page 324)

¾ cup beef stock (page 310)

2 bay leaves

FOR THE SAUCE

1 (7-ounce) can mild diced green chiles

3 tablespoons apple cider vinegar

3 tablespoons freshly squeezed lime juice

4 cloves garlic

1 tablespoon ground cumin

2 teaspoons dried oregano

1 teaspoon dried thyme

1 teaspoon ground coriander

½ teaspoon ground cloves

¼ teaspoon ground chili powder

3 tablespoons chopped fresh parsley, for garnish (optional)

1. Pat the meat dry with paper towels and season with the salt and pepper. Place the ghee in a large skillet over medium-high heat. Add the meat and sear for 2 minutes on each side, or until browned. Transfer to a slow cooker, then add the stock and bay leaves.

2. Place the sauce ingredients in a blender or food processor and blend until smooth. Pour the sauce over the meat and place the cover on the slow cooker. Cook on low for 6 to 8 hours, until the meat is tender.

3. Remove the bay leaves, shred the meat with two forks, and place on a serving platter. Pour the sauce from the slow cooker over the meat and serve.

TRY THIS!

Leftover barbacoa makes a great cold lunch wrap. Take leaves of butter lettuce and pile in as much meat as you like, then add any leftover toppings from the night before. Roll the lettuce around the meat and tie it up with a fresh chive, just like string. Throw it in your bag and you're all set when lunchtime comes around.

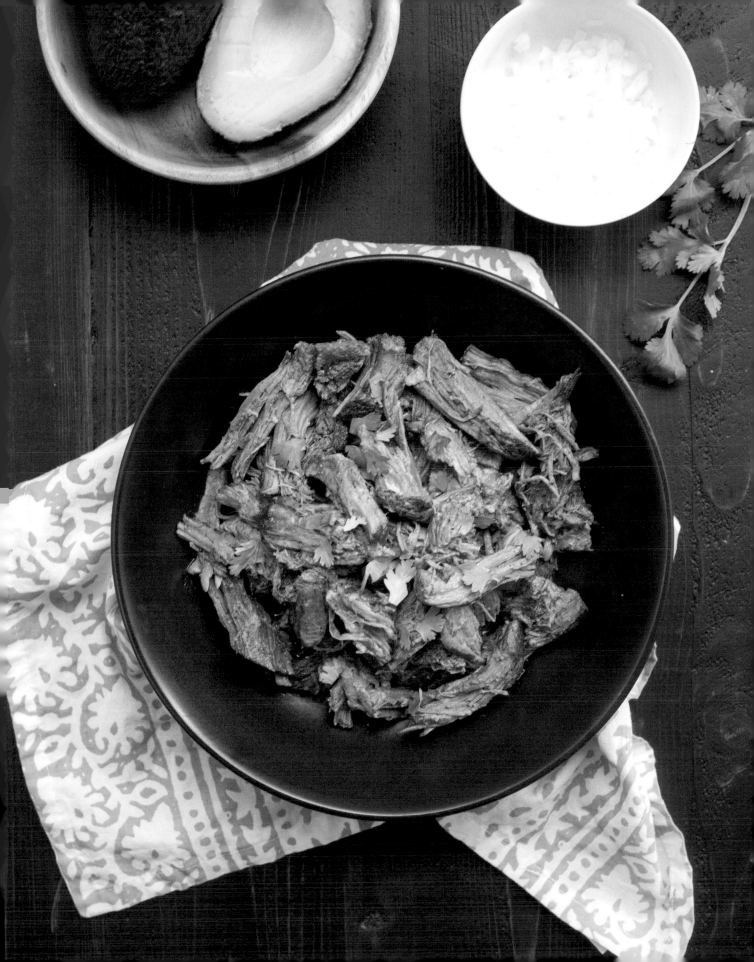

BEEF
OSSO BUCO

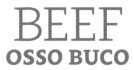

While osso buco is traditionally made with veal, this beef version is just as tender, and the gremolata adds bright citrus notes to this rich and meaty dish. I like to serve this with a simple salad and some Mashed Sweet Potatoes (page 189).

Prep Time: 15 minutes   Cook Time: 1 hour 50 minutes   Yield: 4 servings

FOR THE OSSO BUCO

4 (¾-pound) beef shanks

1 teaspoon fine sea salt

½ teaspoon ground black pepper

⅓ cup tapioca flour or arrowroot flour

⅓ cup ghee (page 320), lard (page 322), or tallow (page 324)

1 large onion, chopped (about 1 cup)

2 medium carrots, chopped (about 1½ cups)

4 cloves garlic, minced

2 tablespoons tomato paste

2 cups beef stock (page 310)

2 sprigs fresh thyme

2 sprigs fresh rosemary

1 bay leaf

FOR THE GREMOLATA

¼ cup tightly packed fresh flat-leaf parsley, finely chopped

2 cloves garlic, minced

1 tablespoon finely grated lemon zest

¼ teaspoon fine sea salt

¼ teaspoon ground black pepper

1. Preheat the oven to 350°F.

2. Pat the beef shanks dry with paper towels and tie each around the middle with kitchen twine. Season with the salt and pepper on all sides.

3. Place the tapioca flour in a medium-sized mixing bowl. Dredge each shank very lightly in the flour, shaking off any excess, and set aside.

4. Melt the ghee in a large Dutch oven over medium-high heat. Add the beef shanks and brown on all sides, about 2 to 3 minutes per side. Remove the shanks from the pan and set aside on a plate.

5. Add the onion, carrots, and garlic to the pan and sauté for about 5 minutes. Add the tomato paste and stir to combine, then add the beef stock and cook for another 10 minutes, or until the liquid has reduced by about half. Add the thyme, rosemary, and bay leaf and stir, then reduce the heat to low. Return the shanks to the pan, cover, and simmer for 1½ hours, or until the meat is soft and tender.

6. While the meat is cooking, make the gremolata: Combine all of the ingredients in a small bowl and stir to mix well.

7. Once the meat is tender, remove the shanks from the pan, cut off the kitchen twine and discard, and transfer the shanks to a serving platter. Discard the bay leaf and pour the juices over the meat. Top with the gremolata and serve.

KITCHEN TIP

To freeze leftover fresh herbs, like the thyme, rosemary, and parsley used here, fill an ice cube tray about two-thirds full with chopped herbs, then pour in your favorite cooking liquids or fats, such as extra-virgin olive oil, bacon drippings, melted ghee, or stock. Once frozen, transfer the cubes to freezer bags or a sealed container, then label and date them. I try to match the liquid I am using with the herbs to whatever I plan on doing with them. For example, if I want to use them for spaghetti sauce, I freeze them in extra-virgin olive oil. If I want to mix them with some chopped sweet potatoes and onions, I use ghee. If I want to use them in a soup or stew, I freeze them in chicken stock.

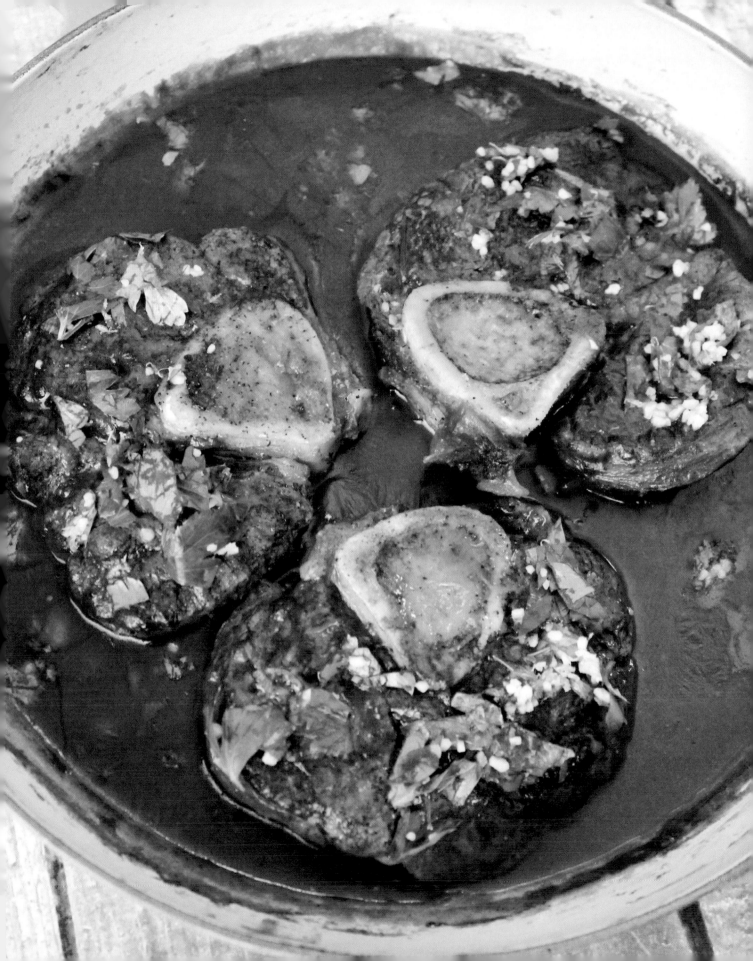

COTTAGE PIE

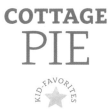

My day job frequently requires me to travel, and on one of my first business trips to Britain I was told by a coworker that what I had been calling shepherd's pie for many years was actually cottage pie. She explained to me that shepherd's pie contains lamb while cottage pie contains beef. She also let me know that when I told my fellow coworkers I needed to go back to my hotel to change my "pants," it actually meant "underpants," and that I should be using the word "trousers." I used the correct term going forward.

Prep Time: 15 minutes   **Cook Time:** 1 hour   **Yield:** 6 servings

FOR THE POTATOES

2 pounds white- or red-skinned sweet potatoes, peeled and cut into 1-inch cubes

¼ cup almond milk (page 318)

3 tablespoons ghee (page 320), lard (page 322), or tallow (page 324)

1 teaspoon fine sea salt

½ teaspoon ground black pepper

1 large egg yolk

FOR THE FILLING

2 tablespoons ghee (page 320), lard (page 322), or tallow (page 324)

1 large onion, chopped (about 1 cup)

2 medium carrots, peeled and chopped (about 1½ cups)

2 stalks celery, chopped (about ¾ cup)

3 cloves garlic, finely chopped

2 pounds ground beef

1 teaspoon fine sea salt

½ teaspoon ground black pepper

1½ teaspoons paprika

2 teaspoons dried rosemary

1 teaspoon dried thyme

2 tablespoons tapioca flour or arrowroot flour

1 tablespoon tomato paste

1 cup beef stock (page 310)

1. Place an oven rack in the middle of the oven and preheat the oven to 400°F.

2. Make the potatoes: Fill a large saucepan two-thirds full with water and bring to a boil. Add the cubed sweet potatoes and boil, uncovered, for 10 to 13 minutes, until fork-tender. Drain the water from the pan. Add the almond milk, ghee, salt, and pepper and blend with a hand mixer on medium speed for 1 to 2 minutes, until the potatoes are smooth. Add the egg yolk and mix for another 30 seconds. Set aside.

3. Prepare the filling: Melt the ghee in a large skillet over medium-high heat. Add the onion, carrots, and celery and sauté for 4 minutes, or until softened. Add the garlic and cook 1 more minute. Add the beef, salt, pepper, paprika, rosemary, and thyme and cook until the meat is browned, about 5 minutes, breaking the meat apart as it cooks.

4. Lightly sprinkle the tapioca flour over the meat and continue to cook for another 2 minutes, stirring frequently. Add the tomato paste and beef stock and stir to combine. Bring to a boil, reduce the heat to low, cover, and simmer for 10 minutes, or until the sauce is slightly thickened.

5. Spread the beef filling into an oven-safe 3-quart baking dish. Top with the mashed sweet potatoes, spreading them evenly across the top and pressing them up against all edges of the pan to prevent the filling from bubbling up. Bake for 25 minutes, or until the potatoes start to brown slightly. Remove from the oven and let cool for 5 minutes before serving.

KITCHEN TIP

You can prep this dish ahead of time and keep it covered in the refrigerator for 1 or 2 days until you're ready to bake it. It also freezes well if you are doing bulk meal-prepping: Make sure it is cooled completely, then tightly cover and store in the freezer. When you're ready to use it, defrost in the refrigerator overnight, then cook in the oven according to the recipe instructions.

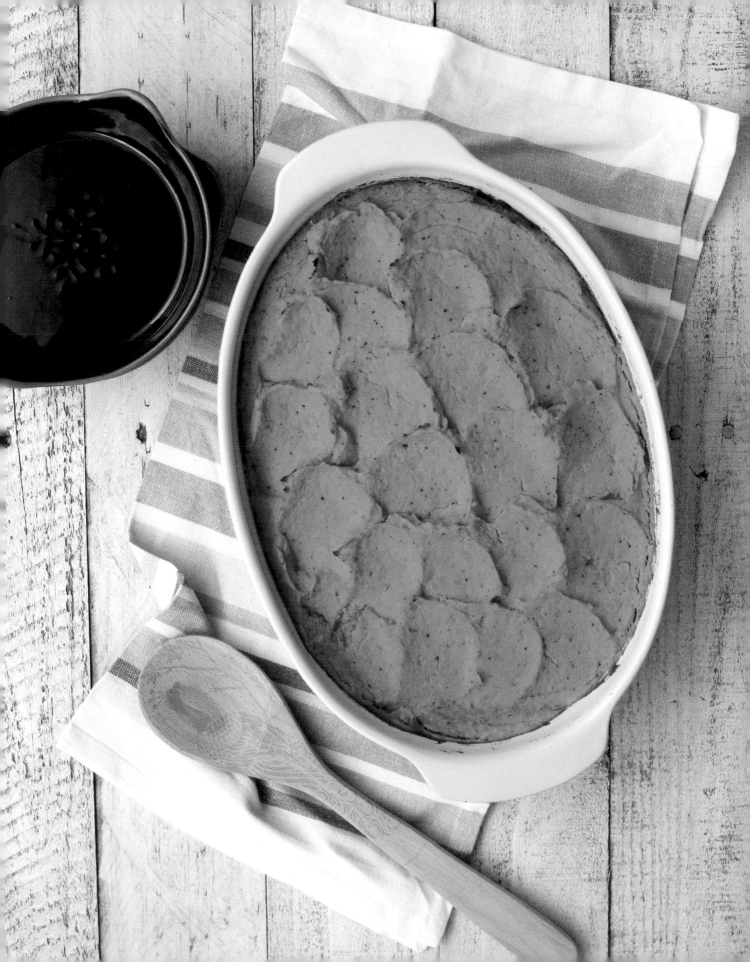

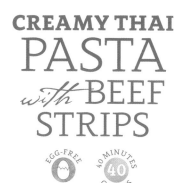

CREAMY THAI PASTA with BEEF STRIPS

This pasta dish requires just a bit of chopping, and you have yourself a meal in 30 minutes. For an even quicker weeknight meal, you can do most of the prep work ahead of time, including making the zucchini noodles and chopping the other vegetables and meat. Just keep the noodles wrapped in paper towels in the refrigerator or on the counter until you are ready to use them. This will also help pull out excess moisture from the zucchini, so it's a win-win!

Prep Time: 20 minutes   **Cook Time:** 10 minutes   **Yield:** 4 servings

FOR THE SAUCE

⅓ cup almond butter

3 tablespoons freshly squeezed lime juice

2 tablespoons coconut aminos or soy sauce substitute (page 283)

1 tablespoon raw honey

1 tablespoon extra-virgin olive oil

2 teaspoons finely grated lime zest

1 teaspoon sesame oil

1 teaspoon ground ginger

2 cloves garlic, minced

¼ teaspoon fine sea salt

¼ teaspoon ground black pepper

1 tablespoon ghee (page 320), lard (page 322), or tallow (page 324)

1 pound flank steak, cut against the grain into 2-inch-long, ½-inch-wide slices

2 cups chopped broccoli florets (1 medium head)

1 cup peeled and chopped carrots (about 2 medium)

1 cup red bell pepper, chopped (about 1 large)

1 batch Zucchini Noodles (page 328), uncooked

2 green onions, chopped, for garnish (optional)

⅓ cup chopped raw cashews, for garnish (optional)

1. Place all the sauce ingredients in a food processor or blender and puree until smooth. Set aside.

2. Melt the ghee in a large skillet over medium-high heat. Add the beef strips and cook for 3 minutes, stirring occasionally. Add the broccoli, carrots, and bell pepper and cook for another 3 to 4 minutes, or until the vegetables are tender. Transfer to a large bowl and cover to keep warm.

3. Reduce the heat to medium, then add the sauce to the pan and cook for 1 to 2 minutes, until it begins to melt. Add the zucchini noodles and cook for another 2 minutes, tossing to coat.

4. To serve, transfer the noodles to serving bowls, top with the beef strip mixture, and sprinkle with the chopped green onions and cashews, if desired.

TRY THIS!
For more heat, try adding ½ teaspoon of crushed red pepper at the same time you add the beef strips to the skillet.

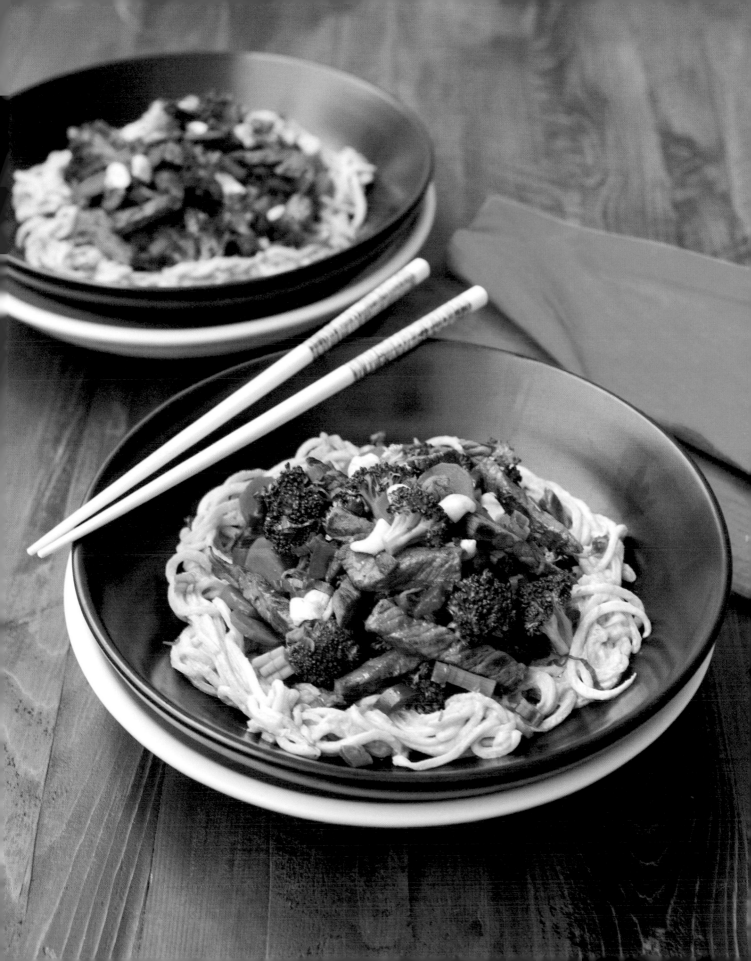

HONEY
CHIPOTLE
MEATBALLS

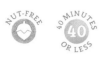

These meatballs make a great appetizer, or you can serve them over zucchini noodles (page 328) or Seasoned Cauliflower Rice (page 200) for a main dish. You can adjust the amount of chipotle powder and dry mustard in the sauce to suit your taste: use less if you are sensitive to heat, or add more if you like things a little spicier!

Prep Time: 15 minutes **Cook Time:** 25 minutes
Yield: 16 to 20 meatballs (8 servings as an appetizer, 4 as a main dish)

FOR THE MEATBALLS

¾ pound ground beef

¾ pound ground pork

½ cup finely chopped onion

2 cloves garlic, minced

1 large egg, beaten

½ teaspoon fine sea salt

¼ teaspoon ground black pepper

2 tablespoons ghee (page 320), lard (page 322), or tallow (page 324)

FOR THE SAUCE

½ cup chicken stock (page 310)

⅓ cup tomato paste

¼ cup raw honey

2 tablespoons freshly squeezed lemon juice

¼ teaspoon chipotle chili powder or chili powder

¼ teaspoon fine sea salt

¼ teaspoon paprika

¼ teaspoon dry yellow mustard

3 green onions, chopped, for garnish (optional)

1. Preheat the oven to 350°F.

2. Make the meatballs: In a medium-sized mixing bowl, mix the ground beef and pork, onion, garlic, egg, salt, and pepper with your hands until just combined. Form the mixture into meatballs 1½ inches in diameter.

3. Melt the ghee in a large oven-safe skillet over medium-high heat. Add the meatballs and cook for 5 minutes, turning frequently, until browned on all sides. Transfer the skillet to the oven and bake for 18 to 20 minutes, until the meatballs are cooked through.

4. While the meatballs are cooking, make the sauce: Place all of the sauce ingredients in a medium saucepan over medium-high heat and whisk to combine. Bring just to a boil, then reduce the heat to low and simmer for 3 to 5 minutes, until the sauce has thickened, stirring occasionally. Taste and add additional chipotle powder or dry mustard if desired.

5. Once the meatballs are done cooking, use a slotted spoon to transfer them to the pan with the sauce and toss to coat. Sprinkle with chopped green onion, if desired, and serve.

TRY THIS!
If you're serving these meatballs as an appetizer, sprigs of fresh rosemary make a great substitute for toothpicks and add a bit of extra flavor.

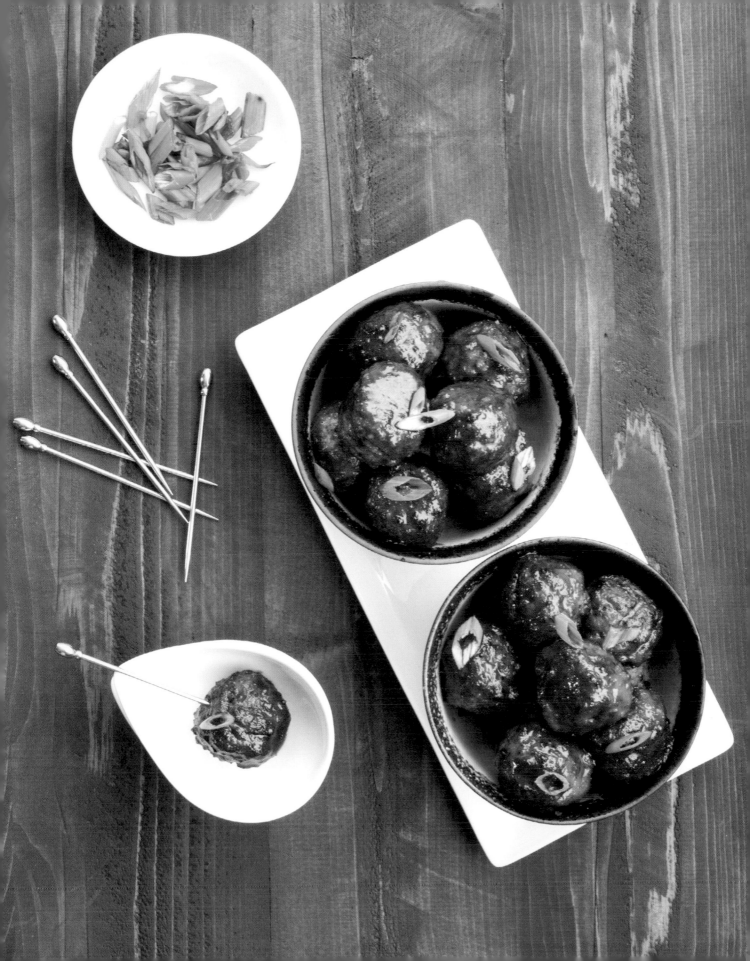

MONGOLIAN BEEF

This is a Paleo-friendly re-creation of one of my favorite takeout recipes. It takes less than 30 minutes to make and tastes better than any restaurant dish. If you like your sauce thick, you can whisk 1½ teaspoons of tapioca flour into the stock before adding it to the pan. You can also increase or decrease the amount of honey and crushed red pepper depending on how sweet and spicy you'd like this dish to be.

Prep Time: 10 minutes   **Cook Time:** 15 minutes   **Yield:** 4 to 6 servings

¼ cup plus 2 tablespoons tapioca flour or arrowroot flour

1 teaspoon ground black pepper

½ teaspoon fine sea salt

2 pounds flank steak, cut against the grain into 2-inch-long, ½-inch-wide slices

FOR THE SAUCE

1 tablespoon plus ½ cup lard (page 322) or tallow (page 324), divided

4 cloves garlic, minced

2 teaspoons ground ginger

¼ teaspoon crushed red pepper

2 tablespoons sesame oil

1 cup coconut aminos or soy sauce substitute (page 283)

1 cup chicken or beef stock (page 310)

½ cup raw honey

3 green onions, chopped, for garnish (optional)

1. Place the tapioca flour, pepper, and salt in a large plastic or paper bag, seal, and shake to combine. Add the steak pieces to the bag and shake to coat. Remove the steak, shaking off any excess coating. Lay the steak pieces on a drying rack and set aside for 10 minutes to let the flour adhere to the steak.

2. While the steak is resting, make the sauce: Heat 1 tablespoon of the lard in a medium-sized saucepan over medium heat. Add the garlic, ginger, and crushed red pepper and sauté for 1 minute.

3. Add the sesame oil, coconut aminos, and stock to the pan and stir to combine. Add the honey, turn the heat up to high, and continue to stir until the sauce boils and reduces slightly, about 4 to 5 minutes. Remove from the heat and set aside.

4. Place the remaining ½ cup of lard in a large skillet over medium heat and heat to 350°F, or until the melted fat bubbles around the handle of a wooden spoon dipped into the pan. Gently drop the beef pieces into the pan, working in batches if needed, and cook for 2 to 3 minutes, until the meat is lightly browned around the edges. Remove with tongs or a slotted spoon and place on a paper towel–lined plate.

5. Discard the fat from the pan, leaving just enough to lightly coat the bottom, and place the pan back over the heat. Add the beef pieces back to the pan and cook for 1 minute, stirring frequently, then add the sauce. Toss to coat and cook for another 3 minutes, or until the sauce and meat are heated through. Transfer to a serving bowl and top with the chopped green onions, if desired.

KITCHEN TIP

If you want your sliced meat to be tender, always cut it against the grain. Whether the meat is cooked or raw, cutting against the grain shortens the fibers within the meat, which lends it more of that melt-in-your-mouth texture (and gives your jaw a bit of a break).

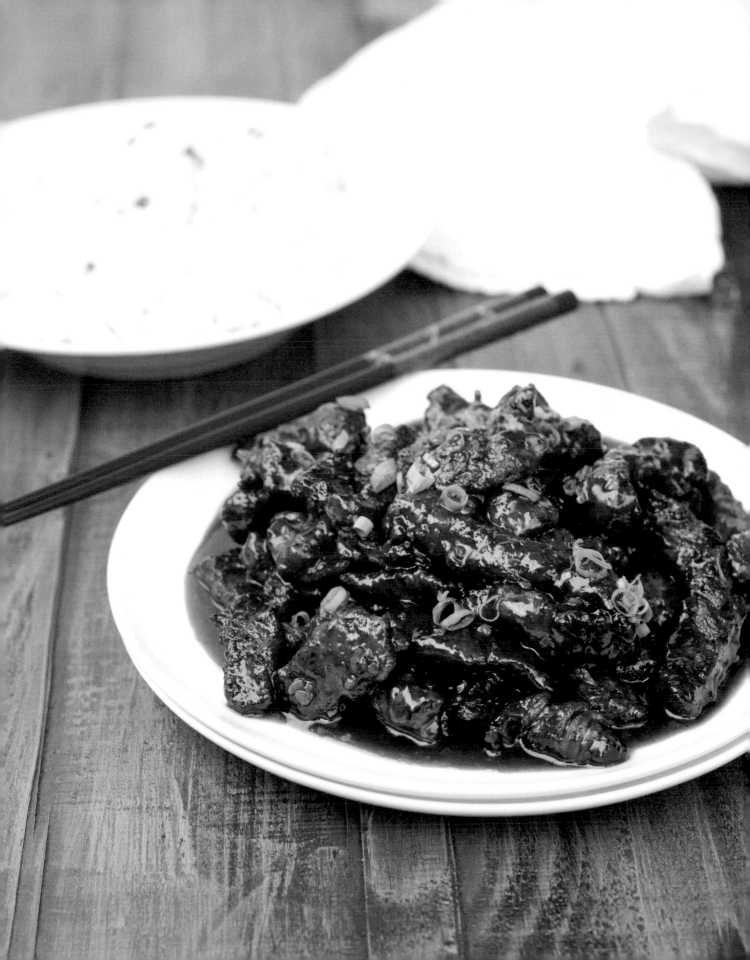

PASTA
BOLOGNESE

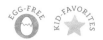

Many people are adamant that if a dish varies even slightly from the traditional recipe, then it must be named something entirely different. Since I enjoy a good controversy, I call this dish "pasta bolognese" and still have the audacity to tell you to serve it over zucchini noodles. (Okay, Paleo-friendly pasta is an option, too.) But at the end of the day, it doesn't really matter what you call this sauce; it's delicious and bursting with fresh flavors. I have been known to stand at the stove and eat it right out of the pan, so feel free to do the same.

Prep Time: 15 minutes   **Cook Time:** 1 hour 45 minutes   **Yield:** 4 to 6 servings

4 tablespoons ghee (page 320), lard (page 322), or tallow (page 324), divided

¾ cup chopped onion (about 1 medium)

½ cup finely chopped carrot (about 1 medium)

½ cup finely chopped celery (about 2 stalks)

3 cloves garlic, minced

3 ounces pancetta, chopped into ½-inch pieces

1 pound ground beef

1 pound ground pork

1 cup beef stock (page 310)

4 large tomatoes (about 2 pounds), seeded and chopped (about 3 cups)

½ cup tomato sauce

1 cup almond milk (page 318)

1 teaspoon dried thyme

1 bay leaf

¼ teaspoon fine sea salt

½ teaspoon ground black pepper

1 batch Pasta (page 194) or Zucchini Noodles (page 328)

3 tablespoons thinly sliced fresh basil, for garnish (optional)

1. Melt 1 tablespoon of the ghee in a large skillet over medium-high heat. Add the onion, carrot, and celery and cook for about 5 to 7 minutes, until the vegetables are tender. Add the garlic and pancetta and cook for 1 minute. Transfer to a bowl and set aside.

2. Melt the remaining 3 tablespoons of ghee in the skillet. Add the beef and pork ¼ pound at a time, allowing the meat to cook for 2 minutes after each addition. Stir and break apart the meat as it cooks. Once all the meat has been added, lower the heat to medium and cook for 15 minutes, or until the meat is fully browned and starting to turn crispy in spots, stirring occasionally.

3. Once the meat has started to caramelize, add the beef stock to deglaze the pan and stir, scraping up pieces that have started to stick to the bottom. Add the vegetable and pancetta mixture back to the pan and add the tomatoes, tomato sauce, almond milk, thyme, bay leaf, salt, and pepper and stir to combine. Bring just to a boil, then cover, reduce the heat to low, and simmer for 1 hour. Remove the bay leaf, taste, and add additional salt and pepper if desired.

4. To serve, ladle over pasta or zucchini noodles and garnish with the sliced basil, if desired.

KITCHEN TIP

Since this sauce needs to simmer for a while to allow the flavors to meld, I like to make a double batch and freeze half of it—frozen sauce is great for days when you don't have a lot of time to cook and want some good comfort food. It will keep in the freezer for up to 2 months; when you're ready to use it, defrost it in the refrigerator overnight and then just heat it in a saucepan until warmed. You can also make the sauce ahead of time and keep it in the refrigerator for 2 to 3 days.

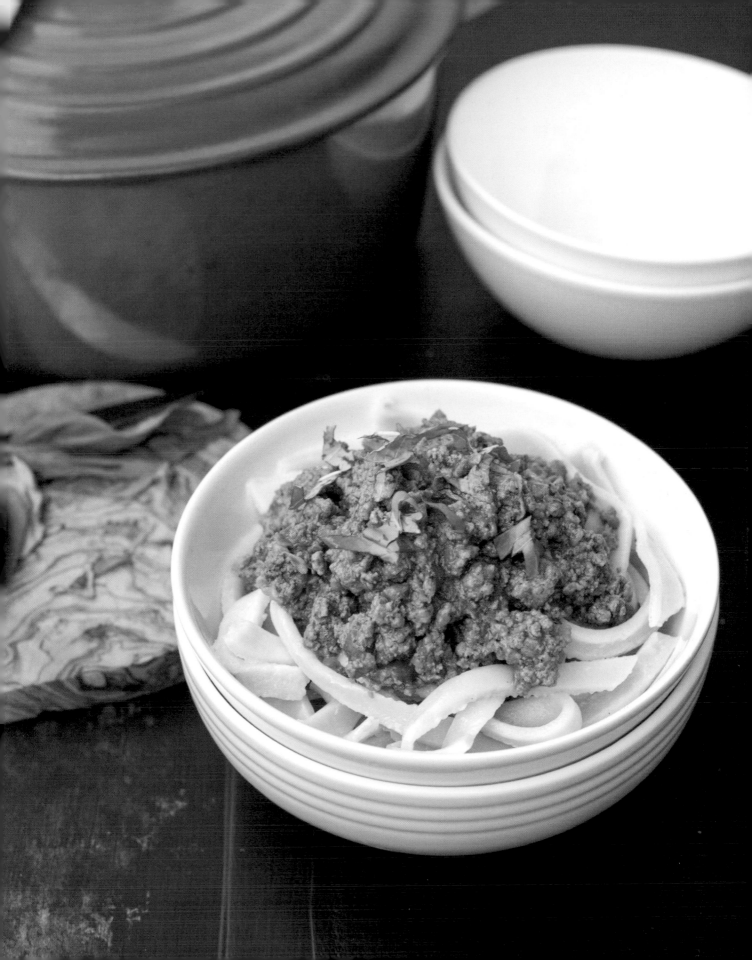

POPCORN CHICKEN-FRIED STEAK and GRAVY

KID-FAVORITES

This is a fun dish for kids or as a party appetizer, but you can use the same recipe to make a traditional chicken-fried steak. To make the traditional version, keep the steak whole instead of cutting it into bite-sized pieces and fill the pan only ½ inch high with lard. Fry for 3 minutes on each side, or until golden brown and cooked through. To reheat leftovers, place the steak in a toaster oven for 2 to 3 minutes, or place in the oven under the broiler for 2 minutes, or until crispy, and heat any remaining sauce in a small saucepan on the stovetop.

Prep Time: 20 minutes   Cook Time: 35 minutes   Yield: 6 to 8 servings as an appetizer, 4 as a main dish

FOR THE GRAVY

2 tablespoons ghee (page 320), lard (page 322), or tallow (page 324)

1 medium onion, sliced (about ¾ cup)

⅓ cup tapioca flour

1½ cups beef stock (page 310)

2 tablespoons almond milk (page 318) or coconut milk (page 314)

¼ teaspoon fine sea salt

¼ teaspoon ground black pepper

FOR THE STEAK

2 large eggs

1 cup almond milk (page 318) or coconut milk (page 314)

1½ cups almond flour (page 316)

3 cups tapioca flour

1½ teaspoons fine sea salt

1 teaspoon ground black pepper

1½ teaspoons paprika

1¾ pounds cube steak, cut into 1-inch pieces

Lard (page 322) or tallow (page 324), for frying

¼ cup chopped fresh parsley, for garnish (optional)

1. Preheat the oven to 200°F. Line a half-sheet baking pan (13 by 18 inches) with paper towels.

2. Melt the ghee for the gravy in a large skillet over medium-high heat. Add the sliced onion and sauté for 15 minutes or until very tender, stirring occasionally. Transfer the onions to a bowl and set aside.

3. While the onions are cooking, prepare the steak pieces: Whisk the eggs and almond milk together in a shallow bowl. In another bowl, combine the almond flour, tapioca flour, salt, pepper, and paprika. Place an empty plate or cooling rack near the bowls to place the breaded pieces on.

4. Working in batches, dip the steak pieces in the flour mixture, making sure to coat lightly on all sides. Move them to the egg mixture and coat thoroughly, then coat with the flour mixture once more. Place the breaded steak bites on a large plate or cooling rack.

5. Once the onions are done and set aside, fill the skillet 1 inch high with lard and place over medium heat. Heat the fat until it reaches 350°F, or until the melted fat bubbles around the handle of a wooden spoon dipped into the pan. Add the breaded steak bites to the pan, working in batches if needed so as not to overcrowd the pan. Cook the meat for about 5 minutes, or until crispy and golden brown on all sides. Use a slotted spoon to transfer the steak bites to the prepared baking sheet and place in the oven to keep warm while you finish the gravy.

6. Make the gravy: Drain most of the fat from the skillet, leaving about 3 tablespoons, and place it back over medium heat. Sprinkle the ⅓ cup of tapioca flour over the fat in the pan. Whisk the flour for about 2 minutes, or until a paste forms and becomes light brown in color. Add the beef stock and almond milk to the pan and stir until the flour has fully dissolved. Add the salt and pepper to the pan and continue to whisk. Taste and add additional salt and pepper if desired. Continue to cook, whisking occasionally, until the gravy is thickened, about 5 minutes. Add the onions back to the pan and stir everything to combine.

7. Transfer the gravy to a blender or food processor and puree until smooth, or use an immersion blender to puree everything directly in the pan. Taste and add additional salt and pepper if desired.

8. Remove the steak bites from the oven, place on a serving tray, and garnish with parsley, if desired. Pour the gravy into a dipping bowl to serve alongside the steak bites.

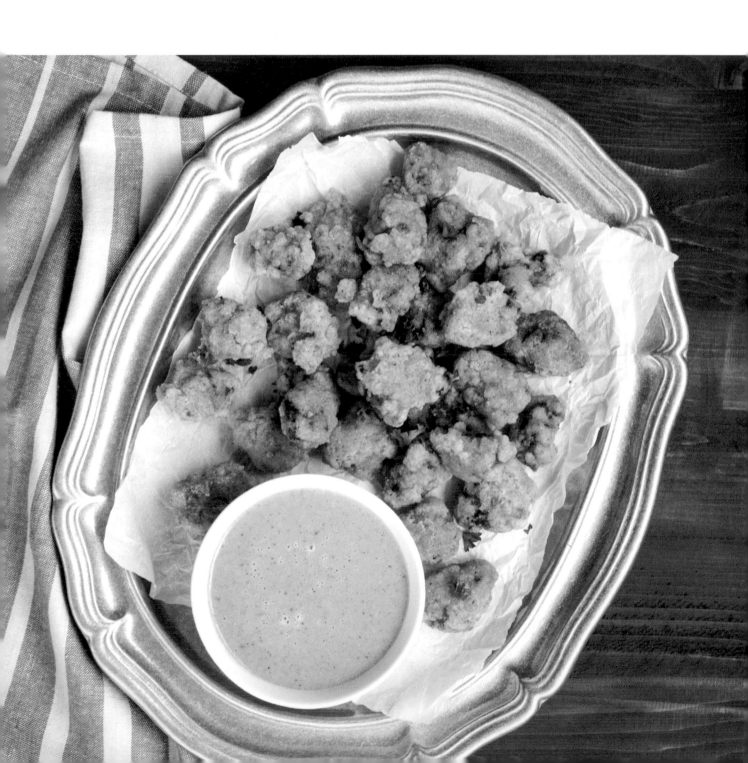

SATAY
with
DIPPING SAUCE

EGG-FREE

Combining oil, salt, and spices in a beef marinade isn't just a great way to use up cupboard ingredients; there's a science behind it, too. The salt in the fish sauce and coconut aminos brines and tenderizes the meat, while the oil intensifies the flavors of the spices and helps them coat the meat evenly. This recipe takes advantage of that trio, and the end result makes a fantastic appetizer or main dish.

Prep Time: 15 minutes, plus 2 hours to marinate   Cook Time: 10 minutes
Yield: 6 to 8 servings as an appetizer or 4 as a main dish

FOR THE MARINADE

3 tablespoons raw honey

3 tablespoons fish sauce

2 tablespoons sesame oil

2 tablespoons coconut aminos or soy sauce substitute (page 283)

4 cloves garlic, minced

1 teaspoon ground ginger

1 teaspoon onion powder

2 pounds beef top sirloin, trimmed of fat and cut into 1-inch-wide, ¼-inch-thick strips

FOR THE DIPPING SAUCE

½ cup almond butter

3 tablespoons chicken stock (page 310)

3 tablespoons coconut aminos or soy sauce substitute (page 283)

2 tablespoons raw honey

2 tablespoons freshly squeezed lime juice

1 clove garlic, minced

½ teaspoon crushed red pepper

2 green onions, sliced, for garnish (optional)

1 lime, quartered, for serving

1. Place the marinade ingredients in a medium-sized mixing bowl and whisk to combine. Add the meat and toss to coat. Cover the bowl, place in the refrigerator, and marinate for at least 2 hours and up to 24 hours.

2. While the meat is marinating, make the dipping sauce: Place all of the sauce ingredients in a blender or food processor and puree until smooth. Cover and store in the refrigerator until ready to serve.

3. Preheat the grill. Soak 10 to 12 bamboo skewers in water for 10 minutes.

4. When the meat has marinated for at least 2 hours, remove it from the bowl and shake off the excess marinade. Thread the meat strips onto the bamboo skewers and grill for about 3 to 5 minutes on each side, until browned and cooked through.

5. Garnish with the green onion slices, if desired, and serve with the dipping sauce and lime wedges.

KITCHEN TIP
Don't hack away at your meat and wind up with sad, misshapen pieces. Freezing it for 20 to 30 minutes before cutting will make the meat firmer, so it's easier to thinly slice.

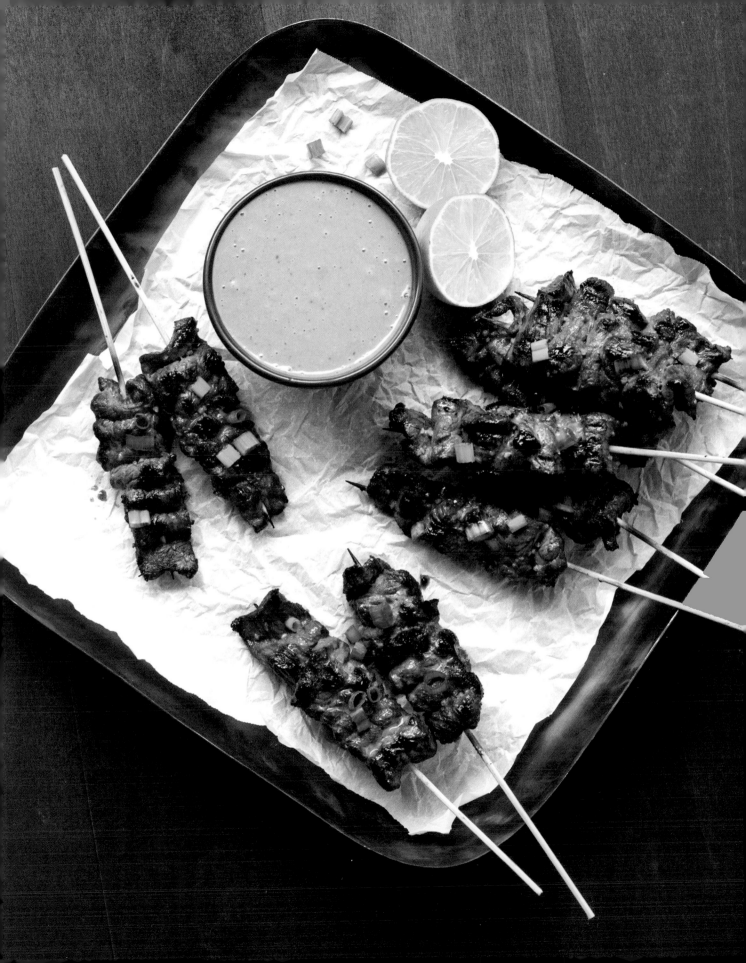

SPICY BEEF and PEPPER STIR-FRY

EGG-FREE *NUT-FREE* *40 MINUTES OR LESS*

This combination of thinly cut strips of beef, fragrant ginger, crisp-tender bell peppers, and a hit of fresh lime juice gives you a fast meal that's tastier and healthier than any takeout around. Because of the short cooking time, it's important to have all of the ingredients prepped and ready to grab before you start cooking. Try serving this dish with Seasoned Cauliflower Rice (page 200).

Prep Time: 15 minutes   Cook Time: 10 minutes   Yield: 4 servings

2 pounds beef sirloin steak, cut against the grain into ½-inch-wide slices

1 teaspoon fine sea salt

½ teaspoon ground black pepper

2 tablespoons ghee (page 320), lard (page 322), or tallow (page 324), divided

1 tablespoon minced fresh ginger

1 teaspoon crushed red pepper

2 cloves garlic, minced

1 medium red bell pepper, cut into thin strips

1 medium green bell pepper, cut into thin strips

½ medium red onion, cut into thin strips

1 cup coconut milk (page 314)

1 tablespoon raw honey

½ teaspoon finely grated lime zest

2 tablespoons freshly squeezed lime juice

1 tablespoon sesame oil

2 green onions, thinly sliced, for garnish (optional)

1. Season the beef strips with the salt and pepper. Heat 1 tablespoon of the ghee in a large skillet over medium-high heat. Add the beef strips and cook for 2 minutes, or until just browned, stirring frequently. Add the ginger, crushed red pepper, and garlic and cook for 1 more minute. Transfer to a bowl and set aside.

2. Melt the remaining 1 tablespoon of ghee in the pan. Add the bell peppers and onion and cook for 2 to 3 minutes, until just tender. Remove from the pan and add to the bowl with the beef strips.

3. Add the coconut milk, honey, lime zest and juice, and sesame oil to the pan and whisk to combine. Bring to a boil, then return the beef and peppers to the pan and cook for 2 more minutes, or until the beef and peppers are heated through. Taste and add additional salt and pepper if desired. Transfer to a serving plate and garnish with the sliced green onions before serving, if desired.

TRY THIS!
If you like a bit of heat, try adding 1 seeded and thinly sliced jalapeño at the same time as the bell peppers and onions.

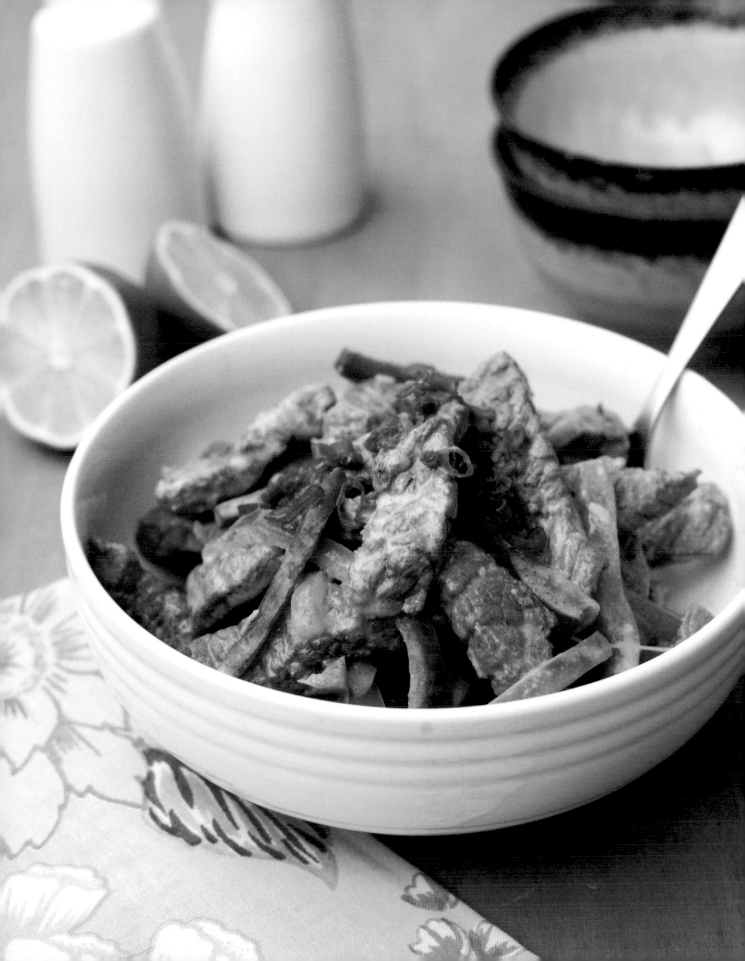

CHILE RELLENOS

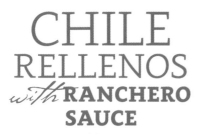

with **RANCHERO** SAUCE

 EGG-FREE NUT-FREE 40 MINUTES OR LESS

Having been born and raised in San Diego, California, I have eaten many chile rellenos in my life, and I love them to this day. If you're roasting chiles for the first time, you might be a little terrified to see them turn from green to black and blistered, but that is exactly what you want to happen, and after you do it a few times you will no longer fret. You can use Anaheim, poblano, or Hatch chiles for this recipe, Anaheim being the mildest and Hatch the hottest. A squeeze of fresh lime juice over the entire plate really brings this dish to life.

Prep Time: 15 minutes   **Cook Time:** 20 minutes   **Yield:** 4 servings

4 large Anaheim, poblano, or Hatch chiles (about 1 pound)

FOR THE SAUCE

¾ pound Roma tomatoes (about 3 large), chopped into ½-inch pieces (about 1½ cups)

⅓ cup finely chopped onion

1 clove garlic, minced

1 medium serrano chile, seeded and chopped

¼ teaspoon fine sea salt

¼ teaspoon ground black pepper

FOR THE STUFFING

1 tablespoon ghee (page 320), lard (page 322), or tallow (page 324)

1 small onion, finely chopped (½ cup)

2 cloves garlic, minced

1 pound ground beef

½ teaspoon fine sea salt

½ teaspoon ground cumin

½ teaspoon chili powder

½ teaspoon dried oregano

¼ cup tomato sauce

Chopped fresh cilantro, for garnish (optional)

1 ripe avocado, sliced, for serving

2 limes, quartered, for serving

1. Roast the chiles over a gas flame stove or under an oven broiler for about 10 minutes, turning occasionally, until the skin is fully blackened and blistering. Place the chiles in a paper bag or a covered bowl and set aside to sweat for at least 10 minutes.

2. While the peppers are sweating, make the sauce: Place the tomatoes, onion, garlic, serrano chile, salt, and pepper in a small saucepan over medium-high heat. Bring to a boil, then reduce the heat to low, cover, and simmer while you prepare the rest of the recipe (about 15 to 20 minutes). If you like a smoother sauce, you can puree it for 20 seconds in a blender or food processor before serving.

3. Make the stuffing for the chiles: Melt the ghee in a large skillet over medium-high heat. Add the onion and garlic and cook for 3 minutes, stirring frequently. Add the ground beef, salt, cumin, chili powder, and oregano and stir to combine, breaking the meat apart into small pieces. Cook for another 5 minutes, or until the meat is browned and cooked through. Add the tomato sauce and cook for 2 more minutes, then remove the pan from heat.

4. Once the chiles are done sweating, use a butter knife to carefully scrape away the skin, leaving the chile intact. Gently slice each chile down the middle lengthwise, from stem to tip. Run the chiles under a trickle of cold water to remove the seeds and any remaining skin, then pat dry with a paper towel. Stuff equal amounts of the ground beef mixture into each chile.

5. To serve, spoon equal amounts of the sauce onto 4 plates and place the chiles on top of the sauce. Sprinkle with fresh cilantro, if desired, and serve each with avocado slices and 2 lime wedges.

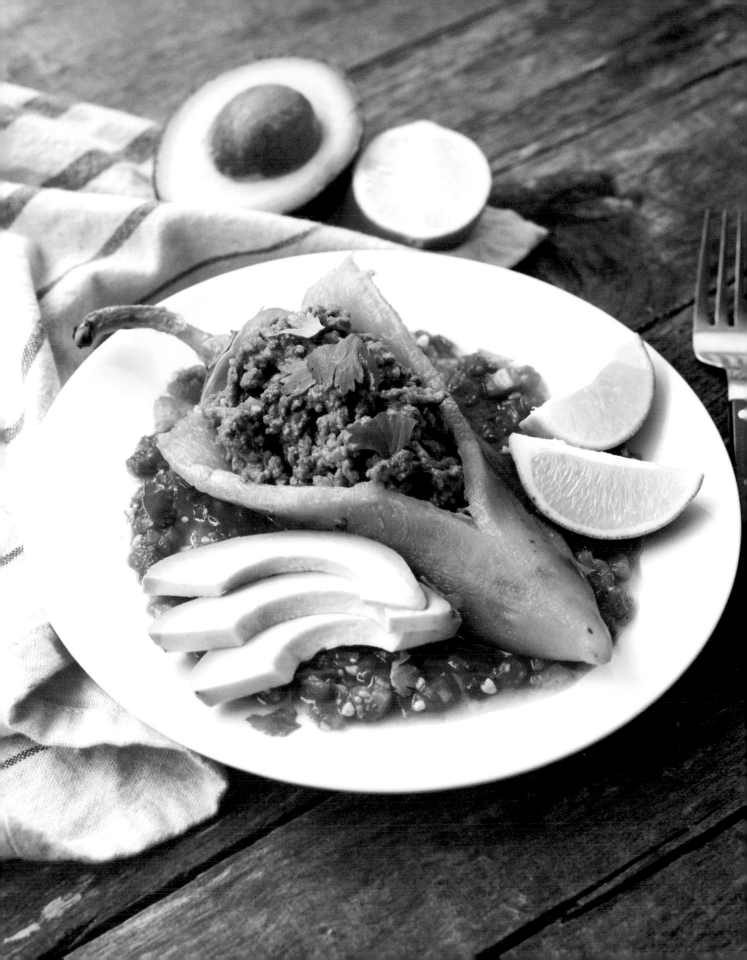

SWEDISH
MEATBALLS

The term "Swedish meatballs" reminds me of a large furniture retailer. One with stores that have a long winding path leading you to showroom after showroom while you try to grasp the smallest pencil ever created and scribble down hard-to-spell coffee table names, the whole time fighting back a serious case of claustrophobia because there are no windows anywhere. Well, no tiny pencils are required for this recipe, only one large skillet that you get to use the whole time, and I guarantee no claustrophobia. Best of all, at the end you get to eat delicious meatballs instead of assemble furniture.

Prep Time: 10 minutes   Cook Time: 40 minutes   Yield: 4 to 6 servings

FOR THE MEATBALLS

3 tablespoons ghee (page 320), lard (page 322), or tallow (page 324), divided

1 small onion, finely chopped (about ½ cup)

2 cloves garlic, minced

1½ pounds ground beef

1 large egg yolk

½ teaspoon fine sea salt

½ teaspoon ground black pepper

FOR THE GRAVY

2 tablespoons ghee (page 320), lard (page 322), or tallow (page 324)

1 small onion, chopped (about ½ cup)

1½ cups sliced white or cremini mushrooms

2 tablespoons tapioca flour

2 cups beef stock (page 310)

1 cup almond milk (page 318) or coconut milk (page 314)

½ teaspoon fine sea salt

¼ teaspoon ground black pepper

3 tablespoons chopped fresh parsley, for garnish (optional)

1. Make the meatballs: Melt 2 tablespoons of the ghee in a large skillet over medium heat. Add the chopped onion and garlic and sauté until the onions are soft, about 2 to 3 minutes. Transfer the onion mixture to a large mixing bowl and set aside to cool for 3 minutes. Add the ground beef, egg yolk, salt, and pepper to the bowl. Using your hands, mix the ingredients together until well combined. Roll into 1½-inch meatballs, making about 24.

2. Heat the remaining 1 tablespoon of ghee in the same skillet over medium-high heat. Add the meatballs to the pan and sauté until golden brown on all sides and almost cooked through, about 8 to 10 minutes. Transfer the meatballs back to the mixing bowl with tongs or a slotted spoon, then cover and set aside.

3. Make the gravy: Melt the 2 tablespoons of ghee in the same skillet over medium heat. Add the onion and cook for 3 minutes, then add the mushrooms and cook for another 3 minutes. Add the tapioca flour and whisk for 10 seconds, then add the beef stock and whisk until sauce begins to thicken. Add the almond milk, salt, and pepper and continue to cook for another 5 minutes, or until the gravy is thickened, stirring frequently.

4. Return the meatballs to the pan and cook for another 5 minutes, or until the meatballs are cooked through. Serve the meatballs and gravy garnished with chopped fresh parsley, if desired.

TRY THIS!

To give these meatballs a bit of a warmer flavor, try adding ¼ teaspoon of ground nutmeg or allspice to the gravy at the same time as the salt and pepper. Using a mix of half ground beef and half ground pork is also a great idea, and the combination makes for earthy but tender meatballs.

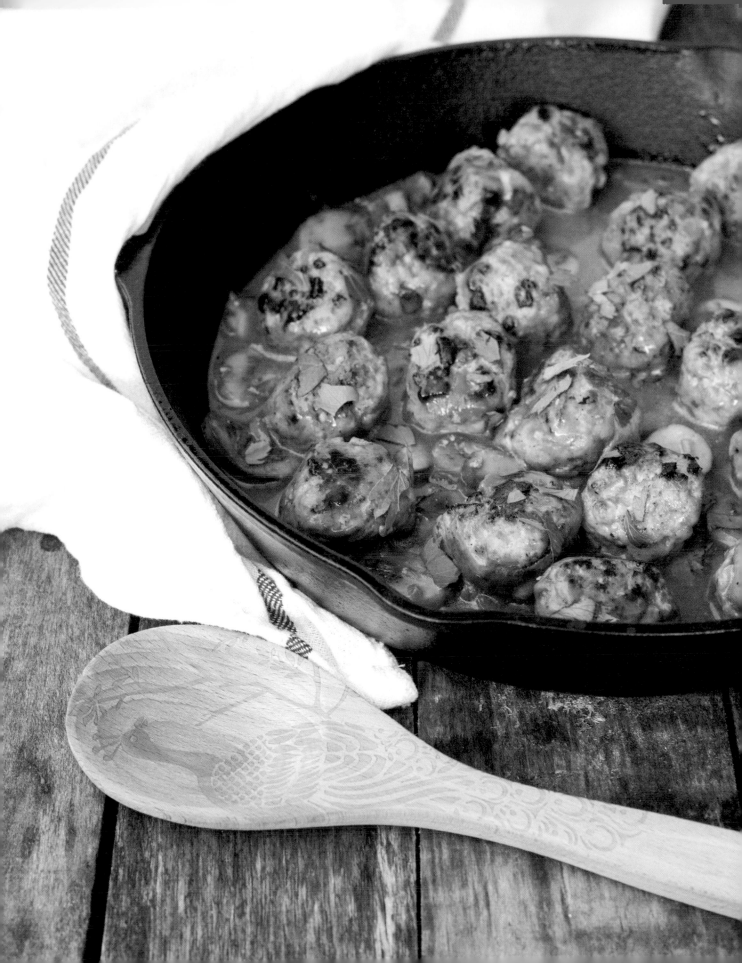

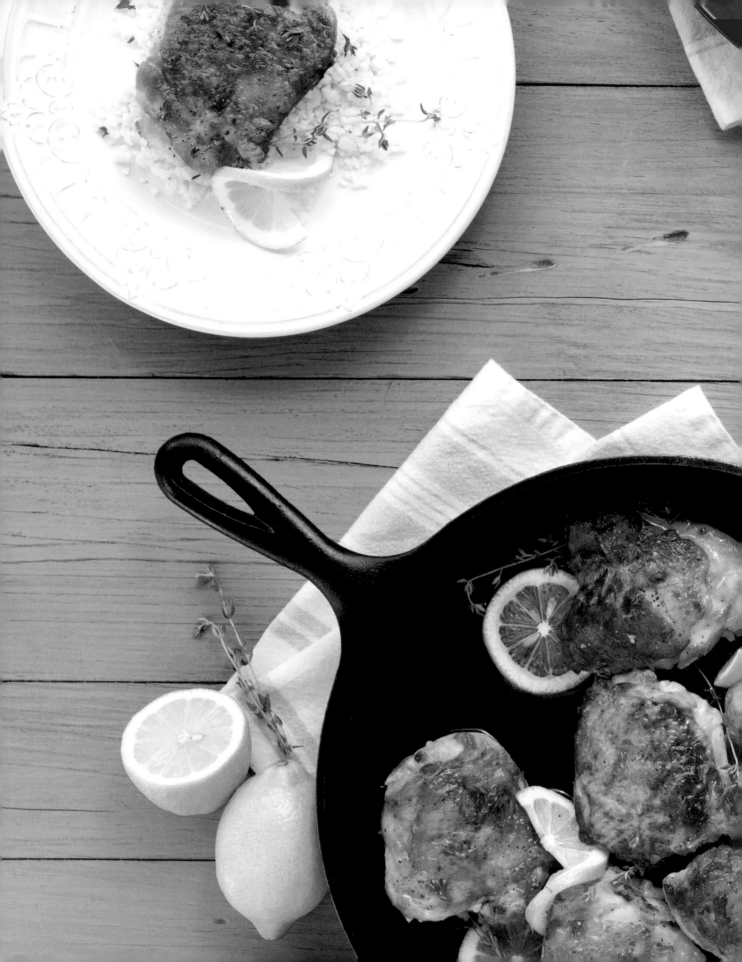

chicken

ALOHA
CHICKEN
DIPPERS

NUT-FREE · KID-FAVORITES · 40 MINUTES OR LESS

This recipe is a hit with both kids and adults, and it makes a great appetizer or main dish. When I was growing up, my parents were often required to travel to Hawaii for work, and my sister and I would spend time there with them when not in school. I remember at a young age being amazed at how many different types of foods were available on the islands, and those flavors make their way into my recipes quite frequently. For this recipe I incorporated pineapple juice, which is very common in Hawaii and provides an awesome tangy, sweet flavor that makes the sauce unique.

Prep Time: 10 minutes   **Cook Time:** 30 minutes   **Yield:** 8 servings as an appetizer, 4 as a main dish

FOR THE SAUCE

1 cup pineapple juice

⅓ cup coconut aminos or soy sauce substitute (page 283)

¼ cup raw honey

½ teaspoon garlic powder

½ teaspoon ground ginger

FOR THE CHICKEN NUGGETS

¼ cup tapioca flour or arrowroot flour

½ teaspoon fine sea salt

½ teaspoon ground black pepper

2 pounds boneless skinless chicken thighs, cut into 1-inch pieces

2 large eggs, beaten

Lard (page 322) or tallow (page 324), for frying

1. Make the sauce: Combine all the sauce ingredients in a small saucepan over medium-high heat. Bring to a boil, then reduce to low and simmer, uncovered, for 10 to 15 minutes, until the sauce has thickened, stirring occasionally. Remove from the heat and set aside.

2. Make the chicken: Place the tapioca flour, salt, and pepper in a large paper or plastic bag, seal, and shake to combine. Add the chicken pieces to the bag and toss until well coated in the flour mixture.

3. Place enough lard in a large skillet to fill it 1 inch up the side. Heat over medium-high heat until the lard reaches 350°F, or until the melted fat bubbles around the handle of a wooden spoon dipped into the pan. Working in batches, dip the chicken pieces into the beaten egg, shake off any excess, then carefully place in the pan. Fry for about 5 to 7 minutes, until the chicken is golden brown and cooked through, and transfer to a paper towel–lined plate.

4. Pour the sauce into a dipping bowl and serve alongside the chicken nuggets.

KITCHEN TIP

I like to start cooking the chicken nuggets while the sauce is simmering to help cut down on cooking time, but if you get nervous with too many pans going at once, then feel free to tackle them back to back, as per the instructions.

TRY THIS!

You can make these chicken nuggets without the sauce or serve them with ketchup (page 275). For a basic nugget recipe without the Hawaiian flavors, add ½ teaspoon of garlic powder and ½ teaspoon of paprika to the tapioca flour mixture and serve with ketchup instead of the sauce.

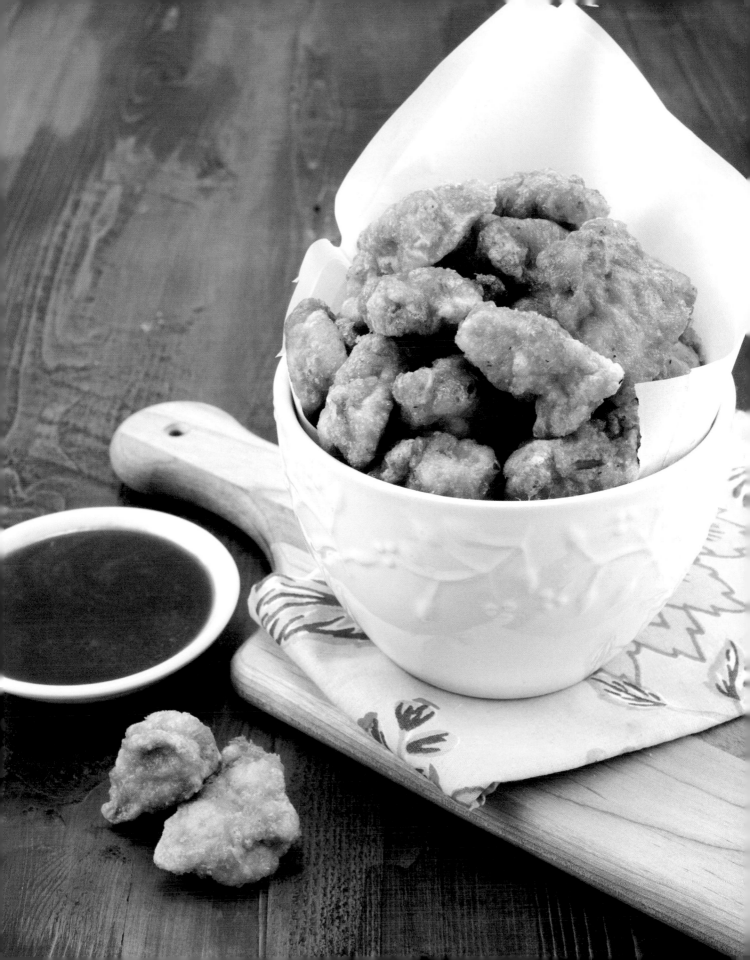

CAJUN CHICKEN PASTA

EGG-FREE · NUT-FREE · KID-FAVORITES

This creamy chicken dish is a favorite of mine, especially because once the prep work is done, the rest comes together quickly and easily. I get a few minutes of chopping time where I can tune out the rest of the world, and then it's just me, a pan, and some seasonings, making magic happen. And don't be intimidated by the word "Cajun"; this dish really doesn't have that much heat to it.

Prep Time: 15 minutes, plus 15 or 25 minutes for the noodles   Cook Time: 15 minutes   Yield: 4 to 6 servings

1 pound boneless skinless chicken thighs, cut into 1-inch chunks

½ teaspoon paprika

½ teaspoon dried oregano

¼ teaspoon cayenne pepper (optional)

¼ teaspoon dried thyme

2 tablespoons ghee (page 320), lard (page 322), or tallow (page 324)

1 small onion, chopped (about ½ cup)

2 cloves garlic, minced

1 small green bell pepper, chopped (about ½ cup)

1 small red bell pepper, chopped (about ½ cup)

6 large white mushrooms, sliced (about 1 cup)

½ teaspoon fine sea salt

¼ teaspoon ground black pepper

Dash of crushed red pepper (optional)

1½ cups coconut milk (page 314)

1 tablespoon tapioca flour

6 fresh basil leaves, thinly sliced, plus 6 more for garnish (optional)

1 batch Pasta (page 194) or Zucchini Noodles (page 328), for serving

1. Place the chicken pieces in a large mixing bowl. Sprinkle the paprika, oregano, cayenne (if using), and thyme over the chicken and toss to coat.

2. Melt the ghee in a large skillet over medium-high heat. Add the chicken and cook for 5 minutes, or until lightly browned, stirring occasionally. Add the onion, garlic, bell peppers, mushrooms, salt, pepper, and crushed red pepper (if using) and cook for an additional 3 to 4 minutes, until the onions start to soften.

3. Whisk together the coconut milk and tapioca flour in a small mixing bowl, then pour into the pan. Add the sliced basil leaves and stir to combine. Cook for another 2 minutes, or until the sauce has thickened and is heated through, stirring frequently.

4. Serve over pasta or zucchini noodles and garnish with additional sliced basil, if desired.

KITCHEN TIP

The last thing you need during food prep is renegade kitchen equipment trying to make a run for it. If you're going to be doing some heavy chopping, placing a dish towel or damp paper towel under your cutting board will keep it from slipping and wobbling on your counter.

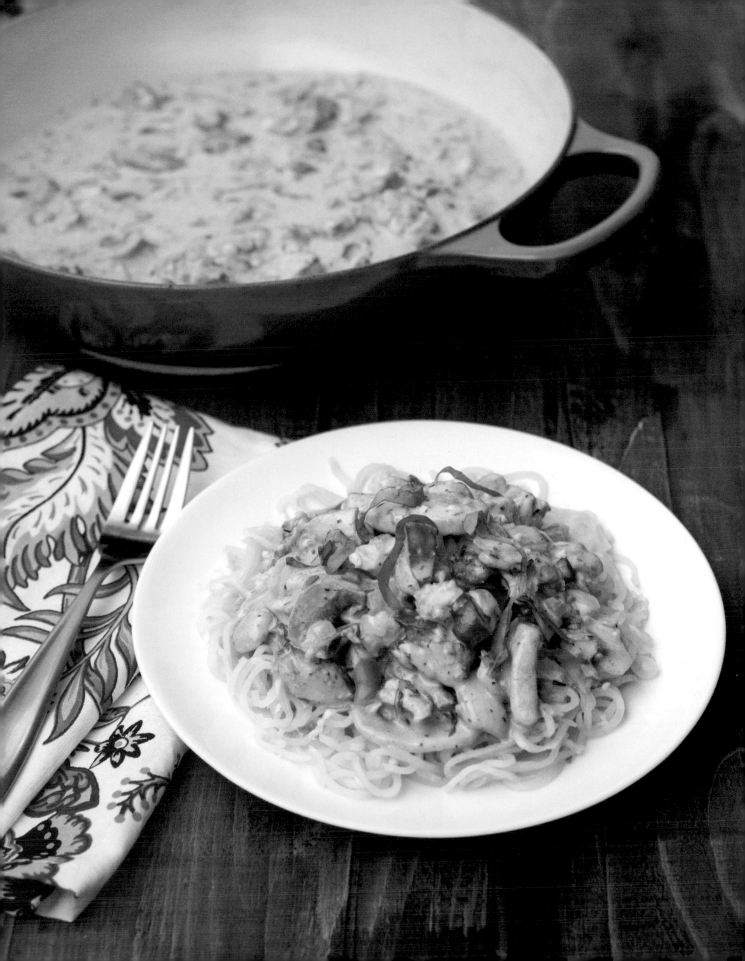

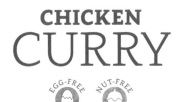

CHICKEN CURRY

EGG-FREE · NUT-FREE

This is a basic curry recipe, but my goal here is to introduce you to the method of cooking rather than just the recipe. Making this dish involves frying spices in a bit of fat, which makes their flavor bolder and more intense—think of it as giving them an ego boost. Remember this trick in the future if you ever want to make the spices in your dishes more pronounced. Try serving this curry with a side of Seasoned Cauliflower Rice (page 200).

Prep Time: 10 minutes   **Cook Time:** 35 minutes   **Yield:** 4 to 6 servings

2 pounds boneless skinless chicken thighs, cut into 1-inch pieces

2 teaspoons fine sea salt

½ teaspoon ground black pepper

⅓ cup ghee (page 320), lard (page 322), or tallow (page 324)

4 teaspoons curry powder

1 teaspoon ground cumin

½ teaspoon turmeric

½ teaspoon ground ginger

¼ teaspoon cayenne pepper

2 cloves garlic, minced

3 tablespoons tomato paste

1 (13.5-ounce) can full-fat coconut milk or 1⅔ cups homemade coconut milk (page 314)

1 small onion, chopped into 1-inch pieces

1 medium green bell pepper, seeded and chopped into 1-inch pieces

1 large tomato, seeded and chopped (about 1 cup)

¼ cup chopped fresh cilantro, for garnish (optional)

1. Season the chicken thigh pieces with the salt and pepper and set aside. Melt the ghee in a large skillet over medium-high heat. Add the curry powder, cumin, turmeric, ginger, and cayenne pepper and cook for 2 minutes, stirring frequently. Add the chicken and cook for 3 minutes, or until browned on all sides. Add the garlic and cook for 1 more minute.

2. Add the tomato paste and coconut milk and stir to combine. Bring to a boil, then reduce the heat to low and simmer for 15 minutes, uncovered. Add the onion, bell pepper, and tomato and simmer for another 10 minutes, or until the chicken is cooked through and the vegetables are tender.

3. Taste and add additional salt and pepper if desired. Sprinkle with chopped cilantro to serve, if desired.

KITCHEN TIP
Adding a teaspoon of raw honey to your dishes will help combat the bitterness of tomato or too much heat from spices.

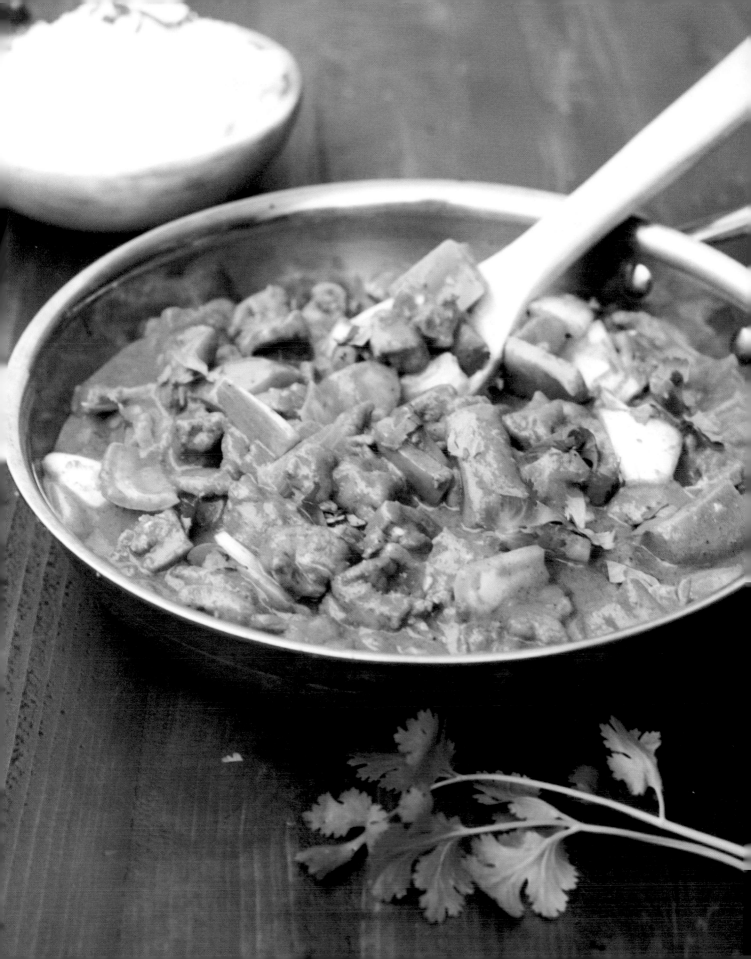

CHICKEN
PICCATA

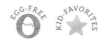

While chicken breasts on their own have a fairly neutral flavor, cooking them piccata—a method that calls for butterflying, sautéing, and serving in a sauce of lemon juice and capers—allows the bursts of lemon and garlic to shine through. Basically, you will have everyone thinking you are a gourmet chef without having to do too much work. Try serving this dish with a side of zucchini noodles (page 328) or other vegetable noodles (pages 326 to 327).

Prep Time: **20 minutes**   Cook Time: **25 minutes**   Yield: **4 servings**

1½ pounds boneless skinless chicken breasts

¼ cup almond flour (page 316)

¼ cup tapioca flour or arrowroot flour

¼ teaspoon fine sea salt

¼ teaspoon ground black pepper

½ cup ghee (page 320), lard (page 322), or tallow (page 324), for frying

1 small white onion, chopped (about ½ cup)

2 cloves garlic, chopped

½ cup freshly squeezed lemon juice

¾ cup chicken stock (page 310)

¼ cup capers, drained and rinsed

⅓ cup fresh parsley, chopped, plus more for garnish (optional)

1 lemon, sliced, for garnish (optional)

1. Cut the chicken breasts in half along the thickness, so you have two thin slices from each breast. Set aside.

2. Mix together the almond flour, tapioca flour, salt, and pepper in a medium-sized mixing bowl. Dredge the chicken breasts in the mixture and set aside on a cooling rack.

3. Melt the ghee in a medium skillet over medium-high heat. Add half of the chicken to the pan and cook for about 3 minutes on each side, until lightly browned. Transfer the chicken to a plate, then repeat with the other half of the chicken. Transfer the second half of the chicken to the same plate.

4. Add the onion and garlic to the pan. Stir for 2 minutes, then add the lemon juice, chicken stock, capers, and parsley and stir to combine. Bring the sauce to a boil and reduce for 3 minutes, stirring frequently. Return the chicken to the pan and decrease the heat to low. Cover and simmer for 5 minutes, or until the chicken is heated through and fully cooked. Taste the sauce and add additional salt and pepper if desired.

5. Place the chicken on a serving platter, pour the sauce over the chicken, garnish with additional parsley and lemon slices, if desired, and serve.

KITCHEN TIP

Before cutting a lime or lemon for juicing, roll it back and forth on the counter while applying pressure with the palm of your hand. This helps break down the citrus flesh so it releases much more juice.

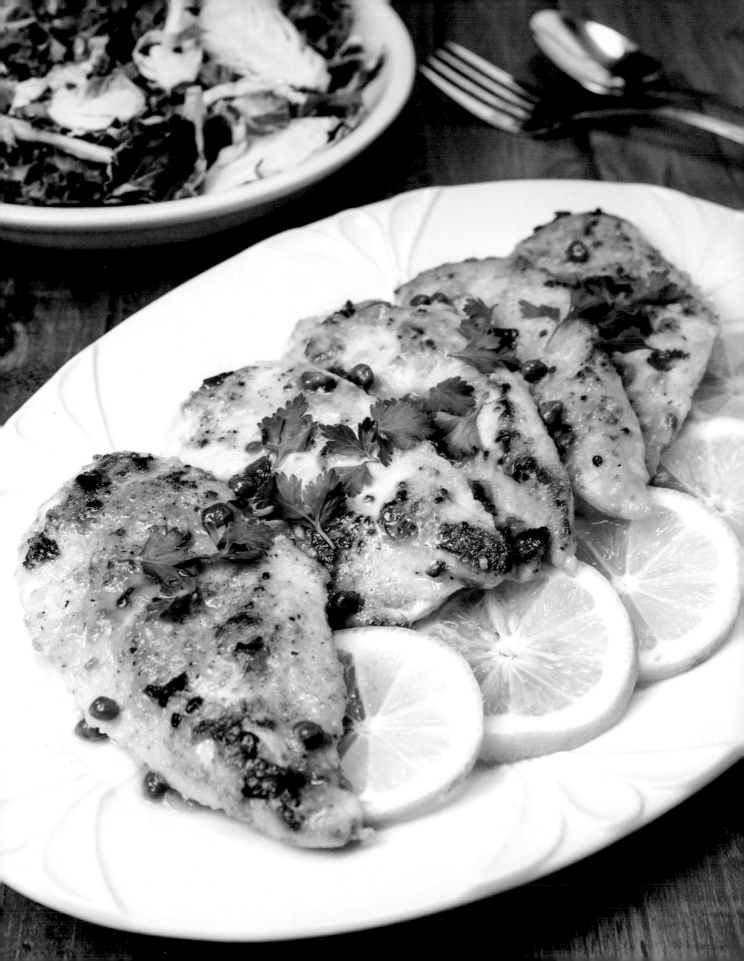

CHICKEN SALAD
on
APPLE SLICES

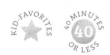

This chicken salad can be made ahead of time, which makes it a great option for an easy appetizer, lunch, or snack. While apple slices aren't required to enjoy chicken salad, they make a great substitute for bread or crackers while also adding flavor and crunch.

Prep Time: 8 minutes   Yield: 4 to 6 servings

1 pound chicken breasts, cooked and cut into ½-inch cubes (about 2 cups)

1 cup chopped celery

1 cup seedless red grapes, halved

½ cup roasted pecans, chopped

½ cup mayonnaise (page 278)

¼ teaspoon fine sea salt

¼ teaspoon ground black pepper

3 small red apples, such as Gala, Fuji, or Red Delicious, cored and cut into ¼-inch-thick slices

1. Place the chicken, celery, grapes, pecans, mayonnaise, salt, and pepper in a medium-sized mixing bowl and stir until well combined. Taste and add additional salt and pepper if desired.

2. Place the apple slices on a serving tray and scoop 2 to 3 tablespoons of chicken salad onto each slice. Store any leftover chicken salad in a sealed container the refrigerator for up to 3 days.

KITCHEN TIP

A quick way to cook chicken breasts for use in a salad like this is to poach them. Place boneless, skinless chicken breasts in the bottom of a large skillet. Fill the skillet with enough water to cover the chicken by 1 inch, then place on the stovetop over medium-high heat. If I have any extra onions, carrots, or celery lying around, I usually throw them in with the chicken. Bring the water just to a boil, then cover the pan and turn the heat to low. Simmer for 10 minutes, or until the chicken is cooked through, then remove the chicken from the pan and place on a cutting board. Let cool for at least 10 minutes before cutting.

TRY THIS!
To spice up this basic chicken salad, try mixing in 3 teaspoons of curry powder and 1 to 2 teaspoons of raw honey. Toasting the pecans also adds an extra nutty taste.

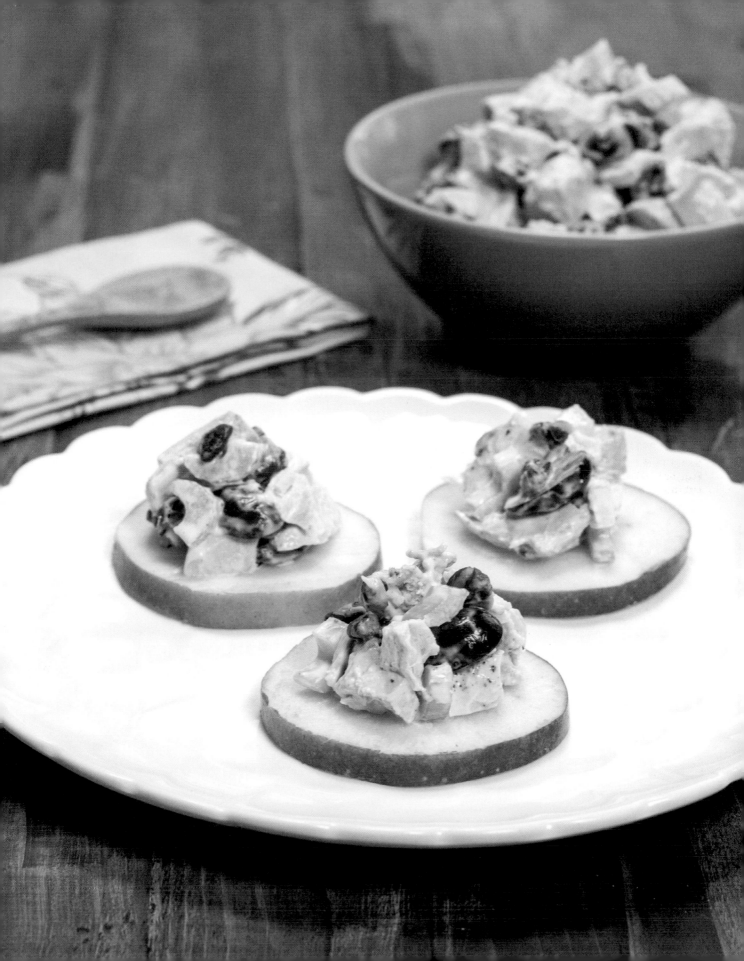

JERK
CHICKEN

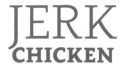

The last time I was planning to make this chicken, I came back from grocery shopping, where I had purchased a large number of onions, pulled into my sloped driveway, and went around to the back of the car to bring in my hoard of groceries. But when I opened the trunk, five onions leapt from my car all at once, rolling down toward the street at top speed. I chased after them, flapping my arms and yelling mean words at the onions, trying to grab them while running at the same time. When I had finally retrieved them, I looked up to see that a lady walking her dog had stopped in her tracks and was staring at me, looking horrified. I gave her a nod and brought my captives back to my car. Luckily for you, this recipe calls for only one onion, so you shouldn't have to worry about any produce mutinies.

Prep Time: 15 minutes, plus 2 hours to marinate   Cook Time: 45 minutes   Yield: 4 to 6 servings

FOR THE MARINADE

6 green onions, chopped

3 cloves garlic, minced

2 kiwis, peeled and quartered (optional)

2 habañero chiles, stemmed (seeded if sensitive to heat)

1 serrano chile, stemmed (seeded if sensitive to heat)

1 small onion, quartered

½ cup coconut aminos or soy sauce substitute (page 283)

⅓ cup extra-virgin olive oil

¼ cup apple cider vinegar

¼ cup freshly squeezed orange juice

3 tablespoons fresh thyme leaves

2 tablespoons raw honey

½ teaspoon fine sea salt

½ teaspoon ground black pepper

¼ teaspoon ground nutmeg

¼ teaspoon ground allspice

¼ teaspoon ground cloves

3 pounds bone-in chicken breasts, thighs, and/or drumsticks

1 tablespoon chopped fresh parsley, for garnish (optional)

1 lime, quartered, for serving

1. Make the marinade: Place all the marinade ingredients in a food processor or blender and blend until smooth. Place the chicken in a large bowl and pour the marinade over the top. Toss the chicken to fully coat, then cover the bowl and place in the refrigerator. Marinate for at least 2 hours and up to 24 hours.

2. **To use a grill:** Preheat the grill to medium heat and remove the chicken from the marinade. Grill the chicken over medium heat for 35 to 45 minutes, turning occasionally, until a meat thermometer reads 165°F or the juices run clear when a knife is inserted and the meat is no longer pink inside.

   To use an oven: Preheat the oven to 400°F. Place the chicken in a large baking dish and bake in for 40 to 45 minutes, until a meat thermometer reads 170°F or the juices run clear when a knife is inserted and the meat is no longer pink inside.

3. Garnish with chopped parsley, if desired, and serve with lime wedges.

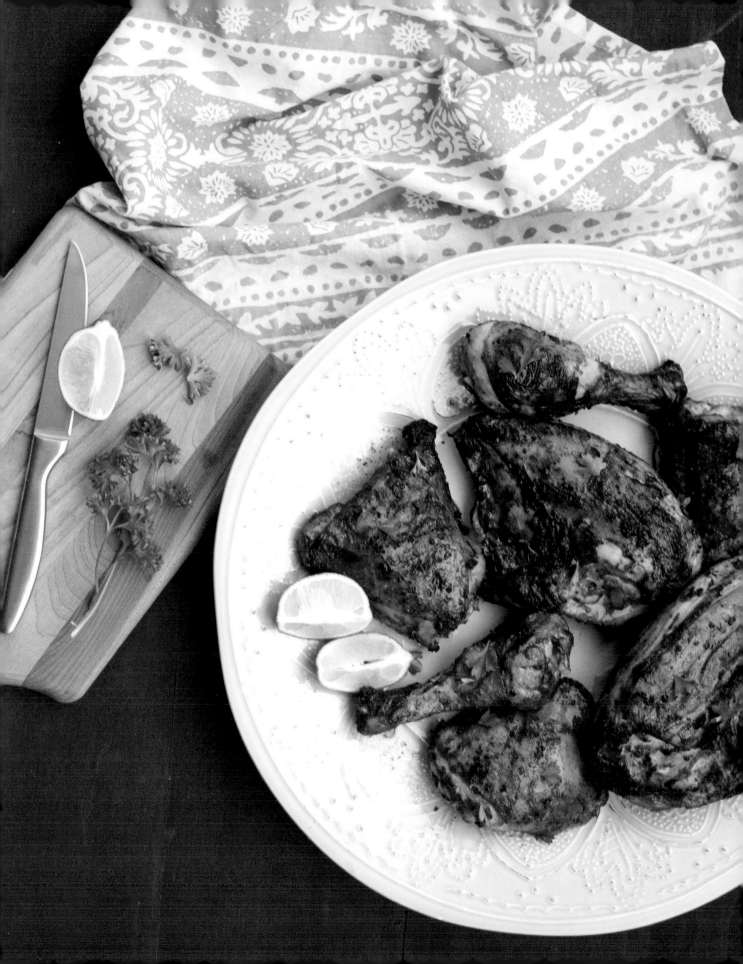

ORANGE
CHICKEN

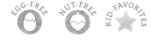

EGG-FREE   NUT-FREE   KID-FAVORITES

This is one of my favorite slow cooker recipes, and it's a big hit with my kids as well. The tangy and sweet flavors of the sauce go great with the tender chicken, and best of all, your whole house will smell amazing by the time it's done cooking. I like to serve this with a side of Sesame Ginger Broccolini (page 206) and some zucchini noodles (page 328).

Prep Time: 15 minutes   **Cook Time:** 5 to 6 hours   **Yield:** 4 to 6 servings

4 pounds bone-in chicken drumsticks and thighs, skin removed

½ teaspoon fine sea salt

½ teaspoon ground black pepper

⅓ cup raw honey

¼ cup coconut aminos or soy sauce substitute (page 283)

3 tablespoons freshly squeezed orange juice

1 tablespoon finely grated orange zest

3 cloves garlic, minced

2 tablespoons minced or grated fresh ginger

1 tablespoon apple cider vinegar

¼ teaspoon crushed red pepper

2 teaspoons sesame seeds, for garnish

1. Rinse the chicken and pat dry with paper towels. Sprinkle with the salt and pepper and place in the slow cooker.

2. In a small mixing bowl, whisk together the honey, coconut aminos, orange juice and zest, garlic, ginger, vinegar, and crushed red pepper. Pour the sauce over the chicken, cover the slow cooker, and cook on low for 5 to 6 hours, until the chicken is cooked through.

3. Transfer the chicken to a serving platter and cover to keep warm. Pour the sauce into a medium-sized saucepan over medium-high heat. Bring to a light boil and cook for 10 minutes, or until the sauce has reduced and formed a thin glaze, stirring occasionally. Pour over the chicken, sprinkle with the sesame seeds, if desired, and serve.

KITCHEN TIP

Fresh ginger will keep in a sealed bag or container in the freezer for up to 6 months. Whenever you need to use it, just grab it from the freezer, use a vegetable peeler to remove the skin around the piece you want to use, and grate the ginger with a Microplane grater. Grating fresh or frozen ginger instead of mincing it is an easy way to get small pieces without spending a lot of time fiddling around with a knife.

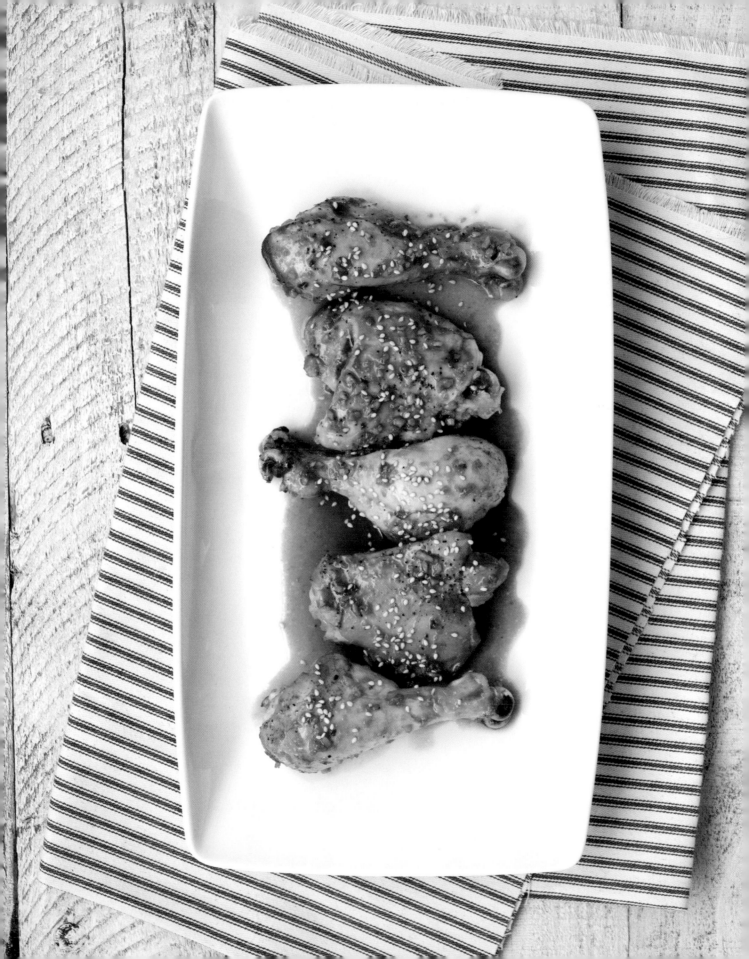

LEMON *and* THYME CHICKEN THIGHS

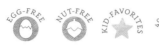

This recipe highlights how great high-quality chicken can taste when combined with just a little seasoning, fresh herbs, and lemon juice. A well-seasoned cast-iron skillet is the perfect pan for this recipe because it prevents the chicken skin from sticking and transfers well between the stovetop and oven. The pan will get very hot and might smoke a bit, so turn on the vent and crack open a window just to be safe.

Prep Time: 5 minutes   **Cook Time:** 30 minutes   **Yield:** 4 servings

6 bone-in, skin-on chicken thighs (2 pounds)

½ teaspoon fine sea salt

½ teaspoon ground black pepper

½ teaspoon garlic powder

1 tablespoon ghee (page 320), lard (page 322), or tallow (page 324)

1 large lemon, sliced

6 sprigs fresh thyme

1 tablespoon freshly squeezed lemon juice

1. Preheat the oven to 450°F.

2. Sprinkle the chicken on both sides with the salt, pepper, and garlic powder. Heat the ghee in a large cast-iron skillet over medium-high heat. Place the chicken thighs in the pan, skin side down, and cook for 2 minutes. Reduce the heat to medium and continue cooking the thighs without touching them for another 10 minutes, or until the skin has released from the pan (the skin will initially stick to the pan and then will release once the fat has rendered). Drain any excess fat from the pan, then transfer the skillet to the oven (remember, the handle will be hot). Cook for 10 more minutes.

3. Remove the skillet from the oven and flip the chicken pieces over. Nestle the lemon slices and thyme sprigs between the chicken pieces, then return the pan to the oven for 5 minutes, or until the skin is crispy and the juices run clear when a knife is inserted and the meat is no longer pink inside, or the internal temperature of the chicken reaches 165°F. Remove from the oven, drizzle with lemon juice, and serve.

KITCHEN TIP

If your food is sticking to your cast-iron pan, there's a good chance it isn't seasoned well—not "seasoned" as in salt and pepper, but "seasoned" as in baked in the oven with a coating of fat or oil to create a protective nonstick surface. Most cast-iron pan manufacturers have information on their websites about how to care for and season their products, so if in doubt, check them out and get your cast iron in tip-top shape!

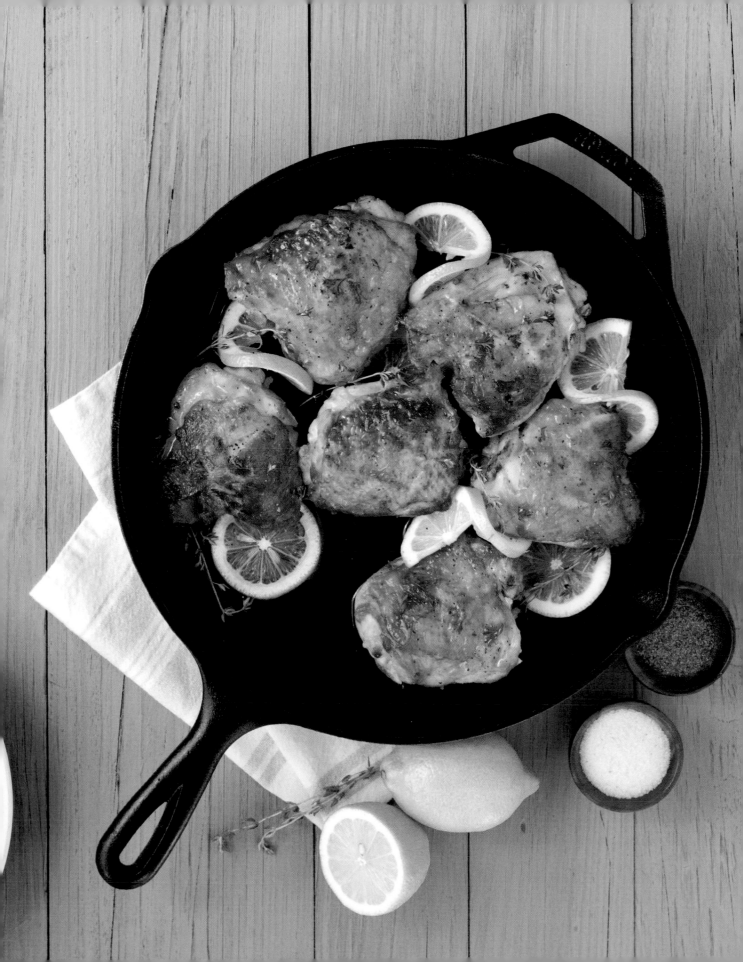

MOROCCAN
CHICKEN

I have to confess that I have never visited Morocco, so I don't know if this recipe is anywhere close to authentic Moroccan cuisine, and I don't even remember how it came to be named, but since it goes by "Moroccan chicken" in my house, that's what it shall be called in this book. I do know that it is a great example of how to blend a variety of spices that will have your taste buds tap dancing, which is much more important than the name of the recipe. I like to serve this chicken with zucchini noodles (page 328) tossed in a batch of Avocado Basil Cream Sauce (page 270). The creaminess of the sauce and noodles helps balance the light spiciness of the chicken.

Prep Time: 10 minutes, plus 2 hours to marinate   **Cook Time:** 35 to 45 minutes   **Yield:** 4 to 6 servings

FOR THE SEASONING MIX

4 teaspoons fine sea salt

4 teaspoons paprika

2 teaspoons ground ginger

1 teaspoon ground black pepper

1 teaspoon ground cumin

1 teaspoon turmeric

1 teaspoon dried oregano

½ teaspoon cayenne pepper

4 pounds bone-in, skin-on chicken legs and thighs

3 tablespoons extra-virgin olive oil

¼ cup freshly squeezed lemon juice

2 lemons, quartered, for serving

1. Combine all of the ingredients for the seasoning mix in a small mixing bowl and set aside.

2. Rinse the chicken, pat dry with paper towels, and place in a large mixing bowl. Pour the olive oil and lemon juice over the chicken and toss to coat, then sprinkle the seasoning mixture over the chicken, making sure to coat the chicken evenly. Cover the bowl, place in the refrigerator, and marinate for at least 2 hours and up to 24 hours.

3. **To use a grill:** Preheat the grill to medium heat and cook the chicken, covered, for 30 to 35 minutes, until the internal temperature reaches 165°F or the juices run clear when a knife is inserted and the meat is no longer pink inside, turning once.

   To use an oven: Preheat the oven to 400°F. Bake the chicken in a large glass baking dish for 30 minutes, then lower the heat to 350°F and bake for another 10 minutes, or until the internal temperature reaches 165°F or the juices run clear when a knife is inserted and the meat is no longer pink inside. Then, if you like a crispier skin, turn the oven to broil and cook for 2 minutes, then turn the pieces over and broil on the other side for another 2 minutes, or until skin is browned and crispy.

KITCHEN TIP

Turmeric can stain your hands a not-so-lovely shade of yellow, so make sure to wash them right away after handling the chicken. (Of course, you always wash your hands anytime you touch raw chicken anyway, right?)

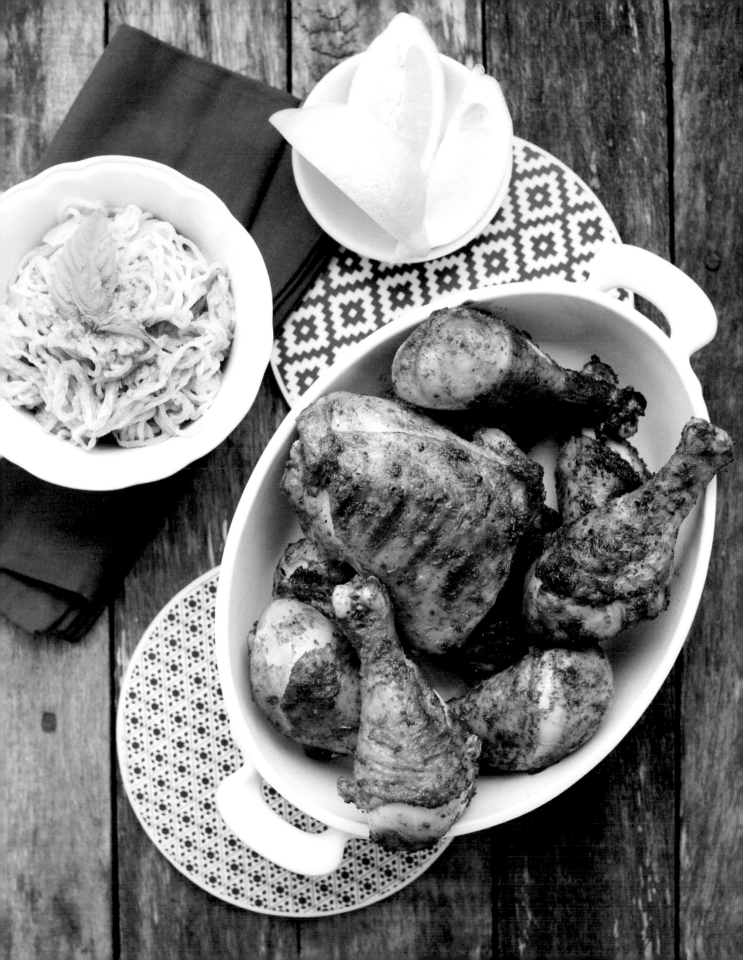

PIRI PIRI CHICKEN

This recipe is inspired by Portuguese and African flavors. The chicken is marinated in a spicy and tangy sauce and then is usually grilled, but I have an oven option for those of you who don't grill or just want to cook it inside. It's hard to find authentic piri piri chiles where I live, so I've used a combination of crushed red pepper and serrano chiles instead. Serving extra sauce on the side allows everyone to add a little more flavor (and heat) if they like. I generally serve this dish with Crispy Sweet Potato Wedges (page 190) and some grilled or roasted vegetables.

Prep Time: 15 minutes, plus 2 hours to marinate
Cook Time: 30 minutes or 1 hour 15 minutes, depending on cooking method   **Yield**: 4 to 6 servings

FOR THE SAUCE

3 cloves garlic

2 serrano chiles or jalapeños, halved and seeded

¼ cup freshly squeezed lemon juice

¼ cup chopped fresh cilantro

¼ cup extra-virgin olive oil

3 tablespoons apple cider vinegar

1 tablespoon paprika

1 tablespoon crushed red pepper

4 pounds chicken leg quarters

1½ teaspoons fine sea salt

¼ teaspoon ground black pepper

2 lemons, quartered, for serving

1. Place all the sauce ingredients in a blender or food processor and blend until smooth.

2. Season the chicken with the salt and pepper and place in a large glass baking dish. Coat with the sauce, reserving ¼ cup for serving. Cover and place in the refrigerator for at least 2 hours and up to 24 hours. Store the reserved sauce in a sealed container in the refrigerator until ready to serve.

3. **To use a grill:** Preheat the grill to medium-high heat. Remove the chicken from the dish and allow the excess sauce to drain off. Place on the grill and cook for 15 minutes on each side, until the internal temperature reaches 165°F or the juices run clear when a knife is inserted and the meat is no longer pink inside.

   To use an oven: Place an oven rack in the middle position and preheat the oven to 375°F, and line a baking sheet with parchment paper. Remove the chicken from the dish and allow the excess sauce to drain off. Place on the prepared baking sheet, skin side up, and bake for 1 hour. Turn the heat up to 400°F and bake for another 15 minutes, or until the skin is golden brown and the internal temperature of the chicken reaches 165°F. Remove from the oven and set aside to rest for 5 minutes before serving.

4. Serve with the lemon wedges and reserved sauce.

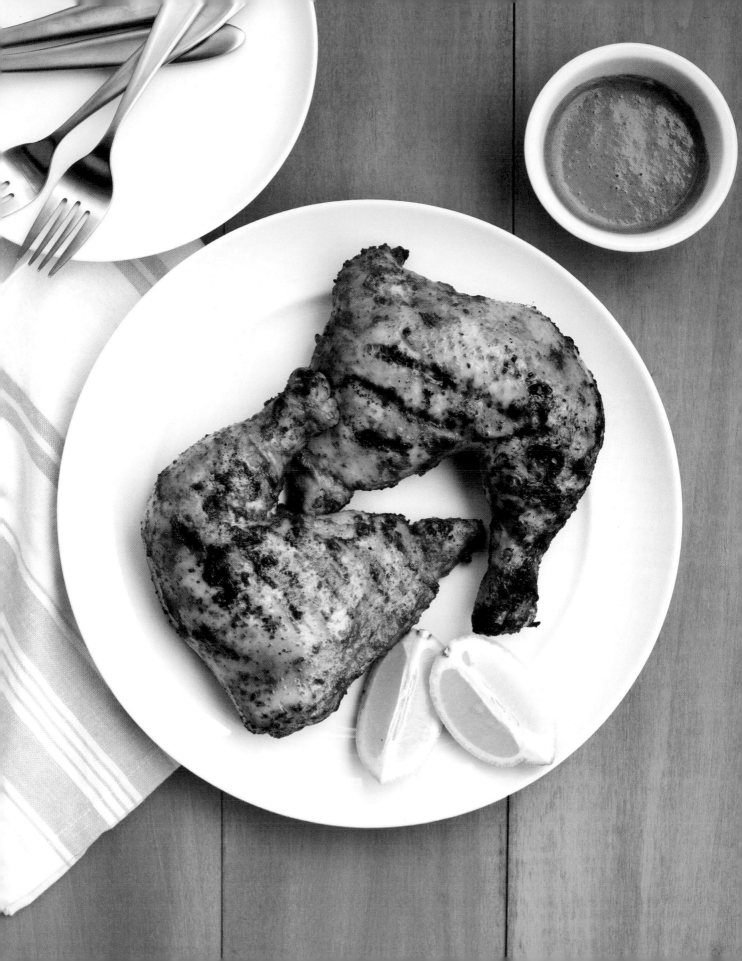

PROVENÇAL CHICKEN

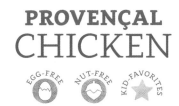

EGG-FREE NUT-FREE KID-FAVORITES

A traditional Provençal-style chicken usually contains olives, but because I am the only one in the house who wants anything to do with them, I usually leave them out or sneak them onto just my plate. If olives are enjoyed in your home, then add ½ cup pitted Kalamata olives at the same time as the thyme, rosemary, and basil. The olives will add a bit of saltiness to the dish, so omit the ½ teaspoon of salt that's added along with the stock and add salt to taste later.

Prep Time: 15 minutes   **Cook Time:** 50 minutes   **Yield:** 4 servings

3 pounds bone-in, skin-on chicken thighs

1½ teaspoons fine sea salt, divided

1½ teaspoons ground black pepper, divided

2 tablespoons ghee (page 320), lard (page 322), or tallow (page 324)

1 medium onion, finely chopped (about ¾ cup)

3 cloves garlic, minced

1½ pounds Roma tomatoes, diced small (about 3 cups)

⅓ cup chicken stock (page 310)

3 tablespoons fresh thyme leaves

1 teaspoon chopped fresh rosemary

¼ cup thinly sliced fresh basil

3 tablespoons chopped fresh parsley, for garnish (optional)

1 lemon, sliced, for serving

1. Place an oven rack in the middle position of the oven and preheat the oven to 375°F.

2. Rinse the chicken and pat dry with paper towels. Rub 1 teaspoon of the salt and 1 teaspoon of the pepper all over the chicken.

3. Heat the ghee in a large Dutch oven over medium heat. Add the chicken pieces, working in batches if needed, and cook for 5 minutes on each side, or until golden brown. Transfer the chicken to a plate and set aside.

4. Add the onion to the pan and cook for 2 minutes, then add the garlic and cook for an additional minute. Add the tomatoes, stock, and remaining ½ teaspoon of salt and ½ teaspoon of pepper to the pan and stir to combine. Turn the heat off and add the chicken back to the pan, skin side up, placing on top of the sauce.

5. Transfer to the oven and bake, uncovered, for 25 minutes, or until the chicken reaches 165°F internally or the juices run clear when a knife is inserted and the meat is no longer pink inside. You may need less time depending on the size of the chicken thighs. Remove the pan from the oven and turn the oven to broil.

6. Place the pan on the stove over medium-high heat and transfer the chicken to a plate. Add the thyme, rosemary, and basil to the sauce and stir to combine. Cook for 5 minutes, or until the sauce has reduced slightly. Add the chicken back to the pan, skin side up, and stick the pan under the broiler for 2 to 3 minutes, until the skin is brown and crispy. Remove from the oven, top with the parsley, if desired, and serve with the lemon slices.

KITCHEN TIP

If you need to chop a variety of fresh herbs and they will all be added to the dish at the same time, put them all on the cutting board and chop them together. It cuts down on prep time and gives the herbs a chance to hang out before you throw them in the pot.

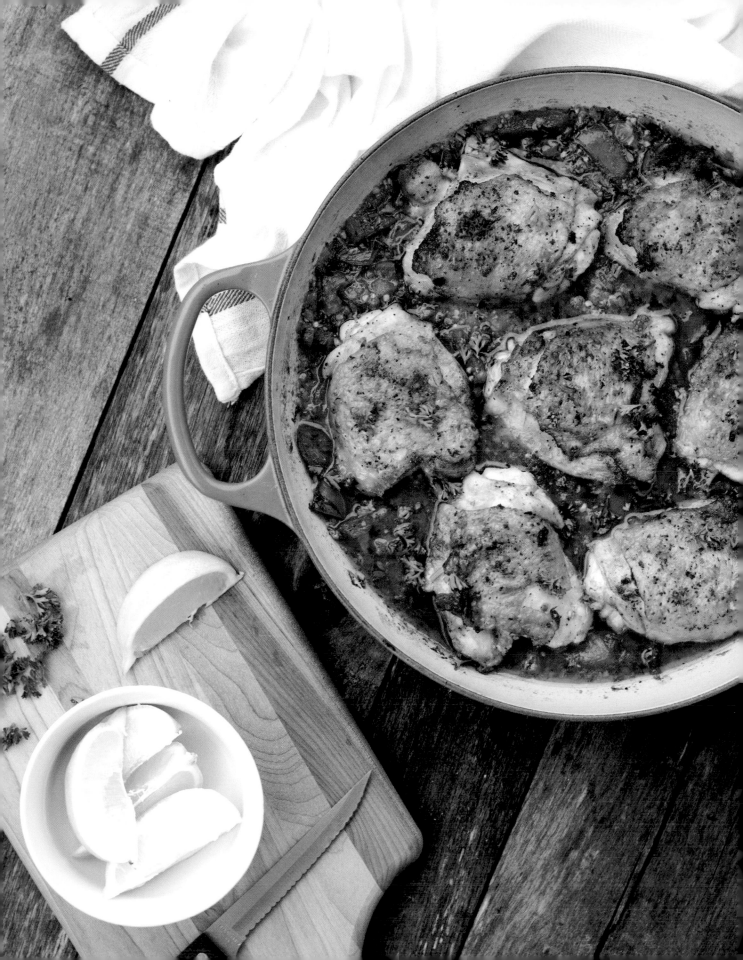

SESAME
CHICKEN
WINGS

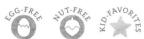

This recipe combines the sweetness of honey, the saltiness of coconut aminos, and just a hint of heat from the crushed red pepper, which leaves you with lick-your-fingers-because-they-taste-so-good chicken wings. These are a great appetizer for parties; make sure to serve them with plenty of napkins.

Prep Time: 15 minutes **Cook Time:** 50 minutes **Yield:** 6 servings as an appetizer, 4 as a main dish

2 pounds chicken wings and drumettes

2 tablespoons ghee (page 320), lard (page 322), or tallow (page 324)

1½ teaspoons crushed red pepper

3 cloves garlic, minced

1½ teaspoons ground ginger

¼ cup apple cider vinegar

¼ cup chicken stock (page 310)

1½ teaspoons sesame oil

¼ cup raw honey

½ cup coconut aminos or soy sauce substitute (page 283)

¼ cup chopped green onions, for garnish (optional)

2 tablespoons sesame seeds, for garnish

1. Place an oven rack in the middle position and preheat the oven to 350°F. Line a 9-by-13-inch baking sheet with parchment paper or a baking mat.

2. Pat the wings dry with paper towels, then place on the prepared baking sheet and bake for 30 minutes, flipping the wings over halfway through.

3. While the wings are baking, melt the ghee in a medium saucepan over medium-high heat. Add the crushed red pepper and garlic and sauté for 2 minutes, stirring constantly. Next, add the ginger, vinegar, stock, sesame oil, honey, and coconut aminos and stir to combine. Bring just to a boil, stirring frequently, then reduce the heat to medium-low. Stir the sauce occasionally and simmer gently for 10 minutes, or until the sauce has thickened slightly and reduced down to about ¾ cup.

4. Once the wings are done cooking, remove the baking sheet from the oven, leaving the oven on, and place the wings in a large mixing bowl. Pour the sauce over the wings and toss to coat. Pour the wings and sauce back onto the baking sheet and separate the wings so they are not touching. Return to the oven and bake for 10 minutes, then flip the wings over and bake for another 10 minutes.

5. To finish the wings, turn the oven to broil and cook for 1 minute, then flip the wings over and broil for another minute, or until the wings are browned and crispy. Place the wings on a serving platter and top with the chopped green onions, if desired, and sesame seeds.

TRY THIS!
For extra tanginess, try stirring 1 tablespoon of freshly squeezed lime juice into the sauce right before tossing it with the wings.

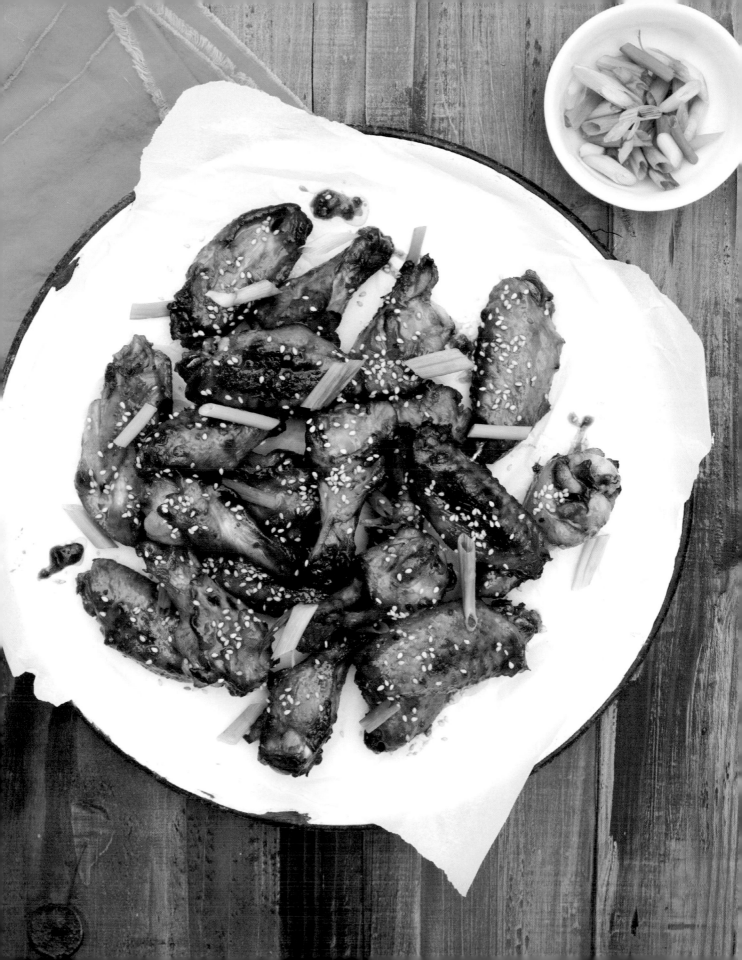

SIMPLE SLOW COOKER CHICKEN

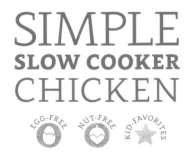

EGG-FREE · NUT-FREE · KID-FAVORITES

If you're thinking, "Really, lady, you're giving me a recipe for just a chicken in a slow cooker?!" then the answer is YES. The leftover chicken from this recipe makes a fantastic stock (see page 310), and it's so easy that even a beginner cook can't mess it up. Not to mention that it gives you a great base recipe that you can experiment with. Think of it as a blank canvas that you can decorate with an unlimited number of flavor combinations. For starters, you can use any of the spice blends in this book (pages 330 to 331): just rub 1½ to 2 tablespoons of your favorite mix on the chicken along with the olive oil, stick it in the slow cooker, and you have the main dish of your meal ready to go.

Prep Time: 15 minutes   **Cook Time:** 6 to 8 hours   **Yield:** 6 servings

1 small onion, quartered

2 large carrots, peeled and chopped into thirds

2 stalks celery, chopped into thirds

1 teaspoon dried thyme

1 teaspoon garlic powder

1 teaspoon paprika

1 teaspoon fine sea salt

1 teaspoon ground black pepper

2 tablespoons extra-virgin olive oil or melted ghee

1 whole chicken (5 pounds), rinsed and patted dry with paper towels

1. Spread the onion quarters, carrots, and celery evenly on the bottom of the slow cooker. This will allow the chicken to stay elevated from the heating element while cooking.

2. Combine the thyme, garlic powder, paprika, salt, and pepper in a small bowl. Rub the olive oil all over the chicken, then rub in the seasoning, making sure the chicken is evenly coated.

3. Place the chicken in the slow cooker on top of the chopped vegetables. Cook on low for 6 to 8 hours, or until the chicken is cooked through.

4. Optional: For a nice finish, place an oven rack in the bottom third of the oven and turn the oven to broil on high. Carefully transfer the chicken to a baking dish and broil for 5 to 7 minutes, until the skin is crispy and brown, then serve.

TRY THIS!

Try drizzling 1 to 2 tablespoons of freshly squeezed lemon juice over the chicken at the same time as the olive oil to give it a refreshing hint of citrus.

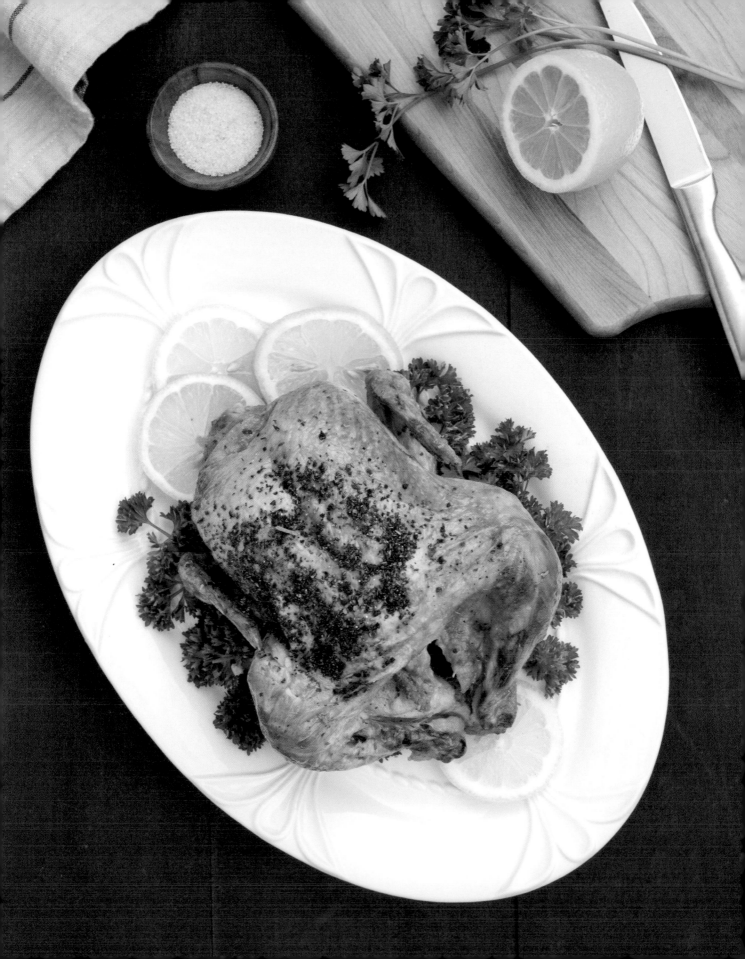

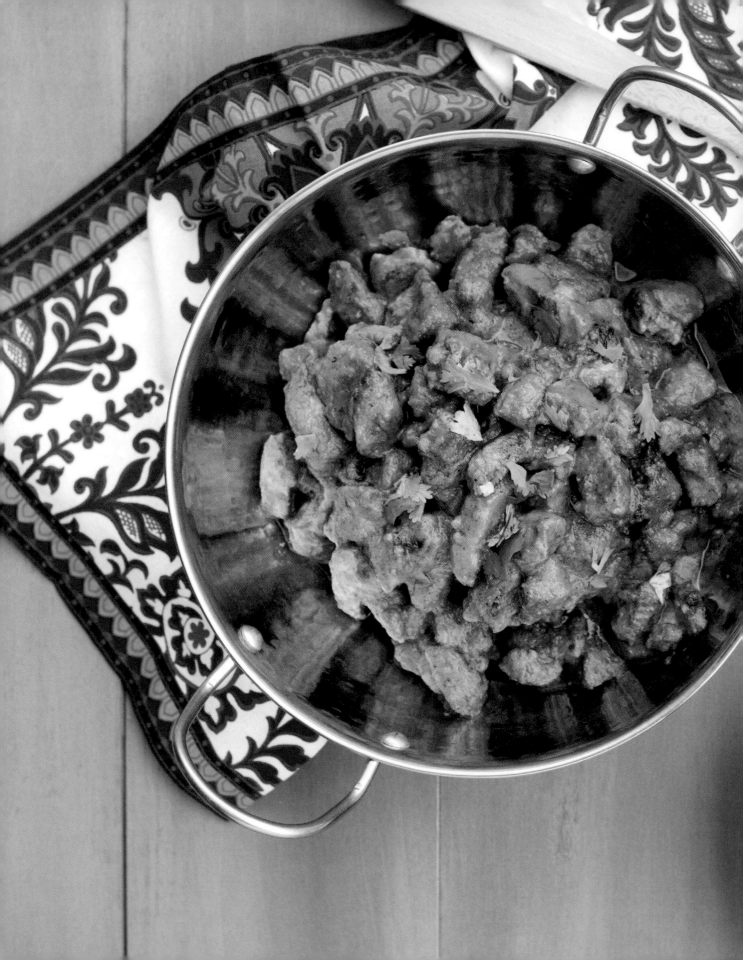

pork

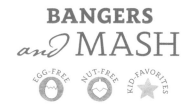

BANGERS and MASH

EGG-FREE NUT-FREE KID-FAVORITES

Bangers and mash, or sausages and mashed potatoes for those in the United States, is not the prettiest dish in the world, but it's a delicious and flavorful comfort food, especially when smothered in onion gravy. Make this for dinner on a cold night, and your friends and family will sing your praises for years to come.

Prep Time: 10 minutes   Cook Time: 40 minutes, plus 30 minutes for the mashed sweet potatoes   Yield: 4 servings

8 pork sausages (2 pounds)

4 tablespoons ghee (page 320), lard (page 322), or tallow (page 324), divided

2 large onions, thinly sliced

1½ teaspoons tapioca flour or arrowroot flour

½ teaspoon dry yellow mustard

¼ teaspoon fine sea salt

⅛ teaspoon ground black pepper

½ cup beef stock (page 310), plus more if needed

2 tablespoons balsamic vinegar

1 batch Mashed Sweet Potatoes (page 189), for serving

1. Bring a large pot of water to a boil over high heat. Drop the sausages in the water, then cover the pot and lower the heat to low. Boil the sausages for 15 minutes, then remove them from the water and place them on a paper towel–lined plate to drain. (If making the mash now, use the hot water to boil the potatoes.)

2. While the sausages are boiling, start the gravy: Melt 2 tablespoons of the ghee in the skillet. Add the onions and stir to coat, then lower the heat to medium-low and cook for 10 minutes without stirring. Toss the onions well, then allow to sit for another 10 minutes without stirring. Toss one more time and leave untouched for 5 to 10 more minutes, or until the onions turn dark brown and are caramelized.

3. While the onions are caramelizing, fry the boiled sausages: Heat 1 tablespoon of the ghee in a large skillet over medium-high heat. Add the boiled sausages and fry for 3 minutes on each side, or until the skin is crispy and browned. Remove from the pan and set aside on a plate.

4. When the onions have been caramelized, add the tapioca flour, dry yellow mustard, salt, and pepper to the onions and toss to coat. Pour the beef stock and balsamic vinegar over the onions to deglaze the pan, and scrape up any bits of onion that may be stuck to the bottom. Bring the mixture to a light boil, then reduce the heat to medium-low, add the remaining 1 tablespoon of ghee, and stir well. If desired, add an additional ¼ cup of stock for a thinner gravy and stir until well combined. Add the sausages to the pan and cook for 5 minutes, or until heated through.

5. To serve, place a scoop of mashed sweet potatoes in a bowl, top with 2 sausages, and cover with gravy.

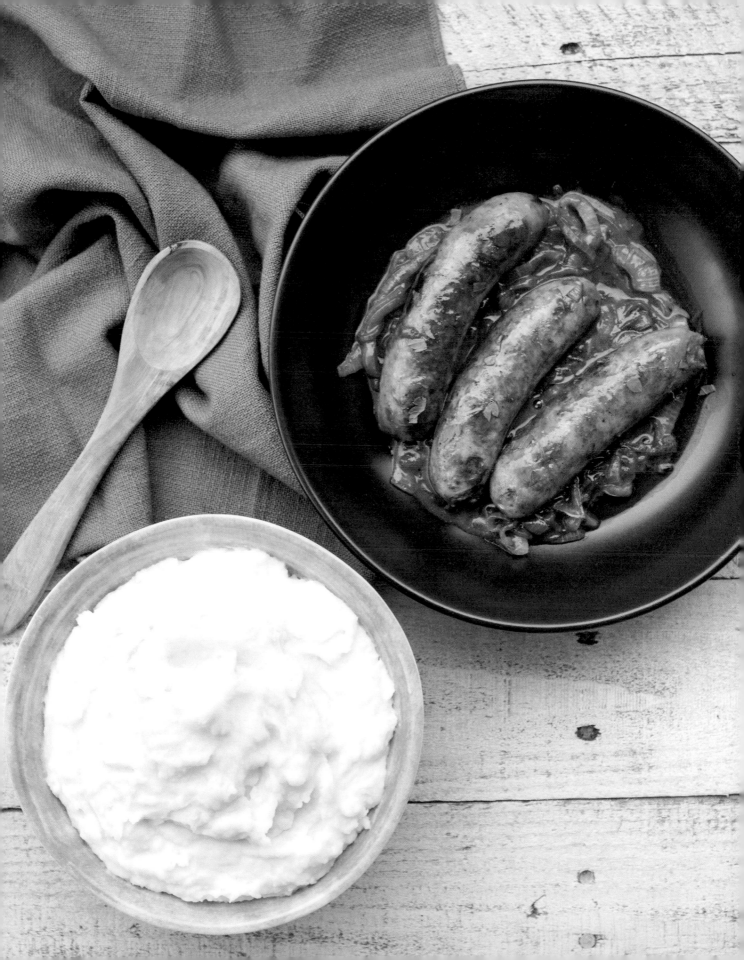

PORK
CHILE VERDE

Pork shoulder just begs to be cooked slow and low with a handful of flavorful ingredients, and this recipe honors that request by pairing the pork with tomatillos, chiles, garlic, onion, and tomatoes. If you can't find fresh tomatillos and chiles or they aren't in season, canned work just as well. Serve this recipe plain, wrapped in tortillas (page 210), or with some Mexican Cauliflower Rice (page 204). Like most slow-cooked foods, this dish is even better next day.

Prep Time: 15 minutes   **Cook Time:** 4 to 8 hours, depending on cooking method   **Yield:** 6 servings

4 pounds pork shoulder or butt, trimmed of fat and cut into 1½-inch cubes

1 teaspoon fine sea salt

1 teaspoon ground black pepper

2 tablespoons ghee (page 320), lard (page 322), or tallow (page 324)

1½ pounds tomatillos, husks removed, quartered

3 cups chicken stock (page 310)

3 poblano or Anaheim chiles (about ½ pound), seeded and chopped

3 cloves garlic, minced

2 yellow bell peppers, seeded and chopped

2 large tomatoes (about 1 pound), chopped (about 1½ cups), or 1 (14.5-ounce) can diced tomatoes

1 cup chopped white onion, plus more for garnish

1½ teaspoons ground cumin

1½ teaspoons ground coriander

¼ cup chopped fresh cilantro, for garnish (optional)

1. Season the pork pieces with the salt and pepper. Melt the ghee in a large skillet over medium-high heat. Add the pork pieces and cook for 5 minutes, or until browned on all sides. Remove the pork pieces from the pan and transfer to a slow cooker turned on low.

2. Place the quartered tomatillos and the chicken stock in a blender and blend for 1 minute. Pour the tomatillo sauce over the pork.

3. Add the remaining ingredients, except the cilantro, to the slow cooker and cook on low for 6 to 8 hours or on high for 4 hours. Taste and add additional salt and pepper if desired.

4. To serve, transfer to bowls and top with a sprinkle of chopped fresh cilantro, if desired, and chopped onion.

TRY THIS!
For extra spice, try adding 1 tablespoon dried oregano and 2 jalapeños, seeded and finely chopped.

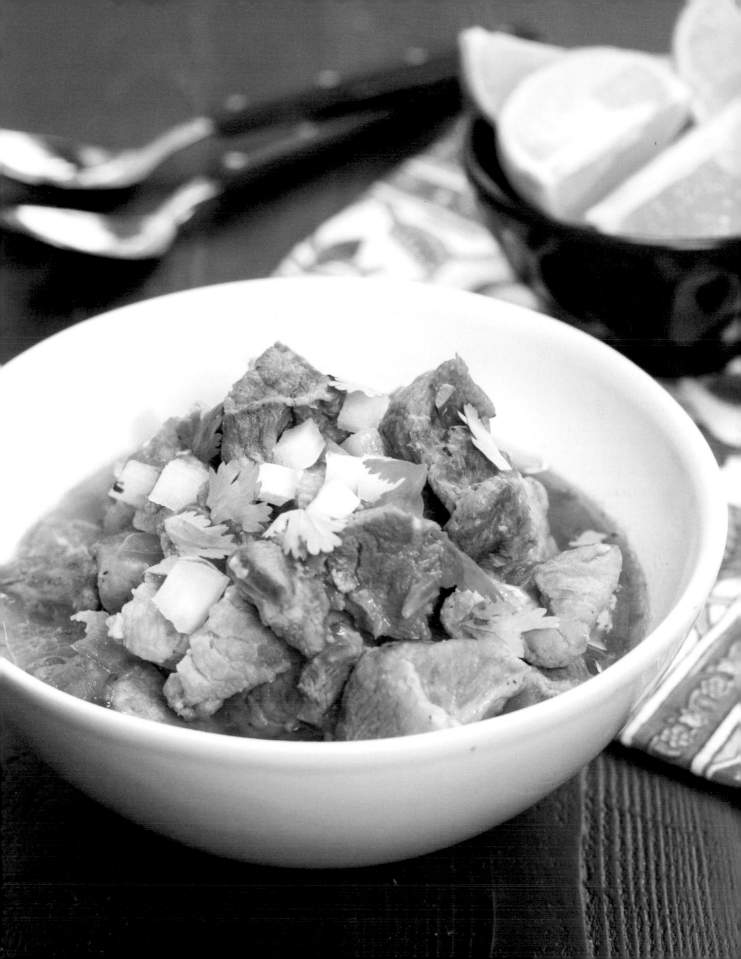

PORK RAGOUT

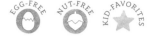

EGG-FREE   NUT-FREE   KID-FAVORITES

This is a great make-ahead dish, and it also freezes and reheats well. This pork ragout is bursting with Italian flavors, can be cooked on the stovetop or in a slow cooker, and is great served over Mashed Sweet Potatoes (page 189) or Pasta (page 194).

Prep Time: 15 minutes   **Cook Time:** 1 hour 45 minutes or 6 hours, depending on cooking method
Yield: 4 to 6 servings

2 pounds boneless pork shoulder, trimmed of excess fat and cut into 1-inch cubes

1 teaspoon fine sea salt

½ teaspoon ground black pepper

3 tablespoons ghee (page 320), lard (page 322), or tallow (page 324)

1 large onion, chopped (about 1 cup)

1 medium carrot, peeled and chopped (about ½ cup)

2 cloves garlic, minced

1 teaspoon dried thyme

1 teaspoon dried basil

1 teaspoon dried rosemary

6 tablespoons tomato paste

6 large Roma tomatoes (about 1½ pounds), chopped (about 3 cups)

1 cup chicken stock (page 310)

3 tablespoons chopped fresh flat-leaf parsley, for garnish (optional)

1 batch Mashed Sweet Potatoes (page 189) or Pasta (page 194), for serving (omit for nut-free)

1. Season the pork with the salt and pepper. Melt the ghee in a large Dutch oven over medium-high heat, then add the pork and cook for 2 minutes per side, or until browned on all sides.

2. Add the onion, carrot, garlic, thyme, basil, and rosemary to the pan and cook for another 3 minutes, stirring frequently. Add the tomato paste and stir to combine, then add the tomatoes and chicken stock and stir again.

3. **To use the stovetop:** Bring just to a boil, then reduce the heat to low, cover, and simmer for 1 hour. Remove the lid and cook for another 30 minutes, or until the sauce has thickened and the pork is tender.

   To use the slow cooker: Transfer to a slow cooker and cook on low for 6 hours.

4. Taste and add additional salt and pepper if desired. Sprinkle with fresh parsley, if desired, and serve over the mashed sweet potatoes or pasta.

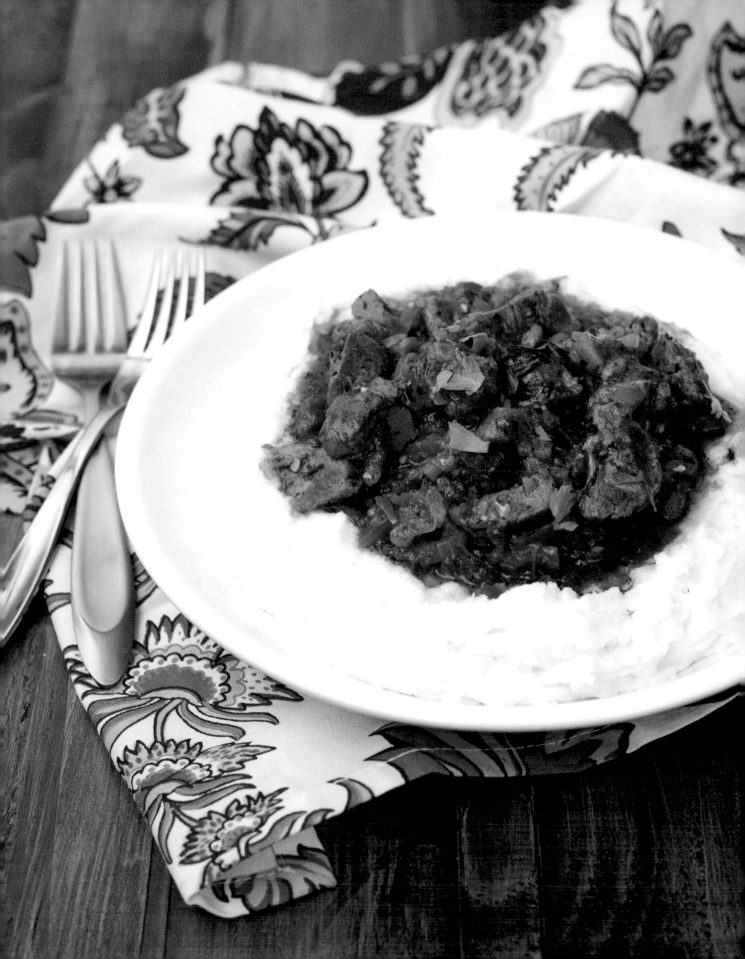

PORK
VINDALOO

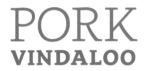

Sometimes you whip up something so good that it makes you want to do a victory lap around the block. For me, this is one of those meals. The combined scents of slow-cooked pork, ginger, garlic, turmeric, vinegar, and honey hitting your nose makes it very hard not to drool while making this dish, so feel free to take the necessary precautions and wear a bib while cooking.

Prep Time: 10 minutes   **Cook Time:** 1 hour 30 minutes   **Yield:** 4 servings

FOR THE SAUCE

1 cup lard (page 322) or tallow (page 324)

2 medium onions, finely sliced (about 2 cups)

4 cloves garlic

1 (1-inch) piece fresh ginger, peeled and chopped

5 tablespoons apple cider vinegar

1 tablespoon ground coriander

2 teaspoons ground cumin

2 teaspoons raw honey

1½ teaspoons fine sea salt

1 teaspoon ground black pepper

1 teaspoon ground cardamom

1 teaspoon turmeric

½ teaspoon dry yellow mustard

½ teaspoon crushed red pepper

2 pounds pork butt, trimmed of excess fat and cut into ¾-inch cubes

1 cup chicken stock (page 310)

2 tablespoons chopped fresh cilantro, for garnish (optional)

1. Heat the lard in a large sauté pan over high heat for 3 minutes. Add the onions and fry until they are slightly crispy and light gold, about 10 minutes. Remove the onions with a slotted spoon and place on a paper towel–lined plate to drain. Keep the fat in the pan and turn the heat to low.

2. Place the cooked onions into a blender or food processor. Add the remaining sauce ingredients and blend until a thin paste forms.

3. Using the same pan that was used to cook the onions, turn the heat to medium-high and brown the pork cubes in batches, making sure to sear on all sides. Remove with a slotted spoon and set aside on a plate. Drain any excess fat from the pan, keeping enough to thinly coat the bottom of the pan. Reduce the heat to medium and add the onion paste. Cook, stirring constantly, for 1 minute.

4. Add the chicken stock to the pan, whisking to combine. Add the pork pieces back to the pan and bring just to a boil, then reduce the heat to low and cover. Simmer for 1 hour, or until the pork is tender. Top with chopped cilantro, if desired, to serve.

TRY THIS!
This pork is even better the next day, and when reheated with some scrambled eggs it makes for an amazingly savory and filling breakfast.

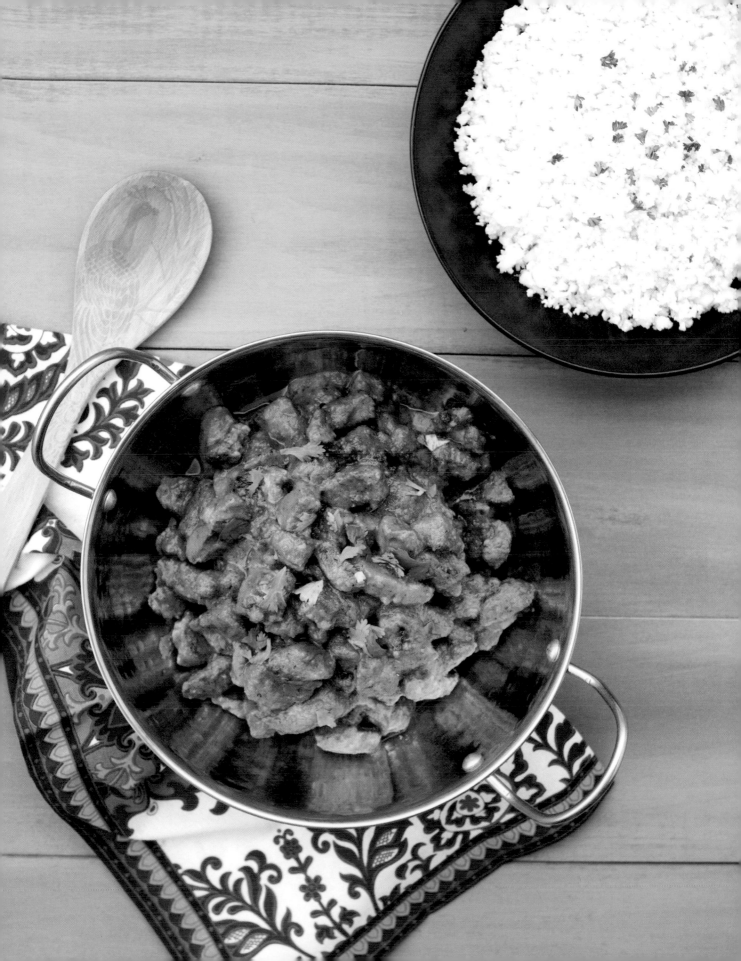

PIZZA STUFFED MUSHROOMS

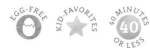

Anytime my mother tries out a new recipe while visiting me, she always starts by threatening to order pizza if it doesn't turn out well. Never once in eighteen years has she had to order pizza, and we avoid takeout pizza anyway now that we follow a Paleo diet, but she still makes the threat with each new dish she attempts. I'd miss pizza more, but luckily these mushrooms help satisfy any cravings. Spices like oregano and thyme give the pork-based sauce a traditional Italian flavor, while toppings like tomatoes, olives, and fresh basil finish off the true pizza experience.

Prep Time: 10 minutes **Cook Time:** 30 minutes **Yield:** 12 mushrooms (about 4 servings)

12 cremini or white mushrooms (about 1½ pounds), washed and dried, stems removed

1 cup tomato sauce

½ teaspoon fine sea salt, divided

½ teaspoon ground black pepper, divided

½ teaspoon dried oregano

½ teaspoon dried thyme

2 tablespoons ghee (page 320), lard (page 322), or tallow (page 324)

¼ cup finely chopped red onion (about ½ small)

1 tablespoon minced fresh garlic

½ pound pork sausage

2 tablespoons almond flour (page 316)

¼ cup sliced black olives

6 cherry tomatoes, halved

3 tablespoons thinly sliced fresh basil

1. Preheat the oven to 375°F. Line a 9-by-13-inch baking sheet with parchment paper or a baking mat. Place the mushrooms bottom side up on the baking sheet, leaving some space between them.

2. In a small saucepan over medium-high heat, combine the tomato sauce, ¼ teaspoon of the salt, ¼ teaspoon of the pepper, the oregano, and the thyme. Bring just to a boil, then reduce the heat to low and simmer for 10 minutes, uncovered.

3. While the sauce is simmering, heat the ghee in a medium skillet over medium-high heat. Add the onion and garlic and sauté for 2 minutes. Add the pork sausage and cook for 3 minutes, breaking the meat apart as you stir. Add the almond flour, remaining ¼ teaspoon of salt, and remaining ¼ teaspoon of pepper and stir, then add half of the tomato sauce mixture from the saucepan and stir again until well combined. Remove from the heat and spoon the mixture into the mushroom caps.

4. Place the stuffed mushrooms in the oven and bake for 20 minutes, or until the meat mixture is cooked through and the mushrooms have started to brown. Remove from the oven and top each mushroom with a dollop of sauce, sliced olives, cherry tomatoes, and finally a sprinkle of fresh basil. Serve right away.

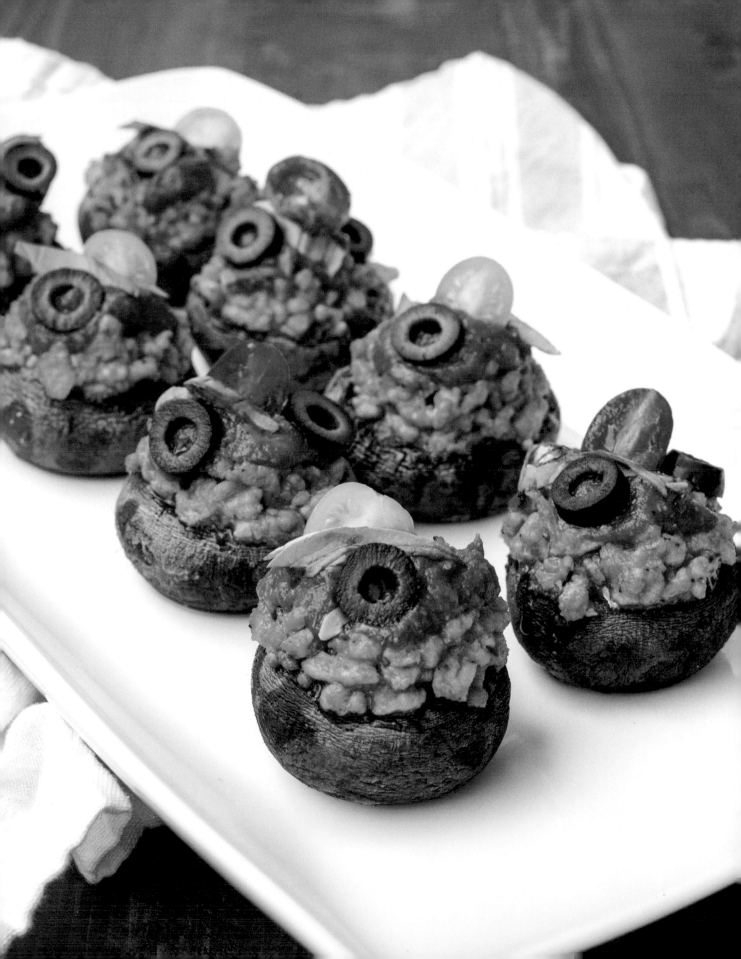

SLOW COOKER
PORK RIBS

EGG-FREE · NUT-FREE · KID-FAVORITES

Sometimes you crave ribs but don't have the time to sit near a grill or oven for hours, and that's when these slow cooker ribs step up and wave their hand. Leave them in the slow cooker to cook most of the way through and serve as is, or finish them off in the oven, bathed in a tasty barbecue sauce. I like to serve these with a side of Creamy Coleslaw (page 188).

Prep Time: 15 minutes · **Cook Time:** 5 or 8 hours, depending on cooking method · **Yield:** 4 servings

3 pounds baby back ribs, membrane removed

½ teaspoon fine sea salt

½ teaspoon ground black pepper

½ teaspoon garlic powder

½ teaspoon paprika

½ cup chicken stock (page 310)

1 small onion, sliced

1 cup BBQ Sauce (page 272)

1. Rinse the ribs and pat dry. Mix together the salt, pepper, garlic powder, and paprika in a small bowl. Rub the spice mixture over the meaty side of the ribs, making sure to massage it into the meat. Slice the ribs between the bones.

2. Pour the chicken stock into the slow cooker and add the ribs so that they are standing upright (one end touching the bottom of the slow cooker and one pointing up). Top the ribs with the sliced onion. Cover and cook on high for 4 to 5 hours or low for 7 to 8 hours, then discard the onion.

3. Preheat the oven to 400°F and line a 9-by-13-inch baking sheet with parchment paper or a baking mat.

4. Place the ribs on the prepared baking sheet, baste with the barbecue sauce, and cook for 10 minutes, or until they begin to get crispy.

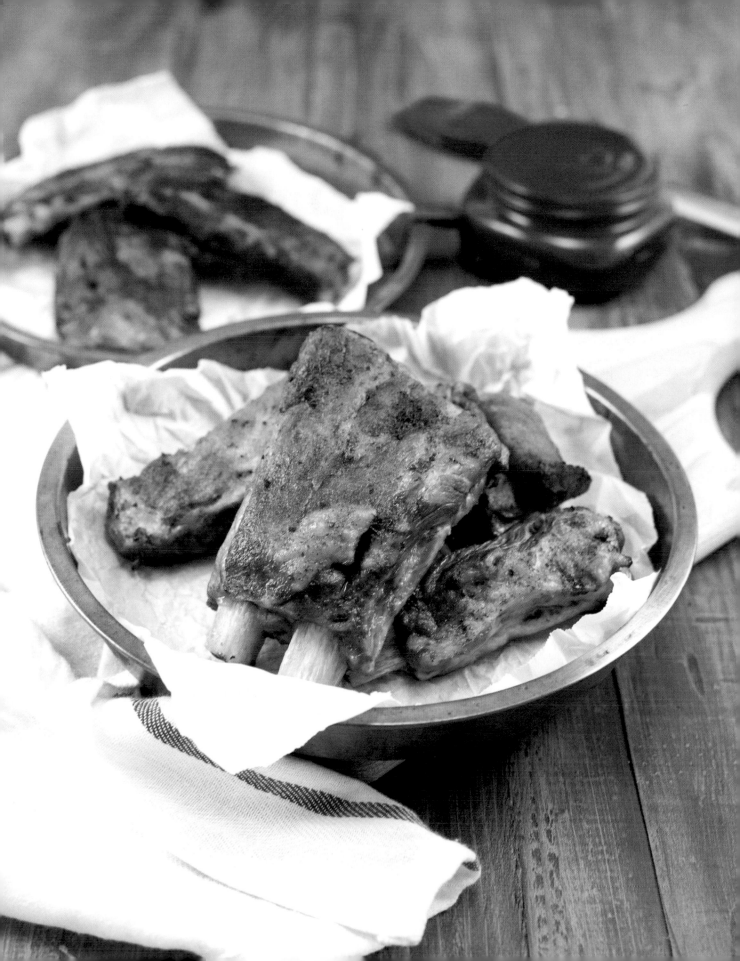

SWEET and SOUR PORK

EGG-FREE · NUT-FREE · KID-FAVORITES · 40 MINUTES OR LESS

Cubed pork sautéed with vegetables and covered in a mouthwatering sweet and sour sauce, that's what I'm talking about! This recipe is kid- and adult-friendly, and you can adjust the sauce to just how you like it. To increase the sweetness, add another teaspoon or two of honey. To increase the sour flavor, add a little more vinegar. If you like a little heat, add a couple dashes of crushed red pepper to the sauce at the same time as the tomato sauce. Try serving with a side of Seasoned Cauliflower Rice (page 200) or Fried Cauliflower Rice (page 202).

Prep Time: 10 minutes   **Cook Time:** 30 minutes   **Yield:** 4 to 6 servings

FOR THE SAUCE

¾ cup chicken stock (page 310)

2 tablespoons tapioca flour

¼ teaspoon fine sea salt

⅓ cup raw honey

¼ cup plus 2 tablespoons apple cider vinegar

¼ cup tomato sauce

⅓ cup pineapple juice

3 tablespoons ghee (page 320), lard (page 322), or tallow (page 324), divided

2 medium green bell peppers, cut into 1-inch pieces

1 medium red bell pepper, cut into 1-inch pieces

1 small onion, cut into 1-inch pieces

2 pounds pork butt, trimmed of excess fat and cut into ¾-inch cubes

1 teaspoon fine sea salt

½ teaspoon ground black pepper

3 tablespoons chopped green onion, for garnish (optional)

1. Make the sauce: Whisk together the stock and tapioca flour in a small bowl and set aside. Place the salt, honey, vinegar, tomato sauce, and pineapple juice in a small saucepan over medium-high heat and whisk to combine. Once the sauce reaches a light simmer, add the tapioca flour mixture and whisk once more. Bring just to a boil, then reduce the heat to low and simmer for 3 minutes, stirring occasionally. Taste and adjust the seasonings as desired. Remove from the heat and set aside.

2. Heat 1 tablespoon of ghee in a large skillet over medium heat. Add the bell peppers and onion to the pan and cook for 3 minutes, or until just tender. Use a slotted spoon to transfer the bell peppers and onions to a bowl.

3. Season the pork with the salt and pepper. Melt the remaining 2 tablespoons of ghee in the skillet used for the vegetables and add the pork. Sauté for 10 minutes, or until the pork is evenly browned on all sides and cooked through. Drain any liquid from the pan, then add the sauce to the pan and cook for another 2 minutes, tossing to coat the pork.

4. Remove the pan from the heat, add the bell pepper and onion mixture back to the pan, and toss to combine. Transfer to a serving platter, sprinkle with the chopped green onion, if desired, and serve.

TRY THIS!

Try adding 1 cup of pineapple chunks during the last 2 minutes of cooking, when you add the sauce back to the pan. Keep in mind that the pineapple chunks will add more sweetness to the dish, so you may want to cut the honey in the sauce down to 2 or 3 tablespoons.

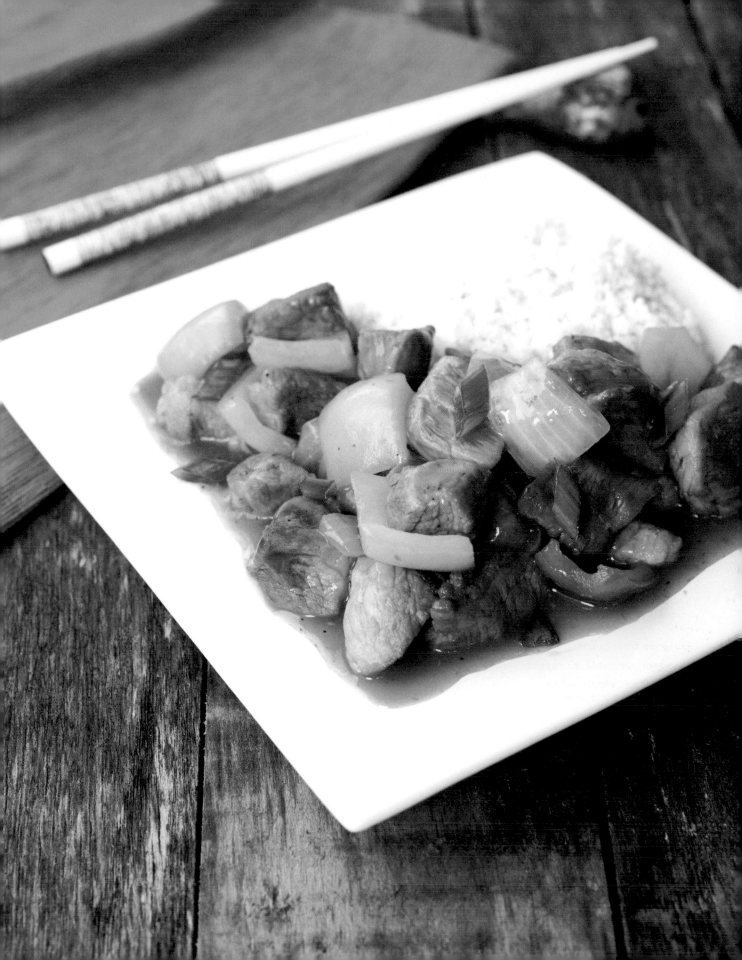

TEX-MEX STYLE
PORK CHOPS

Tex-Mex, as the name hints, is a Texan version of Mexican food that over time has become its own regional cuisine. The predominant ingredients are garlic, chili powder, and cumin, which make for a fantastic flavor combination when mixed with tomatoes and green chiles. This pork chop recipe uses those ingredients in a tasty sauce that is slathered over juicy chops. Serve it with a simple side salad or roasted vegetables, and you have yourself a meal that is great for weeknights or weekends.

Prep Time: 10 minutes   **Cook Time:** 25 minutes   **Yield:** 4 servings

1 teaspoon fine sea salt

1 teaspoon chili powder

½ teaspoon paprika

½ teaspoon ground cumin

¼ teaspoon ground black pepper

4 bone-in pork chops, ¾ inch thick (3 to 4 pounds)

2 tablespoons extra-virgin olive oil

1 tablespoon ghee (page 320), lard (page 322), or tallow (page 324)

1 small onion, sliced (about ¾ cup)

3 cloves garlic, minced

1 (4-ounce) can diced mild green chiles

1 (8-ounce) can tomato sauce

2 medium tomatoes (about ⅔ pound), chopped (about 1¼ cups)

3 tablespoons chopped fresh cilantro, for garnish (optional)

1. Mix together the salt, chili powder, paprika, cumin, and pepper in a small bowl. Pat the chops dry with a paper towel and coat with the olive oil on all sides, then sprinkle half of the spice mixture over the chops. Set aside.

2. Melt the ghee in a medium saucepan over medium-high heat. Add the onion slices and cook for 4 minutes, then add the garlic and cook for another minute. Add the green chiles, tomato sauce, tomatoes, and the remaining half of the spice mixture, stir, and bring to a boil. Reduce the heat to low and simmer for 13 to 15 minutes, uncovered, while you cook the pork chops.

3. **To use a grill:** Preheat the grill to medium heat. Place the chops on the grill and cook for 3 to 4 minutes on each side, until almost cooked through.

   To use an oven: Place an oven rack in the middle position. Place a large cast-iron skillet in the cold oven, then preheat the oven to 400°F. Once the oven has reached 400°F, turn the stove vent on and turn the stove on to medium-high heat. Carefully transfer the hot skillet to the stove. Add the pork chops to the pan and sear for 2 minutes, then flip and sear on the other side for another 2 minutes. Flip once more, then return the pan to the oven. Cook the chops for 6 minutes, or until the internal temperature reaches 145°F or the juices run clear when the chops are stuck with a knife and the center has only a faint pink tint.

4. Transfer the cooked pork chops to a plate, loosely tent with foil, and let rest for 5 minutes. To serve, pour the sauce onto a serving platter, place the pork chops on top, and sprinkle with cilantro, if desired.

TRY THIS!

Pork chops are delicious if cooked correctly, but they're easy to overcook and dry out. If you have the time, I recommend brining your pork chops before cooking them, even if it's just for 30 minutes. There's some science at play here, but basically the salt in the brine is your buddy that is going to help make sure you have a juicy pork chop (and before you ask, no, it doesn't make them taste salty). To make a simple brine, place 1 cup of water in a small saucepan and bring to a boil. Add 2½ tablespoons of fine sea salt and stir to dissolve. Add 5 black peppercorns and 1 bay leaf, then stir in 2 cups of cold water. Place the pork chops in a shallow dish and pour the brine over the chops to cover, adding a little more cold water if needed. Cover and place in the refrigerator for at least 30 minutes and up to 3 hours.

> **KITCHEN TIP**
> The oven method described here is also a great way to cook steak indoors. You may need to increase or decrease the cooking time depending on the thickness of the steak and how you like it cooked.

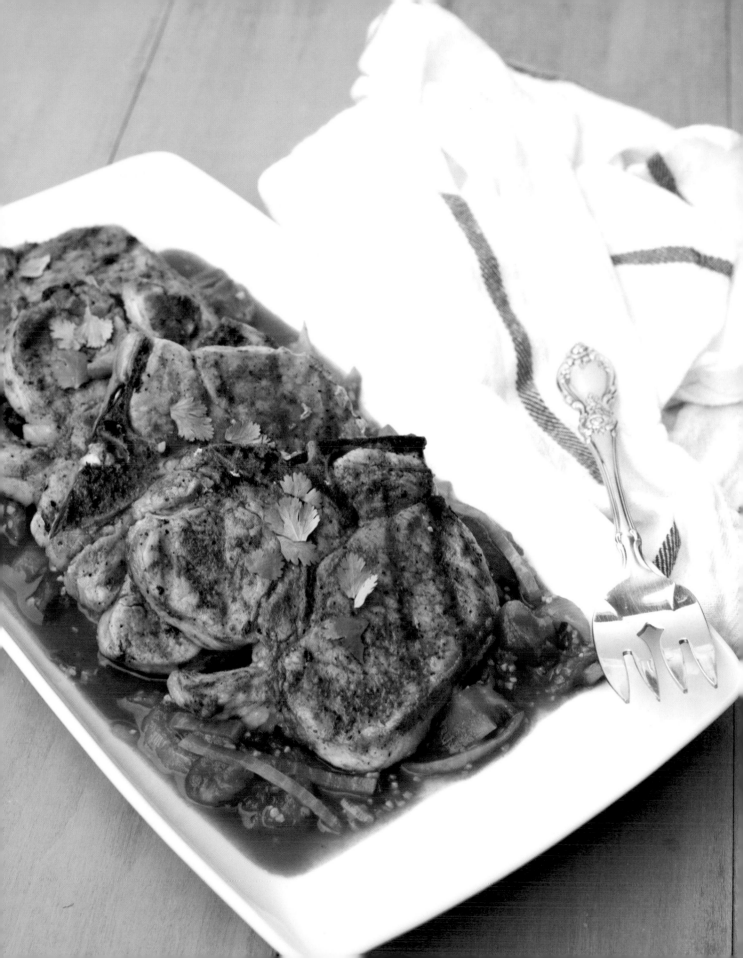

TUSCAN PORK ROAST

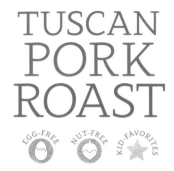

EGG-FREE · NUT-FREE · KID-FAVORITES

This roast recipe highlights fresh herbs, garlic, and lemon, and it's perfect for everything from a dinner party to a simple family meal on the weekend. Once you have the roast in the oven, there's very little to do for a while, which gives you time to cook a side dish, clean your kitchen, or pour a glass of wine and pat yourself on the back for making it through the day and having food in the oven.

Tying the roast with butcher string helps ensure the meat stays round while cooking. You can either tie it yourself, placing the ties about 2 inches apart, or ask someone at the meat counter to wrap it for you. Some roasts come pre-tied, which is even easier.

Prep Time: 10 minutes   **Cook Time:** 1 hour 25 minutes   **Yield:** 4 to 6 servings

6 cloves garlic, minced

2 tablespoons chopped fresh flat-leaf parsley, plus more for garnish (optional)

1 tablespoon fresh rosemary leaves

1 tablespoon chopped fresh sage leaves

2 tablespoons extra-virgin olive oil

1 teaspoon finely grated lemon zest

½ teaspoon fine sea salt

½ teaspoon ground black pepper

1 (3-pound) boneless pork loin roast, tied with butcher string

1¼ cups chicken stock (page 310)

2 tablespoons ghee (page 320), lard (page 322), or tallow (page 324)

2 lemons, sliced, for serving

1. Preheat the oven to 350°F.

2. Combine the garlic, parsley, rosemary, sage, olive oil, lemon zest, salt, and pepper, in a food processor or blender and puree for 30 seconds, or until a paste forms.

3. Use the tip of a small knife to pierce the pork in about 10 different places. Rub the paste over the entire outside of the roast, making sure it gets into the cuts. Place the roast in a 10-by-14-inch roasting pan and cook for 30 minutes, then flip the roast over to brown on the other side. Cook for another 45 minutes, or until a meat thermometer inserted into the middle of the meat registers 145°F or the juices run clear when the roast is stuck with a knife and the center has only a faint pink tint. Remove the roast from the pan and set on a cutting board to rest while you make the sauce.

4. Place the roasting pan over medium-high heat. Add the stock to the pan and stir to loosen any bits from the bottom of the pan. Cook for 5 minutes, or until the sauce has reduced by about half. Add the ghee and melt it into the sauce, stirring to combine. Taste and add salt and pepper if desired.

5. Remove the string from the roast and slice. Place on a serving platter, pour the sauce over the meat, sprinkle with parsley, if desired, and serve with lemon slices.

TRY THIS!

For even more flavor and to save yourself some prep time later on, you can rub the paste over the roast and place it in a sealed container in the refrigerator for 8 hours, or until ready to cook. Remove the roast from the refrigerator 15 minutes before you want to stick it in the oven.

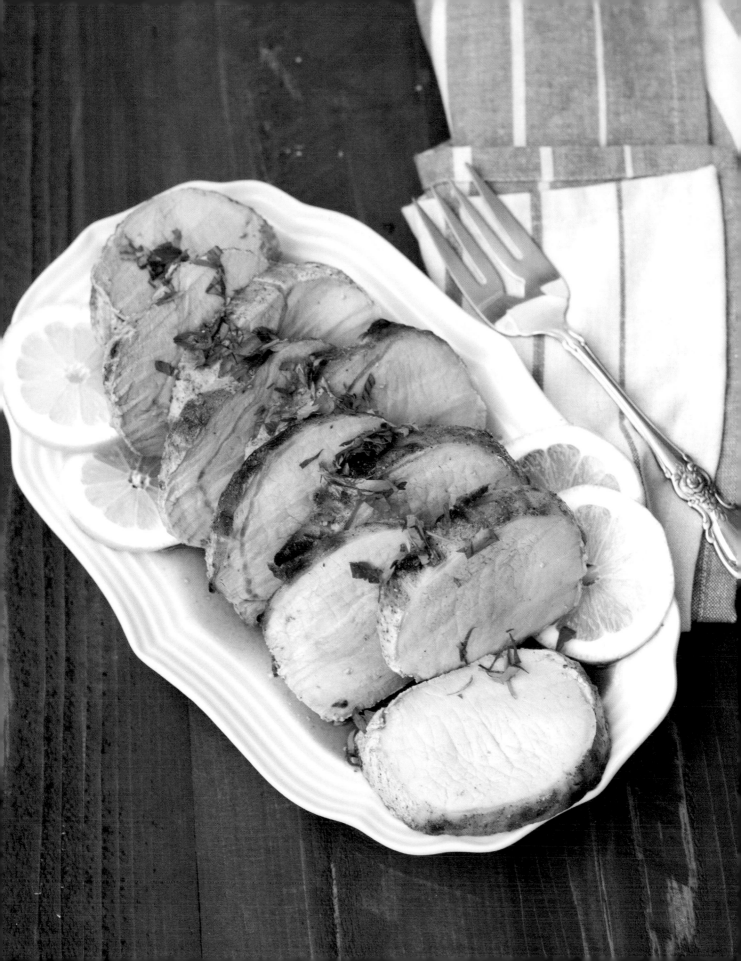

PORK
SCHNITZEL

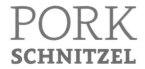
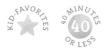

I like this recipe for two reasons. The first is that my family has been making schnitzel my entire life, and it is one of my easy, go-to comfort foods. The second reason is that I get to use a meat tenderizer and beat the pork chops, which can be very therapeutic after a bad day at the office. Not much more than salt and pepper is needed for this dish, and a squeeze of fresh lemon juice right before eating rounds out this simple recipe. Serve with your favorite vegetables or a leafy green salad.

Prep Time: 10 minutes   **Cook Time:** 15 minutes   **Yield:** 4 servings

1½ pounds boneless pork loin chops

¼ cup tapioca flour

1½ cups almond flour (page 316)

1 teaspoon fine sea salt

¼ teaspoon ground black pepper

2 large eggs

1 cup lard (page 322) or tallow (page 324), for frying

3 tablespoons chopped fresh parsley, for garnish (optional)

2 lemons, sliced, for serving

1. Pat the pork chops dry with paper towels, place between two sheets of parchment paper or plastic wrap, and pound to ¼ inch thick.

2. Mix the tapioca flour, almond flour, salt, and pepper together in a shallow bowl or dish. Whisk the eggs in a separate shallow bowl or dish. Dip each chop fully into the eggs and then into the flour mixture, gently shaking off any excess. Place the coated chops on a wire cooling rack or a piece of parchment paper and set aside.

3. Melt the lard in a large skillet over medium-high heat. Once it reaches 350°F or the melted fat bubbles around the handle of a wooden spoon dipped into the pan, place the chops gently in the pan, working in batches if needed. Fry for 2 minutes on each side, or until golden brown and cooked through. Transfer to a paper towel–lined plate to drain.

4. Place the chops on a serving platter, top with chopped fresh parsley, if desired, and serve with lemon slices.

KITCHEN TIP

Pounding boneless meat like chicken breasts and pork chops allows it to cook quickly and evenly. If you don't have a meat tenderizer, use a rolling pin or small, heavy pan to pound the meat.

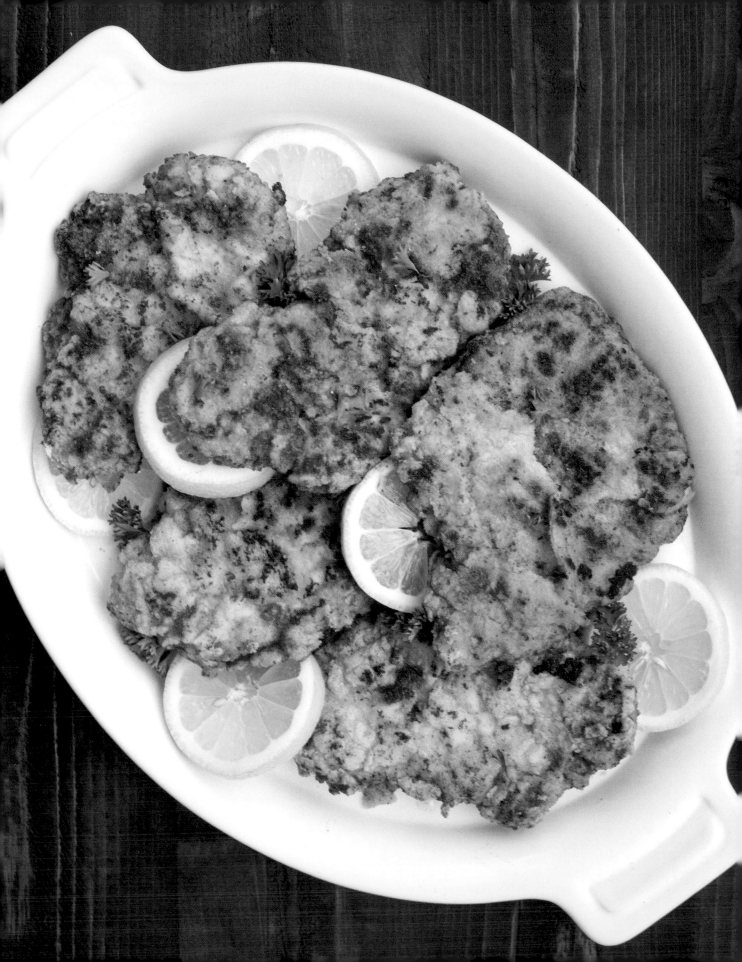

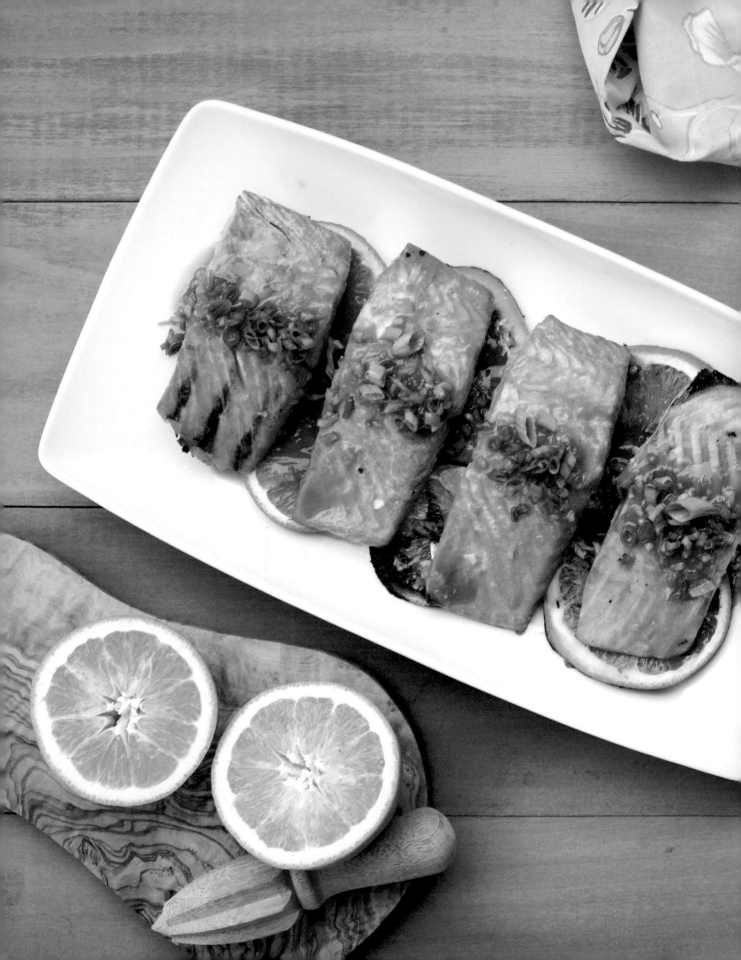

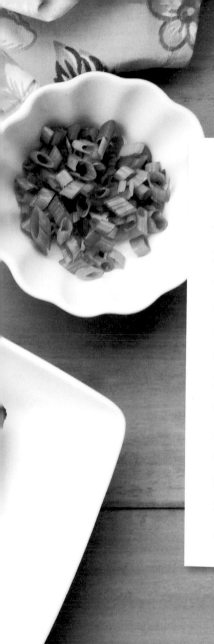

seafood

BLT SCALLOPS *with* **HERB** MAYO

A skewered scallop with bacon, tomato, arugula, and a dollop of herb mayo is basically a perfect bite on a stick. Or maybe two bites if you have a small mouth or take dainty bites. I'm a sucker for anything with bacon on it, and bacon and scallops just beg to be together. These make a fun appetizer or party dish, and a slice of avocado works well if you want a quick but creamy substitute for the herb mayo.

Prep Time: 10 minutes   **Cook Time:** 10 minutes   **Yield:** 6 skewers (3 servings as an appetizer)

FOR THE HERB MAYO

¼ cup mayonnaise (page 278)

⅛ teaspoon ground black pepper

⅛ teaspoon garlic powder

⅛ teaspoon dried oregano

⅛ teaspoon dried thyme

⅛ teaspoon paprika

⅛ teaspoon celery seed

3 slices thick-cut bacon

6 large sea scallops (about ½ pound), patted dry with paper towels

¼ teaspoon ground black pepper

1 tablespoon ghee (page 320), lard (page 322), or tallow (page 324)

¼ cup baby arugula

1 small Roma tomato, cut into 6 slices

1. Make the herb mayo by mixing together all the ingredients in a small bowl. Place in the refrigerator until ready to use.

2. In a large skillet over medium-high heat, cook the bacon until crispy. Place the bacon on a paper towel–lined plate to drain, keeping the drippings in the pan.

3. Sprinkle the scallops with the pepper and cook in the pan for 1 minute, then flip and cook for an additional minute. Melt the ghee in the pan and then add the herb mayo. Gently shake the pan to coat the scallops. Cook for another 30 seconds, then transfer the scallops to a cutting board. Rest for 1 minute, then slice each scallop in half.

4. Cut each cooked bacon strip into 4 pieces. To assemble the skewers, top a scallop half with a bit of arugula, a tomato slice, 2 pieces of bacon, a dollop of herb mayo, and then the other half of the scallop. Gently skewer with a toothpick and serve.

TRY THIS!

The herb mayonnaise in this recipe makes a great base for a chicken salad. Just double the amount to make ½ cup, and then mix with 2 cups cooked diced chicken, ½ cup chopped onion, and ¾ cup chopped celery.

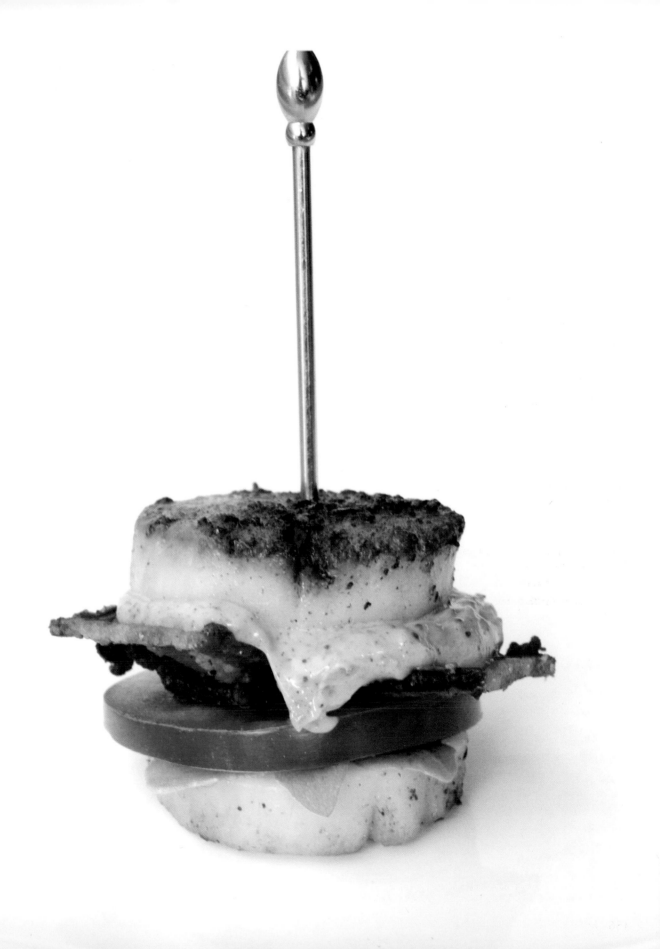

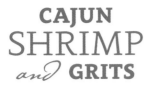

CAJUN SHRIMP and GRITS

EGG-FREE

The Paleo-friendly grits in this recipe are made from cauliflower, and they really do have the taste and texture of traditional grits. This recipe calls for a crumbled bacon topping, and if you cook the bacon ahead of time you can use any leftover strained drippings to cook the shrimp and grits. Mmm, extra bacon flavor!

Prep Time: 25 minutes   **Cook Time:** 35 minutes   **Yield:** 4 servings

FOR THE GRITS

1 medium head cauliflower (about 1 pound), cut into 1-inch pieces

1 tablespoon ghee (page 320), lard (page 322), or tallow (page 324)

½ small onion, finely chopped (about ¼ cup)

2½ cups chicken stock (page 310)

1¼ cups almond flour (page 316)

½ teaspoon fine sea salt

½ teaspoon ground black pepper

¼ teaspoon garlic powder

FOR THE SHRIMP

1 teaspoon paprika

½ teaspoon fine sea salt

½ teaspoon garlic powder

½ teaspoon dried oregano

½ teaspoon dried thyme

¼ teaspoon onion powder

⅛ teaspoon crushed red pepper

⅛ teaspoon cayenne pepper (optional)

1 pound large shrimp, peeled and deveined, tails removed

2 tablespoons ghee (page 320), lard (page 322), or tallow (page 324)

½ small onion, finely chopped (about ¼ cup)

2 cloves garlic, minced

1 tablespoon freshly squeezed lemon juice

4 slices thick-cut bacon, cooked and chopped, for garnish

3 tablespoons chopped fresh parsley, for garnish (optional)

1. Make the grits: Working in small batches, pulse the cauliflower pieces a few times in a food processor or blender, until the pieces are the size and shape of grains of rice, being careful not to overblend. Bigger pieces are better than smaller. Measure out 3 cups of riced cauliflower and store the remainder for another use in a sealed container in the refrigerator for up to 3 days.

2. Melt the ghee in a medium saucepan over medium-high heat. Add the onion and sauté for 3 minutes, then add the 3 cups of riced cauliflower and stir to combine. Add the chicken stock and bring just to a boil, then add the almond flour, salt, pepper, and garlic powder and stir until well combined.

3. Cover the pan, turn the heat to low, and simmer for 20 minutes, stirring occasionally. Check the consistency after about 15 minutes. If grits are too thin for your liking, add another ¼ cup of almond flour; if they're too thick, add another ¼ cup of stock. Once they have reached your desired consistency, remove from the heat. Taste and add more salt and pepper if desired, then cover to keep warm while you cook the shrimp.

4. Make the shrimp: In a medium-sized mixing bowl, combine the paprika, salt, garlic powder, oregano, thyme, onion powder, crushed red pepper, and cayenne (if using). Add the shrimp to the bowl and toss to coat.

5. Melt the ghee in a large skillet over medium heat. Add the shrimp, onion, and garlic to the pan and cook for 3 minutes, or until the shrimp turns pink. Add the lemon juice to the pan and sauté for another 3 minutes. Remove from the heat.

6. To serve, place a scoop of the grits in a bowl and top with a serving of shrimp. Garnish with crumbled bacon and a sprinkle of parsley, if desired.

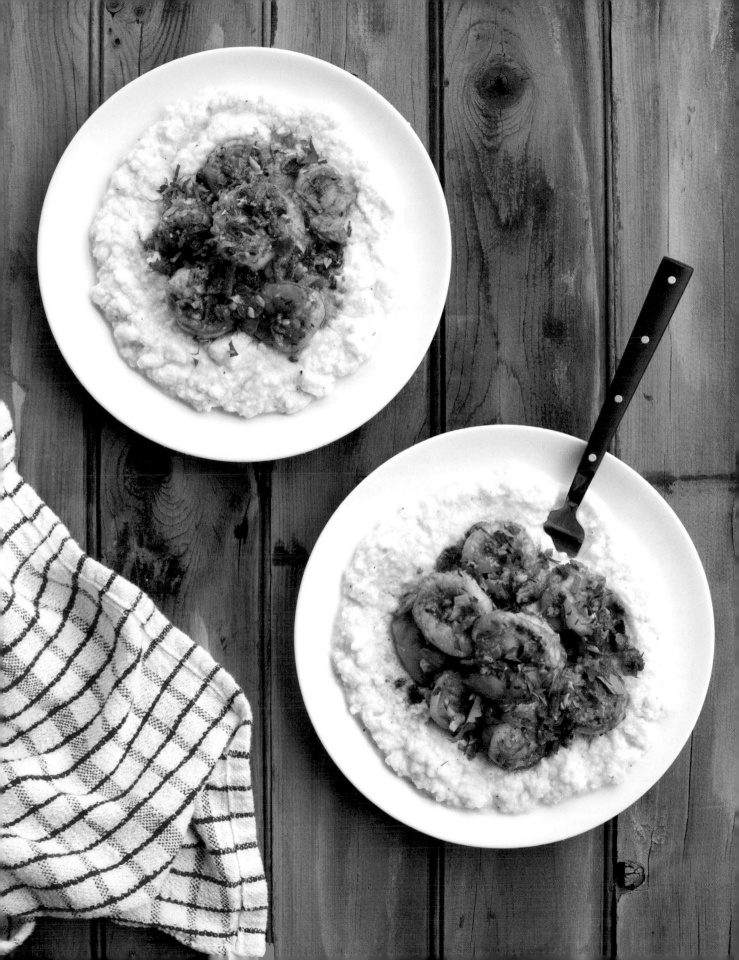

CALAMARI FRITTI *with* TOMATO BASIL DIPPING SAUCE

In Rome, there are gentlemen dressed as gladiators who stand outside the Colosseum. Being a proper tourist, I decided to get my picture taken with one. The fellow decided to be funny and grab my bum right as the picture was being taken, which caused me to scream so loudly that he scurried off in embarrassment. I grabbed my camera and stomped away, but as I was huffing and puffing along, I came across a small restaurant right across from a beautiful old church. I stepped inside and proceeded to try calamari fritti for the first time, and I was hooked. If it hadn't been for that fellow and his wandering hands, it may have taken me years to try this great dish, and that would have been a very sad thing indeed.

Prep Time: 10 minutes   **Cook Time:** 25 minutes   **Yield:** 4 to 6 servings

FOR THE TOMATO BASIL SAUCE

½ tablespoon ghee (page 320), lard (page 322), or tallow (page 324)

1 clove garlic, minced

1 (8-ounce) can crushed tomatoes

¼ teaspoon raw honey

Dash of fine sea salt

Dash of dried oregano

2 fresh basil leaves, chopped

½ cup almond milk (page 318)

1 large egg

½ pound squid, cleaned and cut into ½-inch-thick rings

2 cups almond flour (page 316)

1 cup tapioca flour

1 teaspoon paprika

½ teaspoon fine sea salt

½ teaspoon ground black pepper

Lard (page 322) or tallow (page 324), for frying

1 lemon, quartered, for serving

1. Make the sauce: Melt the ghee in a medium-sized saucepan over medium heat. Add the garlic and cook for 2 minutes, or until soft. Add the crushed tomatoes, honey, salt, and oregano and bring to a boil. Reduce the heat to low and simmer for 10 minutes, stirring occasionally. Add the fresh basil and stir to combine. Remove from the heat and cover until ready to serve.

2. While the sauce is simmering, prepare the calamari: In a medium-sized mixing bowl, whisk together the almond milk and egg until just combined. Add the squid rings to the bowl and place in the refrigerator for 10 minutes. Meanwhile, mix together the almond flour, tapioca flour, paprika, salt, and pepper in another medium-sized mixing bowl and set aside.

3. Fill a large skillet with enough lard to reach 1½ inches up the side of the pan. Place over medium-high heat and heat the lard to 350°F, or until the melted fat bubbles around the handle of a wooden spoon dipped into the pan.

4. Remove the soaking squid from the refrigerator. Working in batches, toss pieces of the wet squid into the flour mixture to coat. Carefully add the squid to the pan and fry until crisp and a light golden color, about 1 to 2 minutes per batch. Using a slotted spoon, transfer the calamari to a paper towel–lined plate to drain. Serve with the lemon wedges and dipping sauce.

KITCHEN TIP

When tomatoes aren't in season, or if I am just making a quick sauce, I usually reach for jarred or canned tomatoes instead of fresh. Most store-bought canned tomatoes are made from fruit that hasn't fully ripened, so they are not as sweet as whole tomatoes, and you may notice that they taste slightly bitter or acidic. You can balance that out by adding a tiny bit of honey to your dish.

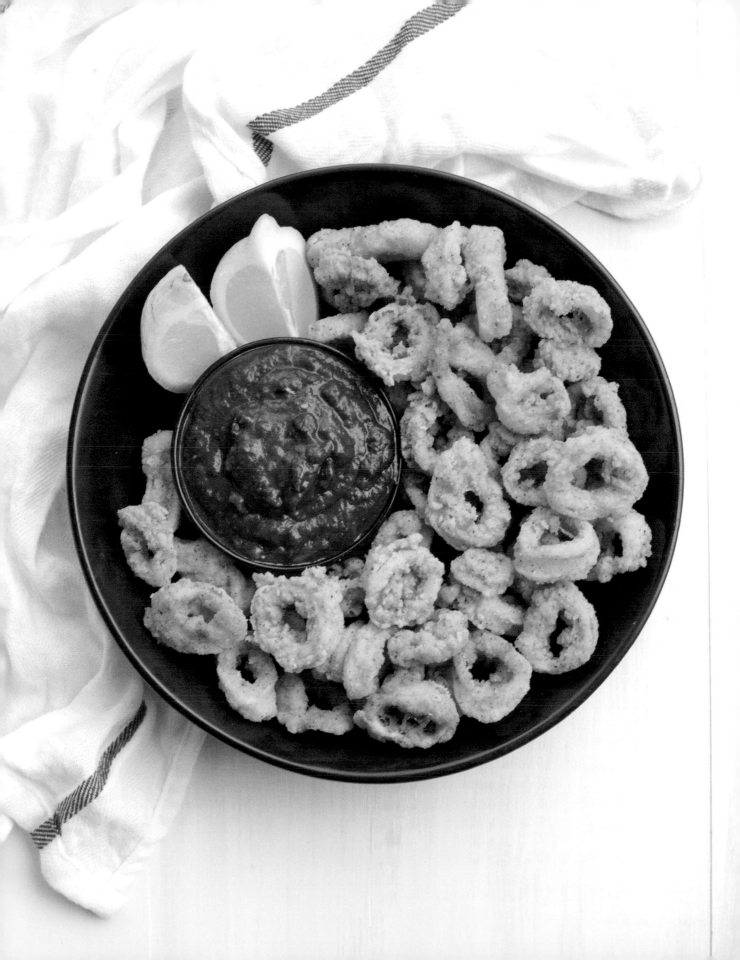

CHIPOTLE SHRIMP TACOS

I was born and raised in San Diego, California, so fish and shrimp tacos are a regular part of my food rotation, and anyone who comes to visit is forced to try them. Even the biggest skeptics are quickly asking for seconds. I serve mine on Paleo-friendly tortillas (page 210), but you can use fresh lettuce leaves or very thin slices of jicama instead.

Prep Time: 15 minutes, plus 30 minutes to marinate the shrimp   Cook Time: 10 minutes   Yield: 4 to 6 servings

FOR THE CREAMY LIME SAUCE

⅓ cup coconut milk (page 314)

1 tablespoon freshly squeezed lime juice

¼ teaspoon chipotle chili powder

¼ teaspoon fine sea salt

FOR THE SHRIMP

½ teaspoon chipotle chili powder

½ teaspoon ground cumin

½ teaspoon fine sea salt

½ pound medium shrimp, peeled and deveined, tails removed

1 tablespoon ghee (page 320), lard (page 322), or tallow (page 324)

SERVE WITH

1 batch Tortillas (page 210)

1 cup finely shredded red cabbage

1 ripe avocado, sliced

1 jalapeño, seeded and sliced (optional)

2 limes, quartered

1. Make the sauce: In a small bowl, whisk together the coconut milk, lime juice, chipotle chili powder, and salt. Place in the refrigerator until ready to use.

2. Make the shrimp: Combine the chipotle chili powder, cumin, and salt in a medium-sized mixing bowl. Add the shrimp and mix with your hands until the shrimp are fully coated in the spices. Cover and place in the refrigerator for 30 minutes or more. Now is a good time to prepare the tortillas and toppings for your tacos.

3. Melt the ghee in a large skillet over medium-high heat. Add the shrimp and cook for 2 minutes on each side, or until cooked through.

4. Assemble the tacos: Place an equal amount of shrimp on each tortilla. Top with the shredded cabbage, avocado slices, jalapeño slices (if using), and a drizzle of the chipotle lime sauce. Serve with the lime wedges.

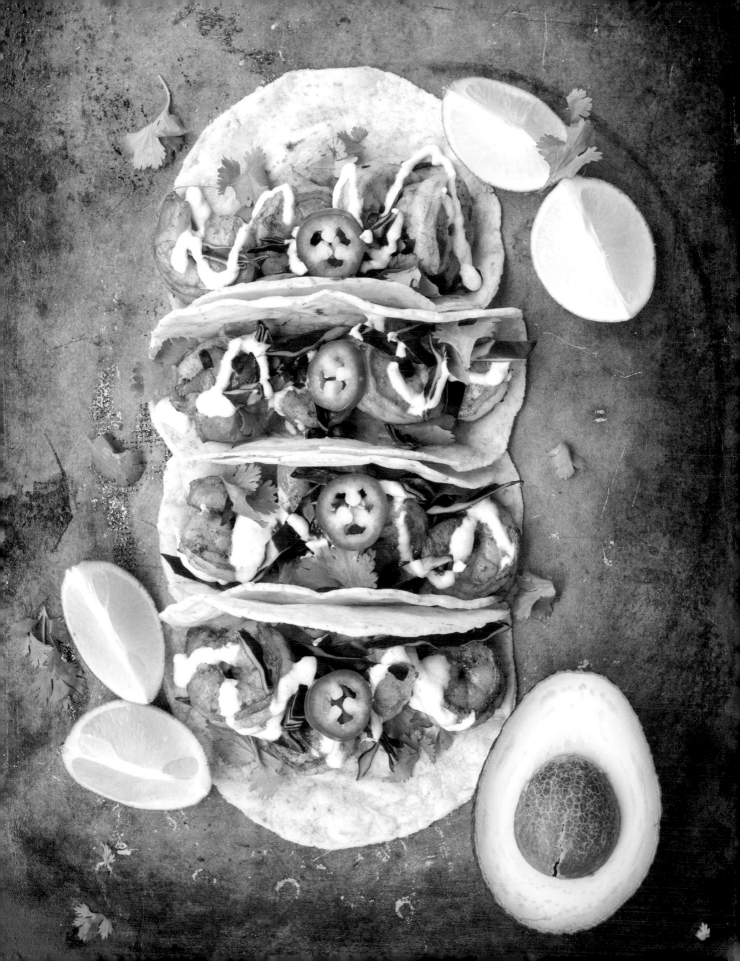

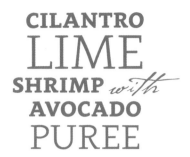

CILANTRO LIME SHRIMP *with* AVOCADO PUREE

EGG-FREE · NUT-FREE · 40 MINUTES OR LESS

These cilantro lime shrimp are so tasty that they flew off the plate the first time I served them. The avocado puree makes a nice dip when these shrimp are served as an appetizer, or you can make them without the dip for a main course.

Prep Time: 15 minutes, plus 10 minutes to marinate the shrimp   Cook Time: 6 minutes
Yield: 6 servings as an appetizer, 4 as a main dish

FOR THE AVOCADO PUREE

2 medium ripe avocados (about ½ pound), halved, pitted, and peeled

½ cup coconut cream (page 315)

1½ tablespoons freshly squeezed lime juice

¼ teaspoon fine sea salt

¼ teaspoon ground black pepper

¼ cup chopped fresh cilantro

½ teaspoon ground cumin

¼ teaspoon garlic powder

¼ teaspoon fine sea salt

¼ teaspoon ground black pepper

1½ tablespoons extra-virgin olive oil

1 pound large shrimp, peeled and deveined, tails on

2½ tablespoons freshly squeezed lime juice

1. Make the avocado puree: Place the avocados, coconut cream, lime juice, salt, and pepper in a blender or food processor and puree for 20 seconds, or until smooth. Place in the refrigerator until ready to use.

2. Combine the cilantro, cumin, garlic powder, salt, pepper, and olive oil in a medium-sized mixing bowl. Add the shrimp and toss to coat, then cover and allow the shrimp to marinate for 10 minutes in the refrigerator. While the shrimp marinates, soak 6 bamboo skewers in water and preheat the grill to medium-high heat.

3. Thread the shrimp onto the skewers and drizzle with the lime juice. Grill for 3 minutes on each side, or until the shrimp is cooked through.

4. Serve the shrimp on a platter with the avocado puree on the side for dipping.

TRY THIS!

Try adding one sliced and seeded jalapeño to the avocado puree before blending. Discarding the seeds from hot peppers reduces the heat a bit and allows the pepper flavor to shine.

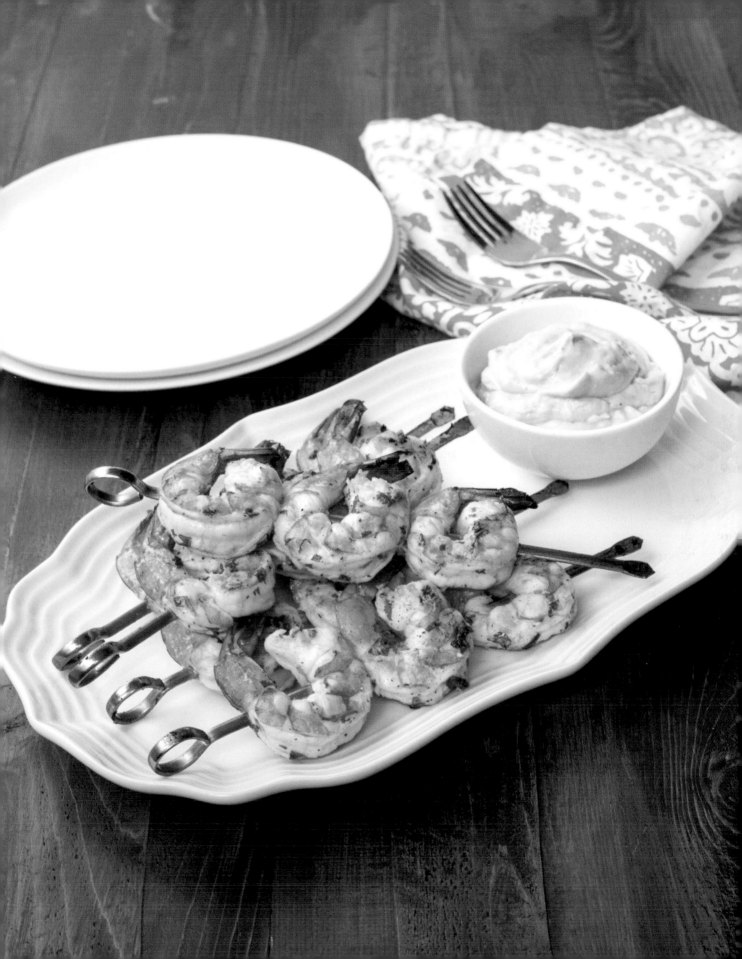

FISH & CHIPS

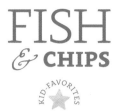

On one of my business trips to England I found myself in a coastal town called Aldeburgh, which the locals told me had the best fish and chips shop in the entire country. The foodie in me jumped for joy, and I waited in the long queue until it was my turn to get my fish and chips. I covered them in a good amount of malt vinegar, as I had seen everyone else do, but as soon as I walked out of the shop to enjoy them by the water, the skies opened up and it started to rain. Being the stubborn person that I am, I was not going to change my mission. I sat there on the rocky beach sheltering my meal with my jacket, getting absolutely soaking wet, and enjoyed every last bite. Nowadays fish and chips are an occasional indulgence around my house, and although I don't have a rocky beach to sit on or any authentic malt vinegar, I do keep tartar sauce (page 284) and ketchup (page 275) around for dipping.

Prep Time: 10 minutes, plus 40 minutes to make the potato wedges   **Cook Time:** 20 minutes   **Yield:** 4 servings

⅓ cup tapioca flour or arrowroot flour

⅔ cup almond flour (page 316), divided

¼ teaspoon fine sea salt

¼ teaspoon ground black pepper

2 large eggs, whisked

⅓ cup beef stock (page 310)

1 cup lard (page 322) or tallow (page 324), for frying

1½ pounds cod or halibut fillets, cut into 1½-inch-wide strips and patted dry with paper towels

1 batch Crispy Sweet Potato Wedges (page 190), for serving

2 lemons, quartered, for serving

1. Combine the tapioca flour, ⅓ cup of the almond flour, the salt, and the pepper in a large mixing bowl and stir to combine. Add the whisked eggs and mix, then add the beef stock and stir until a batter forms. Place the remaining ⅓ cup almond flour in a shallow bowl and set it next to the batter.

2. Heat the lard in a medium-sized skillet over medium-high heat until it reaches 375°F, or until the melted fat bubbles around the handle of a wooden spoon dipped into the pan. Working in batches, dip the fish strips lightly in the almond flour on each side to coat, then fully immerse in the batter. Gently place the battered pieces in the hot lard, making sure they are not touching each other. Fry for 2 to 3 minutes, then turn and fry for another 2 to 3 minutes, or until golden brown and cooked through. Transfer to a paper towel–lined plate to drain.

3. Serve with the sweet potato wedges and fresh lemon.

KITCHEN TIP

To keep the sweet potato wedges warm while you make the fish, place them in a 200°F oven.

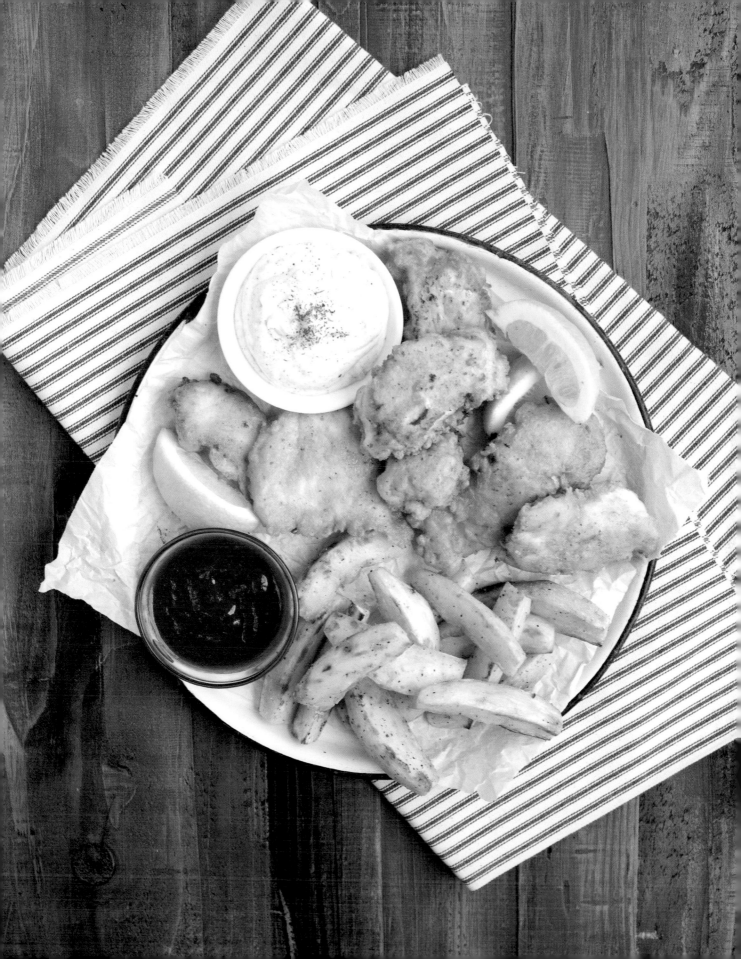

GRILLED SEAFOOD SKEWERS

EGG-FREE   NUT-FREE

Skewers are a quick and easy way to cook vegetables and meat together, but some people like to skewer their vegetables and meat separately to allow for different cooking times. I say go with whatever works best for you.

Which kinds of seafood are most sustainably sourced changes frequently based on fish and shellfish populations. (The Monterey Bay Aquarium Seafood Watch, seafoodwatch.org, is a great resource for the latest recommendations from around the world.) Fortunately, any dense and meaty fish, such as cod, swordfish, mahi mahi, halibut, mackerel, or yellowtail, will work nicely in this recipe.

Prep Time: 15 minutes, plus 20 minutes to marinate the fish   **Cook Time:** 6 minutes   **Yield:** 4 servings

FOR THE MARINADE

3 cloves garlic, minced

3 tablespoons freshly squeezed lemon juice

3 tablespoons extra-virgin olive oil

3 tablespoons chopped fresh flat-leaf parsley

1 tablespoon finely grated lemon zest

1 teaspoon fine sea salt

½ teaspoon ground black pepper

½ teaspoon paprika

2 pounds fresh cod fillets, skin removed, cut into 1½-inch cubes

1 green bell pepper, seeded and chopped into 1½-inch pieces

1 yellow bell pepper, seeded and chopped into 1½-inch pieces

16 small cherry tomatoes

2 lemons, quartered, for serving

Chopped fresh parsley, for garnish (optional)

Seasoned Cauliflower Rice (page 200), for serving (optional)

1. Combine all marinade ingredients together in a large mixing bowl and stir until well combined. Place the cod chunks in the bowl and toss until coated on all sides. Cover and place in the refrigerator for 20 minutes.

2. While the fish marinates, preheat the grill. If using wooden skewers, soak 8 skewers in water for 10 minutes.

3. Thread the marinated fish pieces, bell pepper chunks, and cherry tomatoes onto the skewers.

4. Grill the skewers for 5 to 6 minutes, until the fish is fully cooked, turning once halfway through. Garnish with a sprinkle of chopped fresh parsley and serve with lemon wedges and cauliflower rice, if desired.

KITCHEN TIP

If you have an especially sticky grill, try placing thin slices of lemon over the area you want to grill on. Cook the skewers on top of the lemon slices—they won't stick to the grill, plus you'll get an extra boost of flavor. Look for larger lemons so you don't have to worry about the slices sliding through the grates of the grill.

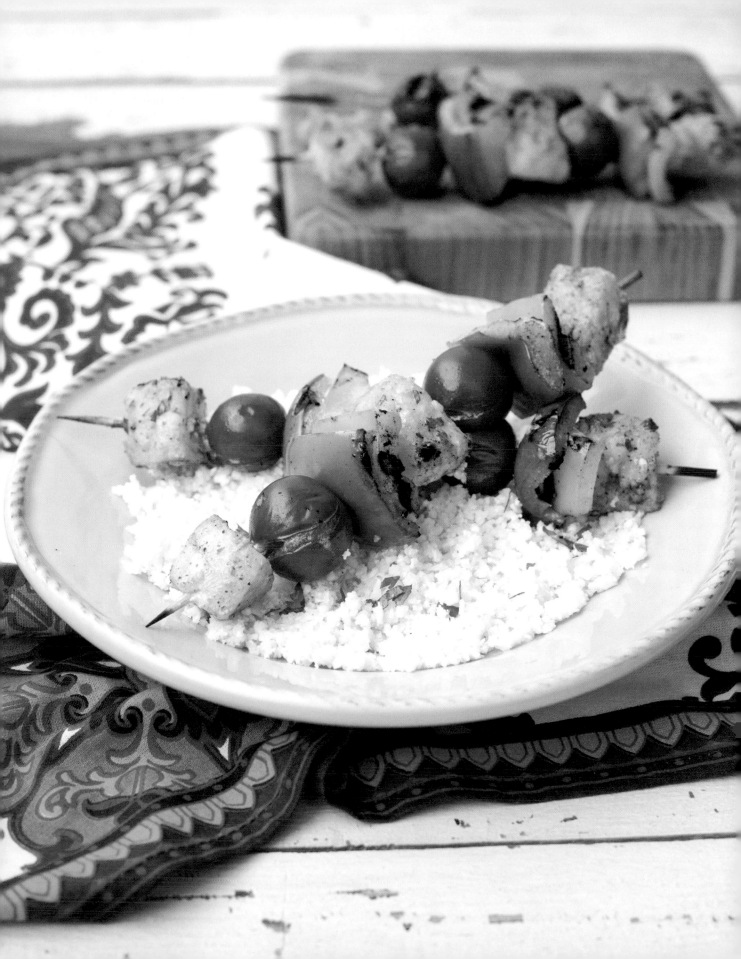

MUSSELS *in* THAI CURRY SAUCE

The best part of this recipe is that everything is cooked in the same pot, which means just one pan to wash, and to me that is a solid victory. These mussels look and taste so elegant, but they take very little effort to make. The broth is fragrant and has just a bit of heat to it, which you can adjust by adding more or less curry paste to your liking. Look for a brand without any preservatives or sugars. Each brand has a different level of heat, so if you're trying a new brand for the first time, add a little bit at a time and taste as you go so you don't overpower your dish.

Prep Time: 10 minutes   Cook Time: 20 minutes   Yield: 4 servings

2 tablespoons ghee (page 320), lard (page 322), or tallow (page 324)

1 small shallot, minced

1 clove garlic, minced

2 tablespoons red curry paste

¼ teaspoon ground ginger

½ cup chicken stock (page 310)

1 (13.5-ounce) can full-fat coconut milk or 1⅔ cups homemade coconut milk (page 314)

2 tablespoons freshly squeezed lime juice

1 teaspoon finely grated lemon zest

2 tablespoons fish sauce

2 pounds mussels, debearded and cleaned

3 tablespoons fresh cilantro or parsley, for garnish (optional)

1. Melt the ghee in a medium skillet over medium heat. Add the shallot, garlic, curry paste, and ginger and cook for 1 minute, stirring frequently.

2. Add the stock, coconut milk, lime juice, lemon zest, and fish sauce, and stir to combine. Bring to a boil, then reduce the heat to medium-low and simmer for 10 minutes.

3. Add the mussels to the pan, cover, and cook for 3 minutes, or until the mussels have opened. Transfer the mussels to serving bowls, ladle the broth over the top, and garnish with the chopped cilantro, if desired.

KITCHEN TIP

Do not store fresh mussels in an airtight container or submerged in water. Place them in a bowl in the refrigerator and cover lightly with a moist paper towel or kitchen towel to help keep them moist. Wait to clean them until right before cooking.

TRY THIS!

I always keep curry paste in my cupboard. In addition to using it in this recipe, I often use it to make a quick and easy soup. Just mix 1 cup of coconut milk, 1 cup of chicken stock, and 2 to 3 teaspoons of curry paste together in a small saucepan, simmer over medium heat until warmed, then pour into a mug or bowl.

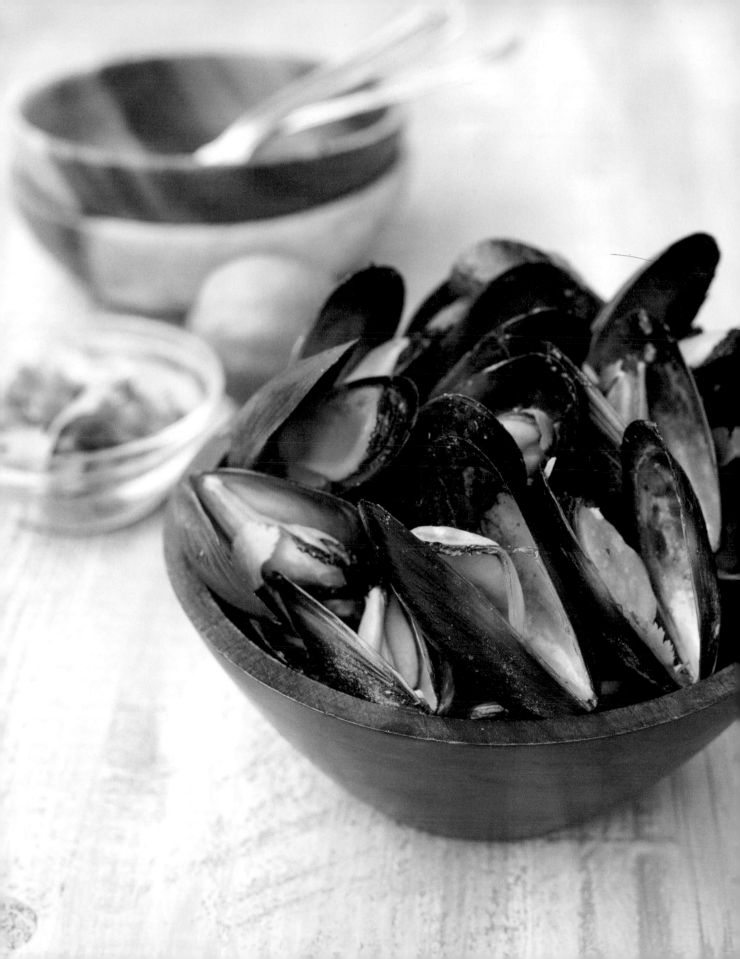

ORANGE
and GINGER
GLAZED
SALMON

Just a bit of orange juice, garlic, and ginger is enough to turn an ordinary piece of salmon into a flavor explosion. This dish is easy enough to make on a weeknight and goes great with your favorite vegetables or served over your favorite greens.

Prep Time: 10 minutes, plus 20 minutes to marinate the salmon   **Cook Time:** 15 minutes   **Yield:** 4 servings

FOR THE MARINADE

1 tablespoon extra-virgin olive oil

1 small shallot, minced

2 cloves garlic, minced

1 teaspoon ground ginger

⅓ cup coconut aminos or soy sauce substitute (page 283)

⅓ cup freshly squeezed orange juice

3 tablespoons raw honey, warmed if solid

1½ pounds skinless salmon fillets, 1 inch thick

1 large orange, sliced

2 green onions, chopped, for garnish (optional)

1. In a small mixing bowl, whisk together the marinade ingredients. Place the salmon fillets in a medium-sized baking dish and pour the marinade over them, cover, and place in the refrigerator for 20 minutes.

2. Drain the marinade from the baking dish into a small saucepan over medium heat. Bring to a boil, then reduce the heat to low and simmer for 15 minutes, or until the glaze has reduced by half and thickened, stirring occasionally.

3. While the glaze is reducing, cook the salmon.

4. **To use the grill:** Preheat the grill to medium heat. Lay the orange slices on the grates and place the salmon on top. Grill for 12 minutes, or until the fish is firm and a knife inserted into the center of the fish shows it is cooked through.

    To use the oven: Preheat the oven to 450°F. Place the orange slices side by side on a baking sheet. Place the salmon on top of the orange slices and bake for 10 minutes, or until cooked through.

5. To serve, transfer the cooked orange slices to a serving platter and place the salmon on top. Drizzle with the glaze and sprinkle with the chopped green onions, if desired.

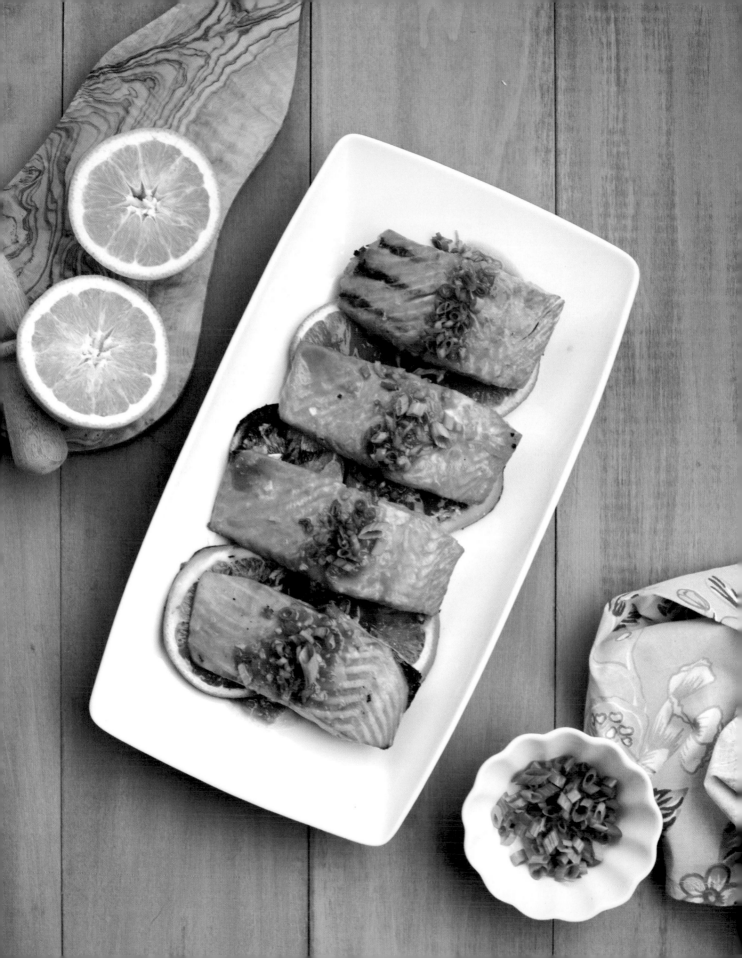

SEAFOOD
FRA DIAVOLO

A bold amount of crushed red pepper gives this recipe a good dose of heat, and the onion, garlic, and tomato bring the heavy-hitting flavor. You can increase or decrease the amount of crushed red pepper to make it more or less spicy, and don't forget that any bitterness or acidity from tomatoes can be balanced with the addition of a tiny bit of raw honey. Taste as you go and adjust as needed. I like to serve this dish with a batch of zucchini noodles (page 328).

Prep Time: 15 minutes   **Cook Time:** 20 minutes   **Yield:** 4 servings

4 tablespoons ghee (page 320), lard (page 322), or tallow (page 324), divided

1 pound large shrimp, peeled and deveined, tails removed

1 large onion, chopped (about 1 cup)

2 teaspoons crushed red pepper

½ teaspoon fine sea salt

3 cloves garlic, minced

1 (14.5-ounce) can diced tomatoes

2 tablespoons tomato paste

¼ cup chicken stock (page 310)

½ pound clams

1 pound mussels, debearded and cleaned

¼ cup chopped fresh basil

Finely grated zest of 1 medium lemon, plus more for garnish (optional)

2 tablespoons fresh flat-leaf parsley, for garnish (optional)

1. Melt 2 tablespoons of the ghee in a large skillet over medium-high heat. Add the shrimp and cook for 2 minutes on each side, then remove from the pan and set aside.

2. Melt the 2 remaining tablespoons of ghee in the pan, then add the onion, crushed red pepper, and salt and cook for 4 minutes. Add the garlic and cook for 1 additional minute.

3. Add the diced tomatoes, tomato paste, and chicken stock to the pan and stir to combine. Bring to a boil, then add the clams, mussels, and basil. Cover and cook for 5 minutes, or until the clams and mussels open.

4. Return the shrimp to the pan, add the lemon zest, and cook for 1 more minute. Sprinkle with parsley and additional zest, if desired, and serve.

KITCHEN TIP

Don't waste that paste! You can freeze any extra tomato paste to use later. Line a baking sheet with parchment paper and use a tablespoon to drop spoonfuls of the paste onto the sheet, evenly spaced, sort of like little tomato cookies. Stick the sheet in the freezer for a few hours and then transfer the frozen tomato paste cookies to a sealed container. They'll keep in the freezer for up to 3 months. Whenever you need tomato paste for a recipe, you will know that each cookie is equal to 1 tablespoon; add it to a hot liquid like a sauce or soup, and it will easily melt.

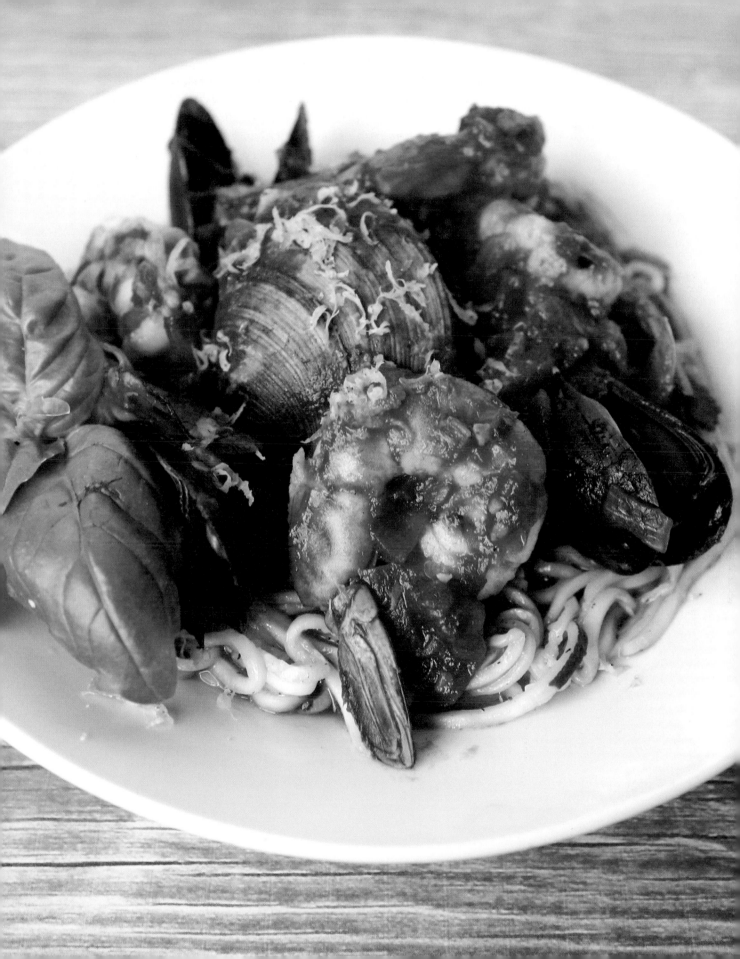

SMOKED SALMON DEVILED EGGS

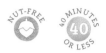

NUT-FREE · 40 MINUTES OR LESS

Deviled eggs are a go-to food around my house, and this version packs a whole lot of texture and flavor into each little egg half. These are fairly quick to throw together and store well in a sealed container in the refrigerator for a few days. You can easily grab a couple when you need a snack or a late-night fix, and they also make a great main dish when served on top of your favorite greens with a drizzle of good olive oil and a sprinkle of salt and pepper.

Prep Time: 10 minutes   Cook Time: 15 minutes   Yield: 12 deviled eggs

6 large eggs

½ teaspoon fine sea salt

3 tablespoons mayonnaise (page 278)

1 tablespoon freshly squeezed lemon juice

2 ounces smoked salmon, finely chopped

2 tablespoons finely minced red onion

2 tablespoons capers, rinsed and roughly chopped

⅛ teaspoon ground black pepper

Dash of paprika, for garnish (optional)

1 tablespoon chopped fresh chives, for garnish (optional)

1. To hard-boil the eggs, place the eggs and salt in a medium-sized saucepan and fill with enough cold water to cover by 1 inch. Bring to a rolling boil over medium-high heat. Turn off the stove, keeping the pan on the burner. Cover the pan and allow to sit for 12 minutes. Transfer the eggs to a bowl of ice water to stop the cooking process. Allow the eggs to cool for 5 minutes, then peel them under a gentle stream of running water.

2. Slice the eggs in half lengthwise. Using a small spoon, scoop the yolks into a medium-sized mixing bowl and mash with a fork until smooth. Add the mayonnaise and lemon juice and stir to combine, then add the salmon, red onion, capers, and pepper and stir again.

3. Spoon the mixture back into the egg whites and garnish with a dash of paprika and a sprinkle of chives, if desired. Keep in a sealed container in the refrigerator for up to 3 days.

TRY THIS!
Lump crab meat makes a great substitute for the salmon.

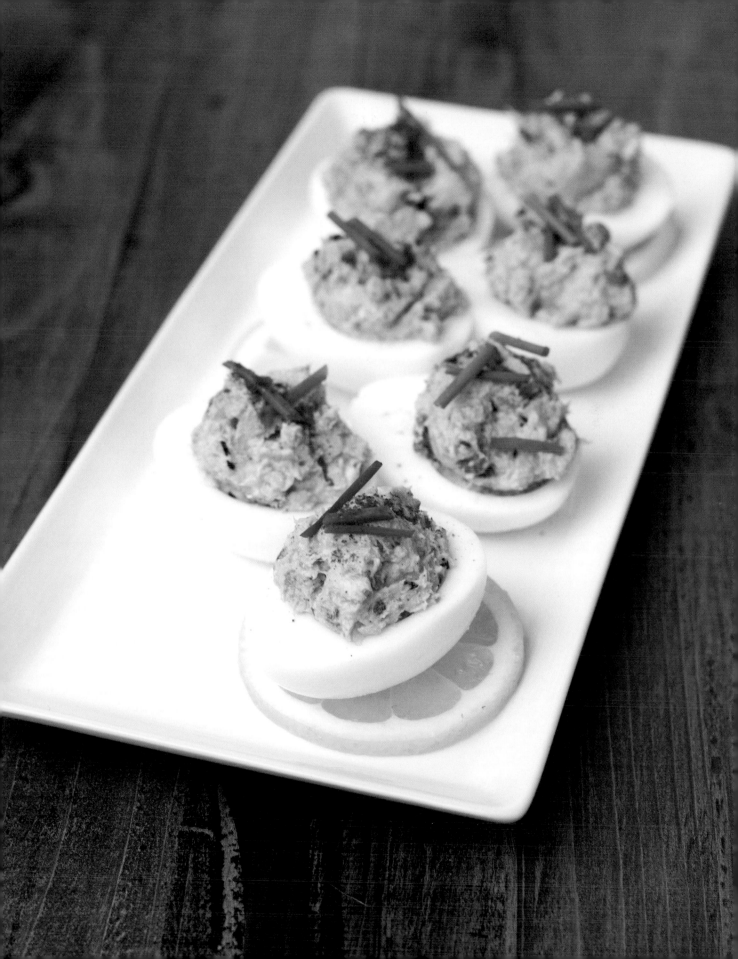

MEDITERRANEAN FISH

EGG-FREE   NUT-FREE

This dish highlights some of the herbs and spices commonly used in the Mediterranean. The fresh squeeze of lemon juice right at the table provides a fantastic burst of flavor, and the winelike flavor of the olives really rounds out this recipe.

Seafood availability is always changing, so the type of fish I use for this recipe has to change to accommodate the supply. I have used halibut, cod, and tilapia and all worked well, which means you have some options when it comes to cost and availability.

Prep Time: 15 minutes   Cook Time: 35 minutes   Yield: 4 servings

4 (6-ounce) halibut fillets

½ teaspoon fine sea salt

¼ teaspoon ground black pepper

1 tablespoon freshly squeezed lemon juice

¼ cup extra-virgin olive oil

1 small onion, chopped (about ½ cup)

2 cloves garlic, minced

1 large tomato, chopped (about ¾ cup)

1 teaspoon dried rosemary

1 teaspoon dried oregano

½ teaspoon dried basil

½ teaspoon dried thyme

¼ cup capers, drained

½ cup pitted Kalamata olives, drained

2 lemons, quartered, for serving

1. Preheat the oven to 350°F.

2. Place the fish in a large glass baking dish and sprinkle with the salt and pepper. Pour the lemon juice over the fish and set aside.

3. Heat the olive oil in a medium saucepan over medium heat. Add the onion and garlic and cook for 2 minutes, stirring occasionally. Add the tomato, rosemary, oregano, basil, and thyme and stir to combine. Cook for another 5 minutes, then remove from the heat and stir in the capers and olives.

4. Spoon the mixture over the fish. Place in the oven and bake for 20 to 25 minutes, until the fish flakes easily with a fork. Thinner cuts of fish will cook faster, so keep an eye on them. Serve with the lemon wedges.

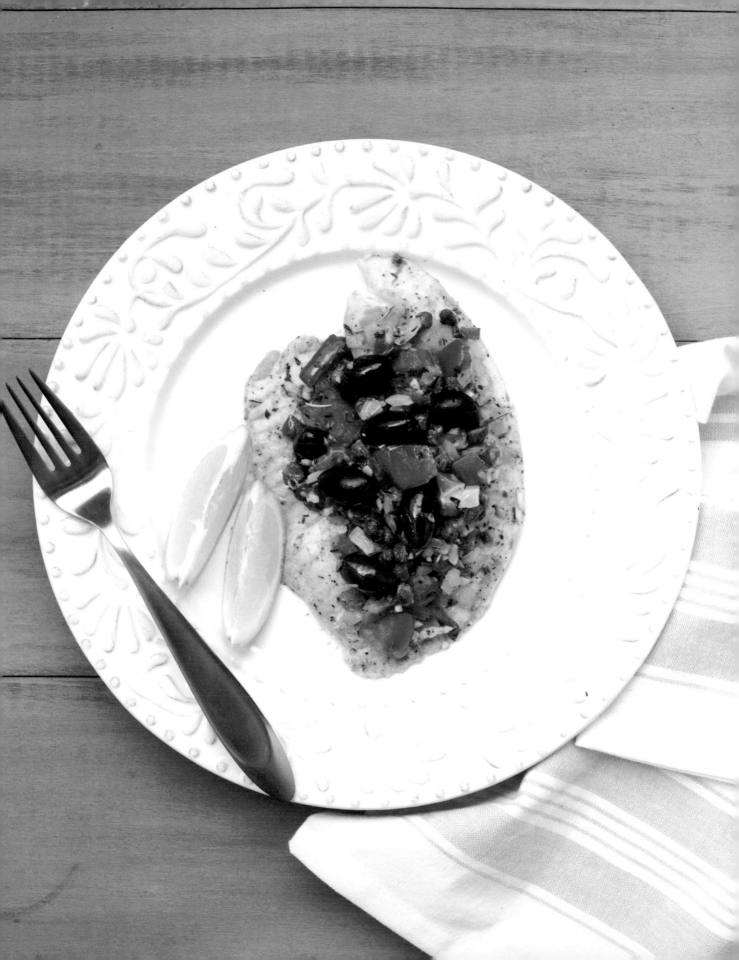

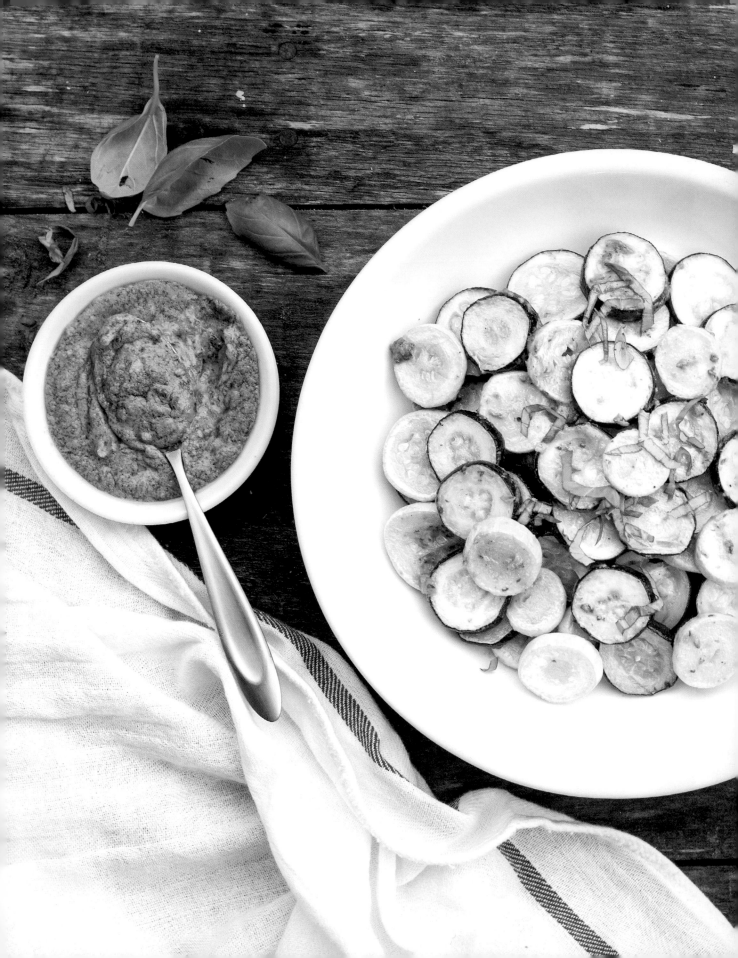

side dishes

BALSAMIC
ROSEMARY
MUSHROOMS

It's a good idea to know a handful of go-to recipes that you can throw together in just a few minutes. This mushroom recipe is one that you should bookmark because it is easy to make and is a great side dish to almost any protein. The fresh rosemary and balsamic vinegar make plain mushrooms pop with flavor.

Prep Time: 5 minutes   **Cook Time:** 10 minutes   **Yield:** 4 servings

1 pound white button or cremini mushrooms

3 tablespoons ghee (page 320), lard (page 322), or tallow (page 324)

1 small white onion, finely chopped (about ½ cup)

2 cloves garlic, chopped

1 tablespoon fresh rosemary leaves

½ teaspoon fine sea salt

¼ teaspoon ground black pepper

1 tablespoon balsamic vinegar

1 tablespoon chopped fresh parsley, for garnish (optional)

1. Wipe the mushrooms thoroughly with a slightly damp paper towel to clean them, then slice in half.

2. Melt the ghee in a large skillet over medium-high heat. Add the mushrooms, onion, and garlic and cook for 6 to 8 minutes, until the mushrooms have released their liquid, stirring frequently.

3. Add the rosemary, salt, pepper, and balsamic vinegar to the pan and stir to coat the mushrooms. Cook for another 3 minutes, or until the mushrooms are tender, then transfer to a serving bowl, sprinkle with the parsley, if desired, and serve.

TRY THIS!

Adding ¼ teaspoon of fish sauce at the same time as the balsamic vinegar will give your mushrooms an extra boost of umami, and you won't even taste any fishiness!

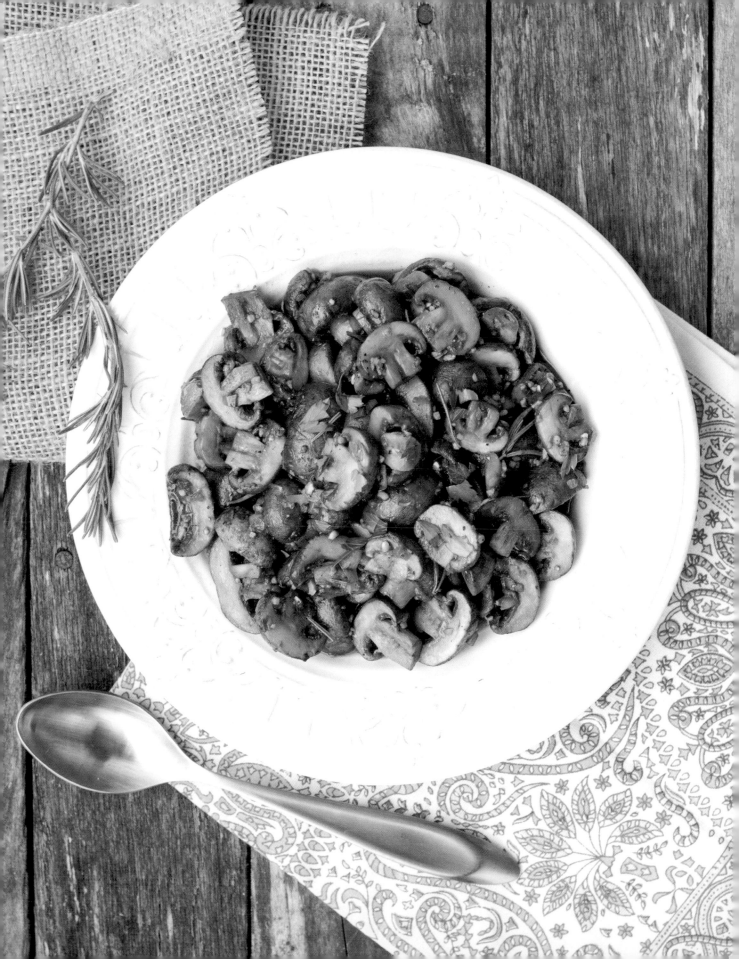

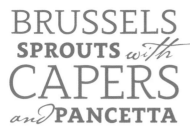

BRUSSELS SPROUTS *with* CAPERS *and* PANCETTA

If you hate Brussels sprouts, it may be because you have only had them when they were overcooked to a mushy mess. It wasn't until a few years ago that I tried roasting and seasoning them, and I instantly fell in love. There's something about the little bits of capers, pine nuts, and pancetta that get picked up with the Brussels sprouts in every forkful that makes this dish totally gratifying. The pancetta and capers add a bit of saltiness, so wait until you are finished cooking to taste and add seasonings.

Prep Time: 5 minutes   **Cook Time:** 20 minutes   **Yield:** 4 to 6 servings

1¾ pounds Brussels sprouts, trimmed and halved

3 tablespoons extra-virgin olive oil

1 tablespoon balsamic vinegar

¼ teaspoon ground black pepper

4 ounces pancetta, chopped into small cubes

¼ cup pine nuts

¼ cup capers, drained

1. Preheat the oven to 400°F. Line a 9-by-13-inch baking sheet with parchment paper or a baking mat.

2. Place the Brussels sprouts in a large mixing bowl, drizzle with the olive oil and balsamic vinegar, and toss until well coated. Spread the Brussels sprouts evenly on the prepared baking sheet. If the baking sheet is crowded the sprouts will not get crispy enough, so use two sheets if needed. Sprinkle the pepper over the sprouts, then place in the oven and bake for 15 to 20 minutes, until the Brussels sprouts are nice and crispy. Larger sprouts will take a little longer to cook than smaller ones.

3. While the sprouts are in the oven, cook the pancetta and pine nuts: Place the pancetta in a medium-sized sauté pan over medium heat and cook until crispy, then use a slotted spoon to transfer to a plate, leaving the fat from the pancetta in the pan. Add the pine nuts to the pan and cook for 1 minute, or until light brown and toasted, stirring frequently.

4. Once the sprouts are done, remove them from the oven and place them in a serving bowl. Add the pancetta, pine nuts, and capers and toss. Taste and add additional salt and pepper if desired.

KITCHEN TIP

When roasting vegetables, make sure to give them some space. Cramming as many vegetables as you can in a roasting pan or on a baking sheet means that they'll release so much liquid and steam that they turn mushy. It's better to use two pans and give them plenty of room than to have your recipe fall flat.

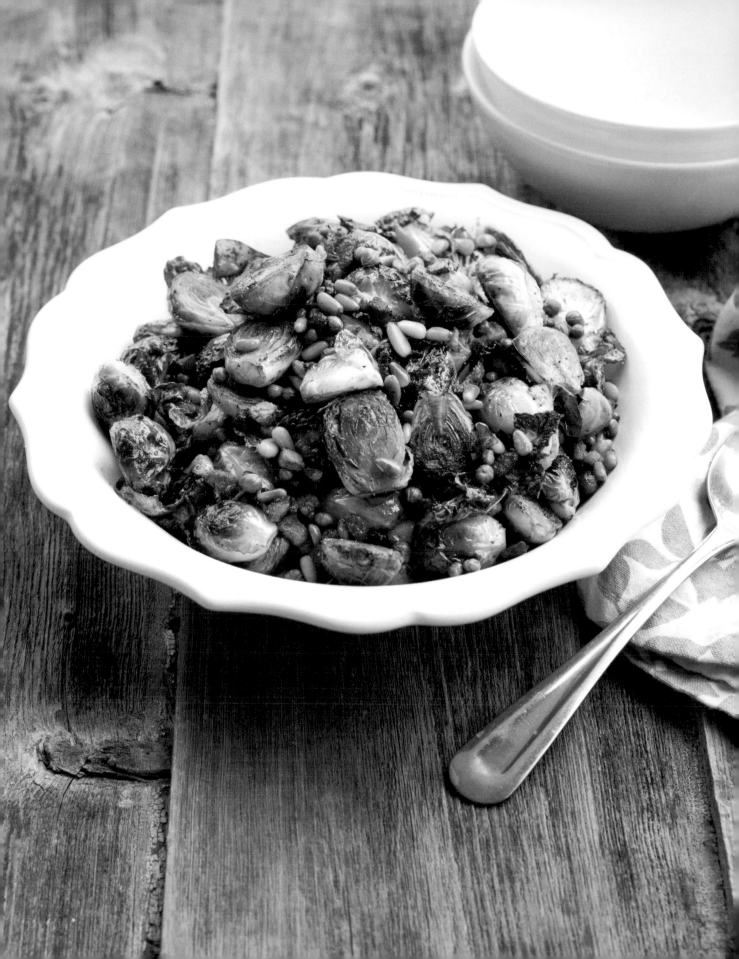

COLCANNON

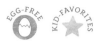

EGG-FREE · KID-FAVORITES

If you're picturing me waving a wooden spoon at you and telling you to eat your cabbage, then you're right, that's exactly what I am doing. To some people the thought of cabbage mixed with mashed potatoes might sound a little strange, but it's actually quite tasty. This recipe is based on a traditional Irish dish, but you can substitute kale for the cabbage or skip the ham and go with a good sprinkle of bacon on top instead. I like to prepare the cabbage and ham mixture at the same time as I'm cooking the mashed sweet potatoes to cut down on cooking time.

Prep Time: 10 minutes   **Cook Time:** 15 minutes, plus 30 minutes for the mashed potatoes
Yield: 4 to 6 servings

3 tablespoons ghee (page 320), lard (page 322), or tallow (page 324)

1 large onion, chopped (about 1 cup)

2 cloves garlic, minced

1 head cabbage (about 2 pounds), shredded

1 pound cooked ham, chopped into bite-sized pieces

1 batch Mashed Sweet Potatoes (page 189)

1. Melt the ghee in a large skillet over medium-high heat. Add the onion and sauté for 4 minutes, then add the garlic and sauté for 1 more minute, or until onions are tender. Add the shredded cabbage and chopped ham and cook until the cabbage is tender, about 8 minutes.

2. Place the mashed sweet potatoes in a large bowl, add the cabbage and ham mixture, and stir to combine.

TRY THIS!
Try adding 3 tablespoons of chopped fresh chives to the sweet potatoes at the same time as the cabbage and ham mixture.

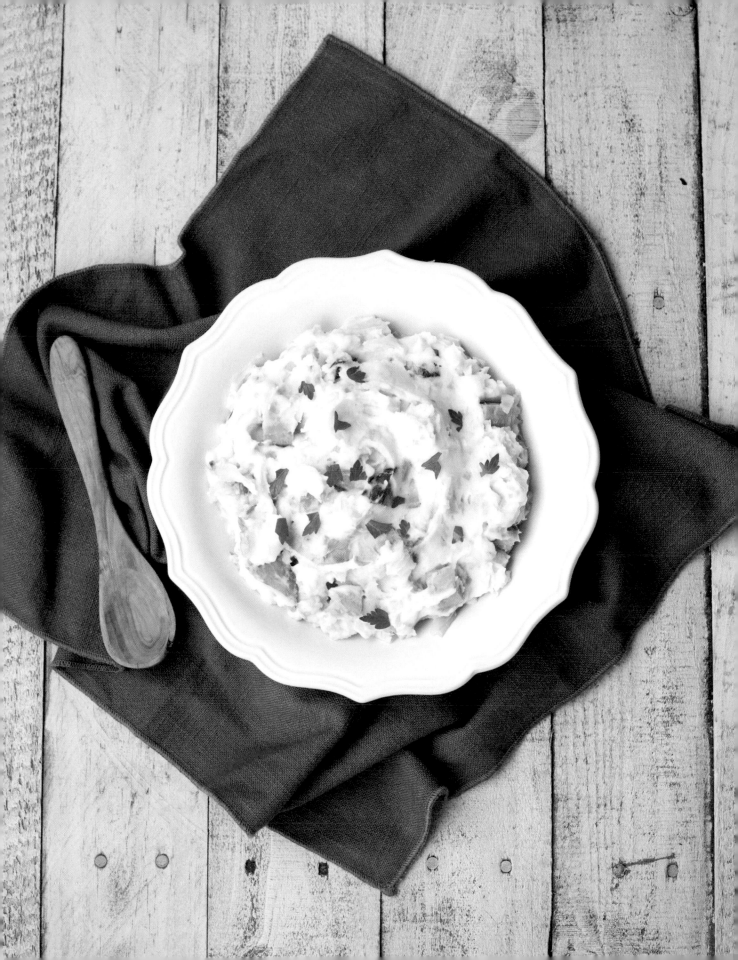

CREAMY
COLESLAW

Coleslaw is the traditional American side dish for any picnic or barbecue, and this recipe highlights the creamy, tangy, and sweet flavors of a traditional slaw—nobody will be able to tell it's Paleo-friendly. If you like, you can use a 1-pound bag of coleslaw mix instead of the cabbage and carrots.

Prep Time: 10 minutes, plus 30 minutes to chill   **Yield:** 4 to 6 servings

FOR THE DRESSING

1 cup mayonnaise (page 278)

2 tablespoons apple cider vinegar

2 tablespoons raw honey, warmed if solid

½ teaspoon dry yellow mustard

½ teaspoon celery seed

¼ teaspoon fine sea salt

¼ teaspoon ground black pepper

1 head cabbage (about 1 pound), shredded

2 large carrots, peeled and shredded (about 1¾ cups)

Fine sea salt and ground black pepper

1. Make the dressing: In a small mixing bowl, whisk together all the dressing ingredients.

2. Place the shredded cabbage and carrots in a large mixing bowl. Pour the dressing over the shredded vegetables and toss to coat. Taste and add additional salt and pepper if desired. Chill in the refrigerator for 30 minutes or until ready to serve.

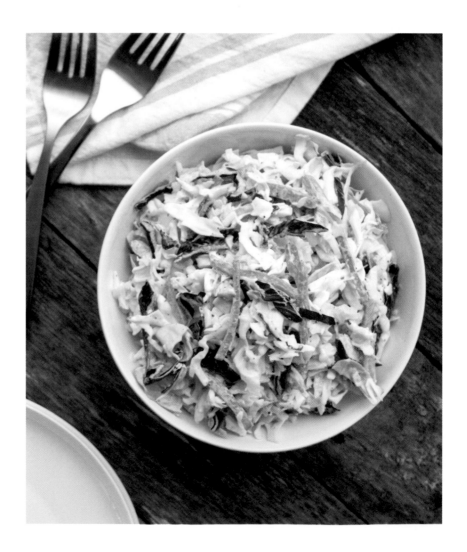

MASHED SWEET POTATOES

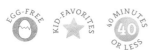

Sweet potatoes come in white- and red-skinned varieties, though in the United States, many stores label red-skinned sweet potatoes as yams. Both varieties make a great Paleo-friendly mashed potato, but red-skinned sweet potatoes are generally softer and cook down to a creamier consistency. You may need to give the white-skinned varieties a few extra minutes to boil or chop them into smaller pieces before boiling.

Prep Time: 10 minutes   Cook Time: 20 minutes   Yield: 4 to 6 servings

2 pounds white- or red-skinned sweet potatoes, peeled and chopped into 1-inch cubes

½ cup almond milk (page 318)

¼ cup ghee (page 320), lard (page 322), or tallow (page 324)

1 teaspoon fine sea salt

½ teaspoon ground black pepper

1 tablespoon chopped flat-leaf parsley, for garnish (optional)

1. Bring a large pot of water to a boil over medium-high heat. Add the potatoes and boil for 15 minutes, or until tender.

2. Drain the potatoes and add the almond milk, ghee, salt, and pepper. Using a hand mixer on medium speed, blend until smooth. Top with parsley, if desired, and serve.

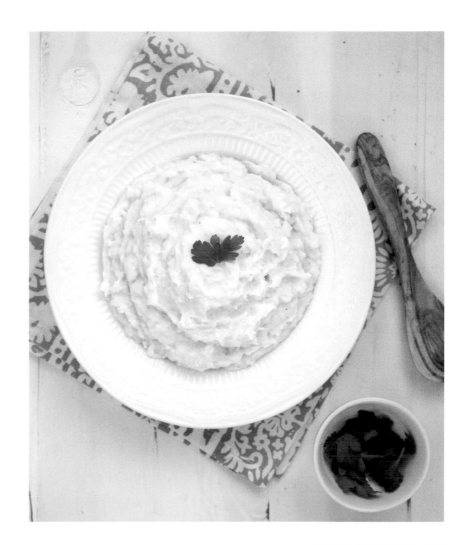

CRISPY
SWEET POTATO
WEDGES

These crispy potato wedges make a great side dish for almost any protein. Look for sweet potatoes that are the same length and width so you can cut your wedges to the same size. This allows them to cook evenly, so you're not left with any soggy stragglers. A small apple slicer is a great tool for cutting a peeled potato, and it also helps make sure the wedges are evenly sized. Don't crowd the wedges on the pan—give those fries their space and they should crisp up nicely for you.

Prep Time: 10 minutes   **Cook Time:** 25 minutes   **Yield:** 4 to 6 servings

4 medium white-skinned sweet potatoes (about 1¼ pounds), peeled and cut into ¾-inch-thick wedges (about 10 wedges per potato)

3 tablespoons extra-virgin olive oil

1 teaspoon garlic powder

½ teaspoon onion powder

½ teaspoon fine sea salt

¼ teaspoon ground black pepper

1. Preheat the oven to 425°F. Line two baking sheets with parchment paper or baking mats.

2. In a large mixing bowl, toss the sweet potato wedges with the olive oil until fully coated. In a separate small bowl, combine the garlic powder, onion powder, salt, and pepper. Sprinkle half the seasoning mixture over the potatoes and toss, then sprinkle the remaining seasoning mixture over the potatoes and toss again, until well coated.

3. Spread the sweet potato wedges in a single layer on the prepared baking sheets, making sure they are not touching each other. Bake for 15 minutes, or until golden brown on top. Remove the baking sheets from the oven, flip all of the wedges over, then return to the oven and bake for another 10 minutes, or until golden brown. For extra-crispy wedges, turn the oven to broil and bake for another 1 to 2 minutes.

TRY THIS!

For chipotle lime sweet potato wedges, add ½ teaspoon of paprika and ½ teaspoon of smoked chipotle to the seasoning mixture, and drizzle 1½ teaspoons of freshly squeezed lime juice over the wedges right after coating them with olive oil.

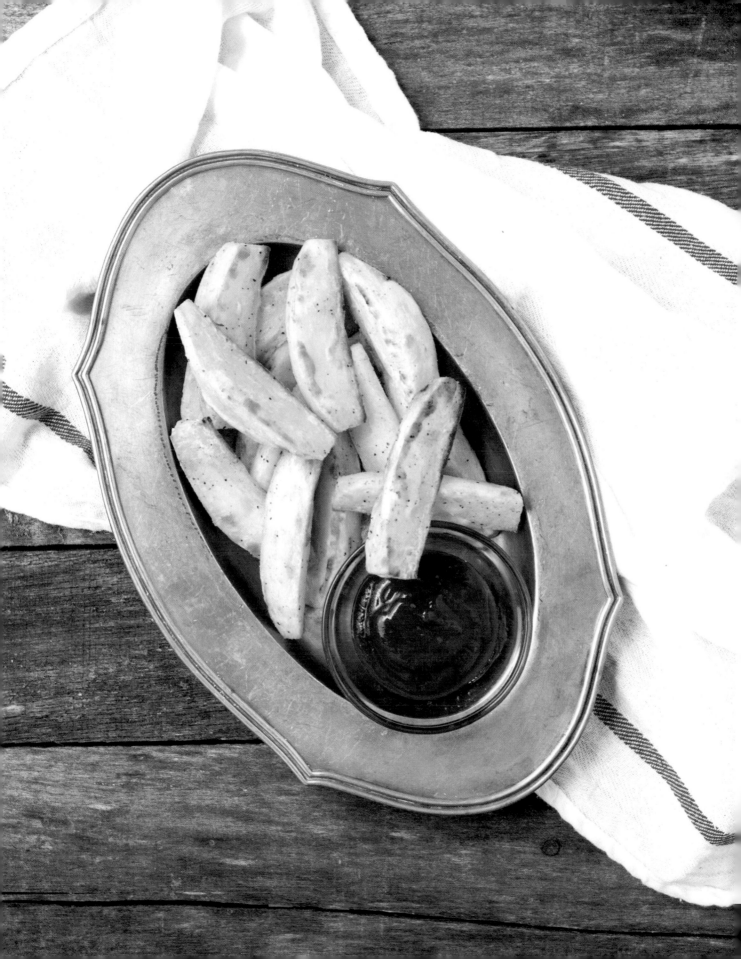

PAN-ROASTED CARROTS *with* GREMOLATA

EGG-FREE · NUT-FREE · 40 MINUTES OR LESS

If you're saying, "You want me put gremo-WHAT on my carrots?" don't worry, it's not anything crazy. Gremolata is just lemon zest, garlic, and parsley combined to make a fresh and tasty condiment. You can use it on top of almost any protein or vegetable. Just make sure to add it near the end of cooking to highlight all the fresh flavors.

Prep Time: 10 minutes   **Cook Time:** 20 minutes   **Yield:** 4 servings

2 tablespoons ghee (page 320), lard (page 322), or tallow (page 324)

1½ pounds carrots, peeled and halved lengthwise

½ cup chicken stock (page 310)

¼ teaspoon fine sea salt

¼ teaspoon ground black pepper

FOR THE GREMOLATA

¼ cup tightly packed fresh flat-leaf parsley, finely chopped

2 cloves garlic, minced

1 tablespoon finely grated lemon zest

¼ teaspoon fine sea salt

¼ teaspoon ground black pepper

1 tablespoon extra-virgin olive oil

1. Melt the ghee in a large skillet over medium-high heat. Add the carrots and chicken stock. Bring to a boil, then reduce the heat to low and cook for 12 to 14 minutes, until carrots are just tender and most of the liquid has evaporated. Season with the salt and pepper.

2. Make the gremolata: Combine the parsley, garlic, lemon zest, salt, and pepper in a small mixing bowl. Add the olive oil, stirring to combine. Add the mixture to the carrots, toss to coat, and then serve.

TRY THIS!

If you just can't get enough of fresh herbs and want this dish to pack even more of a bright flavor punch, try adding 2 tablespoons finely chopped fresh dill to the gremolata mixture.

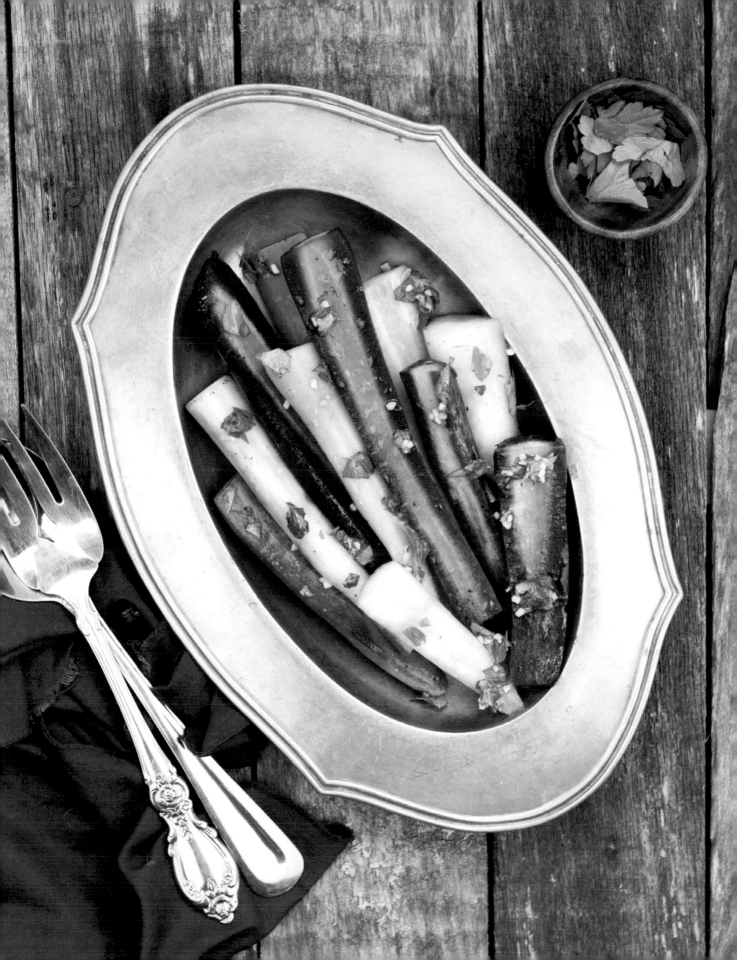

PASTA

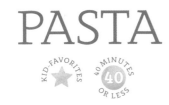

While I usually use vegetable noodles for a pasta base, such as zucchini noodles (page 328) or spaghetti squash (page 326), every now and then you want something that tastes like the wheat-based pasta you may have been used to before going Paleo. This recipe delivers. It's best when you want a thicker pasta, such as a fettuccine or lasagna (no need to cook it ahead of time if you're making lasagna). The dough also works well for stuffed pasta, such as ravioli.

Prep Time: 20 minutes   Cook Time: 5 minutes   Yield: 4 servings

1 cup almond flour (page 316)

1 cup tapioca flour, plus more for kneading

⅔ cup arrowroot flour, plus more for kneading

2 teaspoons fine sea salt

2 large eggs, room temperature

4 large egg yolks

2 tablespoons extra-virgin olive oil

1. In a large mixing bowl, combine the almond flour, tapioca flour, arrowroot flour, and salt. Make a well in the center of the mixture and add the eggs and egg yolks. Begin beating the eggs with a fork, pulling the dry mixture in as you do so to combine it with the eggs. Continue blending with the fork little by little until the flours and eggs are almost fully combined.

2. Dust a work surface generously with arrowroot or tapioca flour and place the dough on the surface. Knead the dough for 3 minutes, or until smooth and no longer sticky. If the dough is too dry at the end, add a teaspoon of water; if it's too wet, add 1 tablespoon of almond flour until the dough is moist but not sticky.

3. Divide the dough into 4 equal balls. One at a time, roll them out to ⅛ inch thick. Make sure to keep the remainder of the dough balls covered with a dishcloth until you are ready to use them or they will begin to dry out. Use a sharp knife to cut the pasta to the desired shape. I recommend a fettuccine-style shape, but the dough also works well for ravioli and lasagna noodles. Repeat with the remainder of the dough, sprinkling the work surface with arrowroot or tapioca flour each time.

4. To cook the pasta, fill a medium saucepan two-thirds full with water and place over medium-high heat. Add the olive oil to the water and bring to a boil. Place about a quarter of the noodles in the boiling water (cooking them in about 4 batches prevents the noodles from sticking to each other). Cook for 1 to 2 minutes, or until all of the noodles are floating at the top. Transfer the cooked noodles to a colander or strainer and repeat with the rest of the noodles.

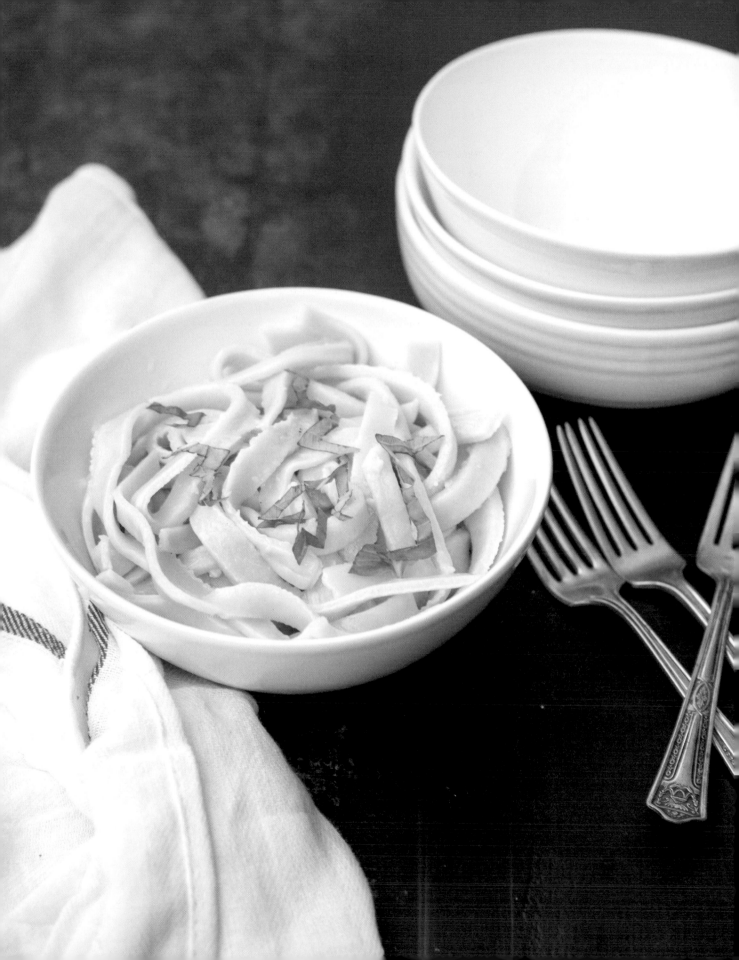

ROASTED ASPARAGUS
with LEMON SAUCE

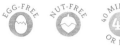

Everyone likes their asparagus a little different. Some like it cooked all the way through, and some like it to have a bit of crunch. Thinner stalks of asparagus can be cooked through in 9 minutes or less, but thicker stalks may take up to 20 minutes or longer to become tender. Whether you're using thick or thin asparagus, try to choose stalks that are about the same thickness so they will cook evenly. Most asparagus will be crisp-tender at around 12 minutes, which is generally when I take mine out of the oven. And by "take it out of the oven," I mean "reach into the oven and start eating it directly off the pan." Try to resist doing that, though, because sometimes being too eager can result in a happy stomach but a fairly burnt tongue.

Prep Time: 10 minutes   Cook Time: 9 to 20 minutes   Yield: 4 to 6 servings

1 pound asparagus, trimmed

3 tablespoons melted ghee (page 320), lard (page 322), or tallow (page 324)

½ teaspoon fine sea salt

¼ teaspoon ground black pepper

¼ teaspoon onion powder

FOR THE SAUCE

3 tablespoons freshly squeezed lemon juice

½ teaspoon finely grated lemon zest

½ teaspoon prepared Dijon mustard

2 tablespoons extra-virgin olive oil

1. Preheat the oven to 375°F. Line a 9-by-13-inch baking sheet with parchment paper or a baking mat.

2. Lay the asparagus on the prepared baking sheet, then pour the ghee over the top. Sprinkle with the salt, pepper, and onion powder, then use the palms of your hands to roll the asparagus back and forth until the stalks are coated on all sides. Make sure that the asparagus stalks are evenly spaced on the pan and there is a bit of room between them, and roast for 9 to 20 minutes (see headnote), until tender enough for your liking. Thinner stalks will cook faster, so keep an eye on them to make sure that they aren't overdone.

3. While the asparagus is cooking, make the sauce: Place the lemon juice, zest, and mustard in a blender or food processor. Turn the blender on low speed, then very slowly drizzle in the olive oil, drop by drop, until the sauce is thoroughly combined and creamy.

4. Place the asparagus on a serving platter, pour the sauce over the top, sprinkle with salt and pepper, and serve.

KITCHEN TIP

Thicker stalks of asparagus sometimes have a tough outer layer of skin, but you can use a vegetable peeler to remove it. Press lightly from right below the tip down to the bottom of the stalk, then turn the asparagus and repeat until all of the skin is removed. Apparently you can also purchase an asparagus trimmer that is designed just for the peeling of this one vegetable. I do not own one.

TRY THIS!

Try sprinkling a couple tablespoons of toasted slivered almonds or pine nuts over the top of the asparagus right before serving to give your dish a little extra crunch and texture. You can also grill the asparagus instead of roasting it, to add a bit of a charred flavor that mixes nicely with the tangy lemon sauce. Just prepare the asparagus with the ghee and spices as you would if roasting, then place it directly onto a preheated grill and cook over high heat for about 5 minutes.

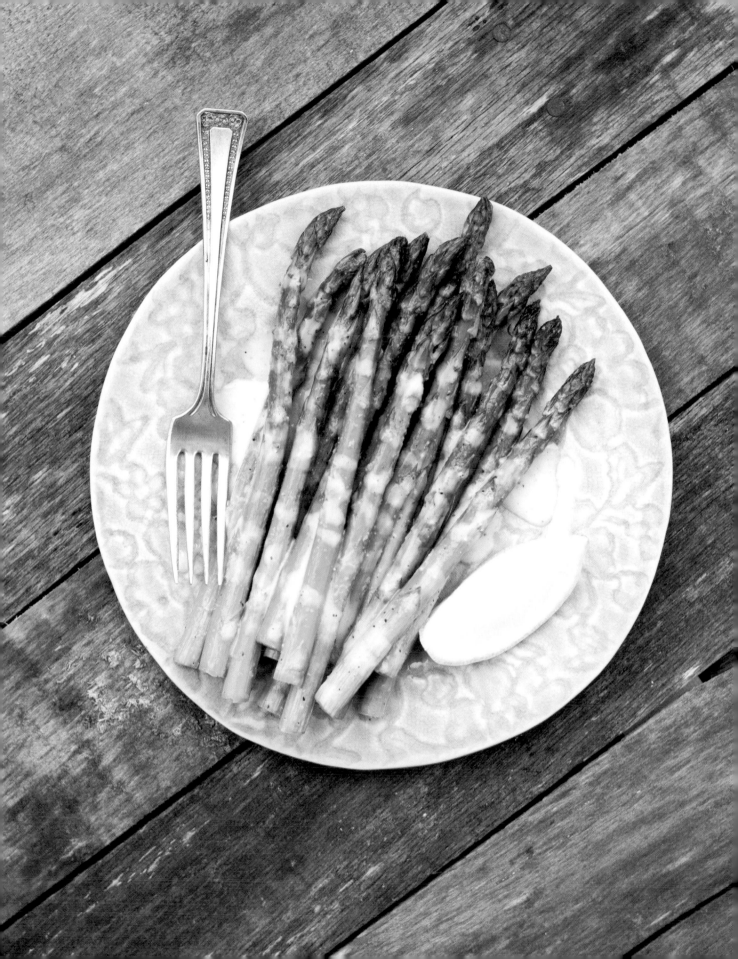

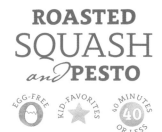

ROASTED SQUASH and PESTO

EGG-FREE · KID-FAVORITES · 40 MINUTES OR LESS

In the world of Paleo cooking, we just love to turn zucchini into noodles, but for this recipe you and I are giving the noodles a break and going with traditional zucchini slices. Both zucchini and yellow squash make great side dishes because you can cook them with just about any fresh herb and they will taste delicious. The vibrant flavor of the basil in the fresh pesto combined with the delicate flavors of zucchini and yellow squash make this a perfect summertime dish.

Prep Time: 8 minutes, plus 10 minutes for the pesto   **Cook Time:** 12 minutes   **Yield:** 4 servings

2 large zucchini (about 1 pound), cut into ¾-inch-thick rounds

2 large yellow summer squash (about 1 pound), cut into ¾-inch-thick rounds

1 tablespoon ghee (page 320), lard (page 322), or tallow (page 324), warmed if solid

3 tablespoons pesto (page 280)

4 fresh basil leaves, thinly sliced, for garnish (optional)

1. Preheat the oven to 400°F. Line a 9-by-13-inch baking sheet with parchment paper or a baking mat.

2. Place the sliced zucchini and squash in a large bowl and drizzle the ghee over the top. Gently toss to coat.

3. Spread the squash evenly on the prepared baking sheet. Roast for 5 minutes, then flip the slices over and cook for another 5 to 7 minutes, until the squash just begins to turn tender.

4. Return the squash to the bowl and toss with the pesto. To serve, place in a serving bowl and top with the sliced basil, if desired.

KITCHEN TIPS

If you have time, salting your squash before you begin will help remove excess liquid so it doesn't get soggy. Place the sliced squash in a colander, sprinkle with ½ teaspoon of salt, and toss. Place the colander over a larger bowl and allow the squash to drain for 20 minutes, then line a cutting board with paper towels or a clean kitchen towel and layer the squash slices on top. Press each slice gently with additional paper towels to remove as much liquid as possible, then follow the recipe as instructed.

Roasting is an easy way to cook vegetables, especially vegetables that you have never tried before. Almost all vegetables taste great tossed with a little ghee or extra-virgin olive oil, seasoned with salt and pepper, and cooked in a 400°F oven until they are just tender. Best of all, you can work on other parts of the meal while the vegetables are in the oven.

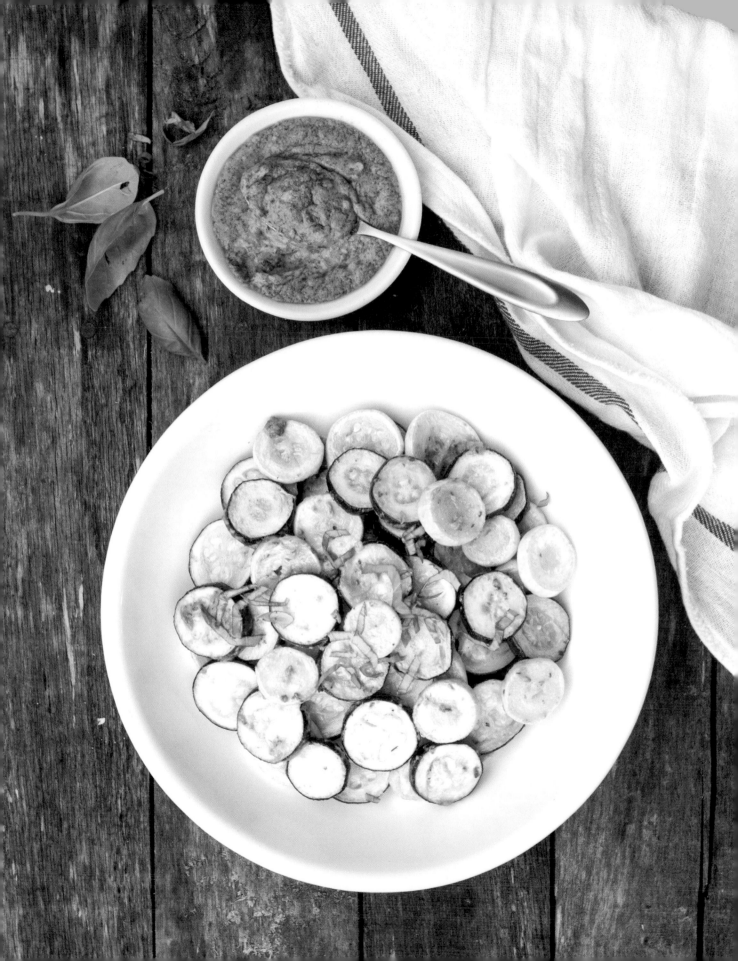

SEASONED CAULIFLOWER RICE

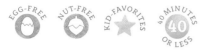

EGG-FREE · NUT-FREE · KID FAVORITES · 40 MINUTES OR LESS

Cauliflower rice is the Paleo version of white rice, and no, it does not taste like rice. It tastes like cauliflower shaped like rice. If you don't like the taste of cauliflower, then adding seasonings can help, or try making a heavily seasoned dish like Mexican Cauliflower Rice (page 204) or Fried Cauliflower Rice (page 202). You don't want to cook cauliflower rice as long as you would regular rice, so if you're incorporating it into one of your favorite recipes, make sure to cook the other ingredients first and add the cauliflower close to the end of the cooking process.

Prep Time: 15 minutes   Cook Time: 10 minutes   Yield: 4 to 6 servings

1 large head cauliflower (about 2 pounds), chopped into 1-inch pieces

2 tablespoons ghee (page 320), lard (page 322), or tallow (page 324)

½ cup chopped white onion

2 cloves garlic, minced

¼ teaspoon fine sea salt

⅛ teaspoon ground black pepper

3 tablespoons chopped fresh parsley, for garnish (optional)

1. Working in small batches, pulse the cauliflower pieces a few times in a food processor or blender, until the pieces are the size and shape of grains of rice, being careful not to overblend (bigger pieces are better than smaller). After each batch, transfer the riced cauliflower to a large mixing bowl. If your riced cauliflower is damp, wrap it in a few paper towels or a clean kitchen towel and wring out any excess moisture, then return it to the mixing bowl.

2. Heat the ghee in a large skillet over medium-high heat. Add the onion and sauté for 3 minutes, then add the garlic and cook for another minute, or until the onions are just softened. Add the riced cauliflower and stir, sprinkle with the salt and pepper, and stir to combine. Sauté for another 3 minutes, or until the cauliflower is slightly tender but not mushy. Taste and add additional salt and pepper if desired.

3. To serve, transfer the cauliflower to a serving bowl and top with chopped fresh parsley, if desired.

TRY THIS!
To make a cilantro lime version of this cauliflower rice, add the juice and zest of 1 large lime at the same time as the salt and pepper, and swap the parsley for chopped fresh cilantro.

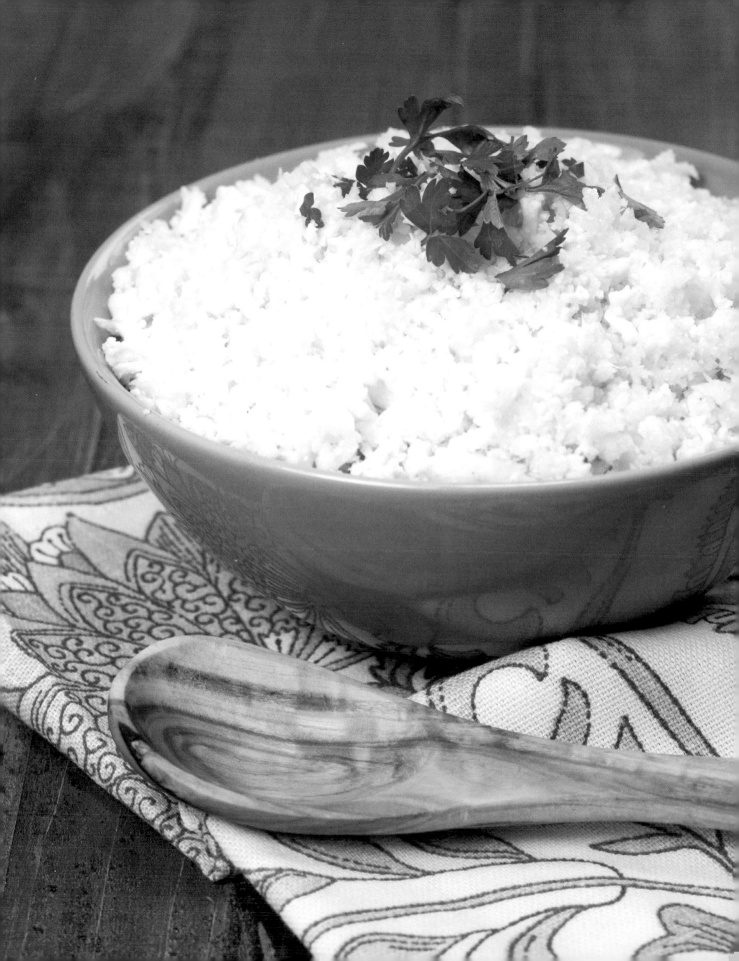

FRIED CAULIFLOWER RICE

If you want all the flavors of fried rice in a Paleo-friendly form, then this is the recipe for you. Most of the people I have made this for can't even tell that they aren't eating rice! If you have picky eaters in your house who won't touch regular cauliflower rice, they may just fall in love with this dish. And if they don't, that's okay—that just means there's more for you to enjoy.

NUT-FREE KID-FAVORITES 40 MINUTES OR LESS

Prep Time: 10 minutes   **Cook Time:** 15 minutes   **Yield:** 4 to 6 servings

1 medium head cauliflower (about 1½ pounds), chopped into 1-inch pieces

4 tablespoons ghee (page 320), lard (page 322), or tallow (page 324), divided

1 small onion, chopped (about ½ cup)

4 medium carrots, peeled and chopped (about 2 cups)

2 cloves garlic, minced

4 large eggs, beaten

¼ teaspoon fine sea salt

¼ teaspoon ground black pepper

½ teaspoon sesame oil

¼ cup plus 2 tablespoons coconut aminos or soy sauce substitute (page 283)

½ teaspoon fish sauce

2 green onions, chopped, for garnish (optional)

1. Working in small batches, pulse the cauliflower pieces a few times in a food processor or blender, until the pieces are the size and shape of grains of rice, being careful not to overblend (bigger pieces are better than smaller). After each batch, transfer the riced cauliflower to a large mixing bowl. If your riced cauliflower is damp, wrap it in a few paper towels or a clean kitchen towel and wring out any excess moisture, then return it to the mixing bowl.

2. Melt 2 tablespoons of ghee in a large skillet over medium-high heat. Add the onion and carrots and cook for 3 minutes. Add the garlic and cook for 1 more minute. Transfer the vegetable mixture to a large mixing bowl.

3. Melt 1 tablespoon of ghee in the pan, then add the beaten eggs and scramble until they are lightly browned. Sprinkle the salt and pepper over the eggs, then transfer the eggs to the bowl with the vegetables.

4. Melt the remaining 1 tablespoon of ghee in the pan. Add the riced cauliflower and toss to coat. Cook for 5 to 7 minutes, stirring only every couple minutes so that the pieces on the bottom are allowed to get brown and crispy. Add the vegetable and egg mixture back to the pan and stir to combine. Add the sesame oil, coconut aminos, and fish sauce and cook for 1 more minute, stirring frequently. Remove from the heat and add additional salt and pepper to taste. Top with the chopped green onions, if desired, and serve.

TRY THIS!

The sky is the limit when it comes to variations for this recipe. Chopped mushrooms, bell peppers, asparagus, broccoli, and broccoli slaw are all great vegetable additions. A sprinkle of toasted sesame seeds or chopped cashews will add a little crunch. For added protein, try mixing in 12 ounces of ground beef or chopped cooked chicken, pork, or shrimp right before serving.

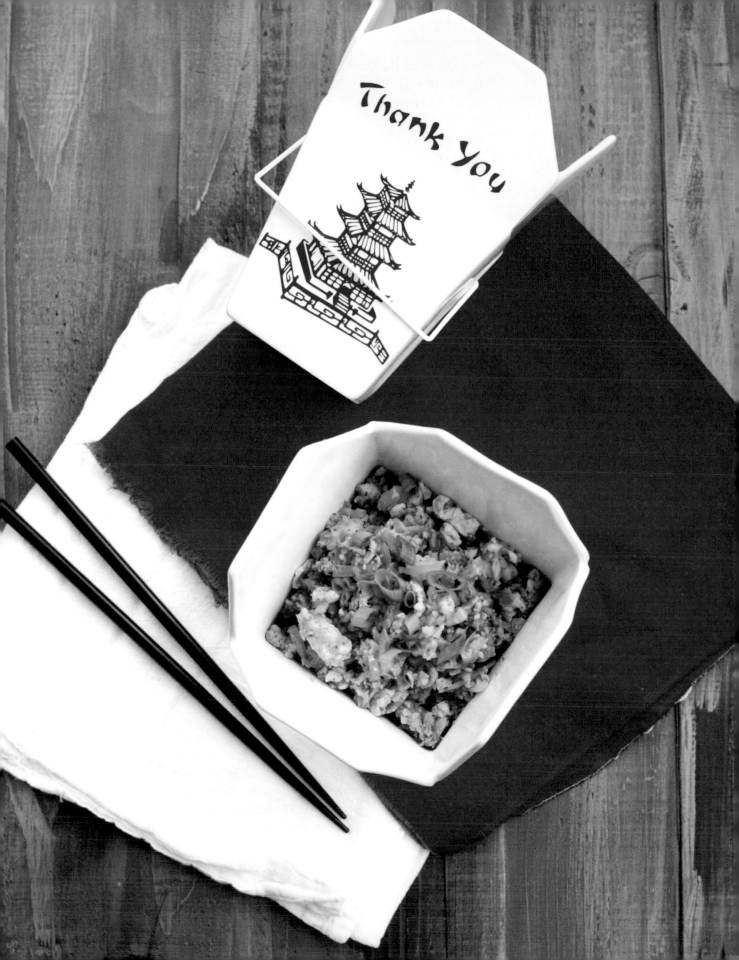

MEXICAN CAULIFLOWER RICE

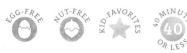

EGG-FREE · NUT-FREE · KID-FAVORITES · 40 MINUTES OR LESS

If you are craving the rice that is served at your favorite Mexican restaurant, then this dish is for you! In this recipe, tomatoes, garlic, onion, and a good helping of spices come together to make a flavorful and tasty side dish. Serve it alongside Tex-Mex-Style Pork Chops (page 148) or Barbacoa (page 80).

Prep Time: 10 minutes   Cook Time: 10 minutes   Yield: 4 servings

1 large head cauliflower (about 2 pounds), chopped into 1-inch pieces

3 tablespoons ghee (page 320), lard (page 322), or tallow (page 324)

1 small white onion, chopped (about ½ cup)

3 cloves garlic, minced

½ teaspoon fine sea salt

¼ teaspoon ground black pepper

½ teaspoon ground cumin

½ teaspoon paprika

¼ cup tomato paste

¼ cup chopped fresh cilantro, plus more for garnish (optional)

1 large tomato, chopped (about ¾ cup)

2 limes, quartered, for serving

1. Working in small batches, pulse the cauliflower pieces a few times in a food processor or blender, until the pieces are the size and shape of rice, being careful not to overblend (bigger pieces are better than smaller). After each batch, transfer the riced cauliflower to a large mixing bowl. If your riced cauliflower is damp, wrap it in a few paper towels or a clean kitchen towel and wring out any excess moisture, then return it to the mixing bowl.

2. Melt the ghee in a large skillet over medium-high heat. Add the chopped onion to the pan and sauté for 4 minutes. Add the garlic and sauté for another minute.

3. Add the riced cauliflower to the pan and stir. Add the salt, pepper, cumin, and paprika to the pan and stir to combine. Cook for another 2 to 3 minutes, stirring occasionally.

4. Add the tomato paste, cilantro, and chopped tomato and stir until all of the liquid is absorbed. Cook for another 2 to 3 minutes, then taste and adjust the seasonings as desired. Serve with a sprinkle of fresh cilantro, if desired, and some lime wedges.

TRY THIS!
For a chunkier version with more veggies, add ½ cup chopped carrots, ½ cup chopped red bell pepper, and/ or 1 seeded and diced jalapeño at the same time as the onion.

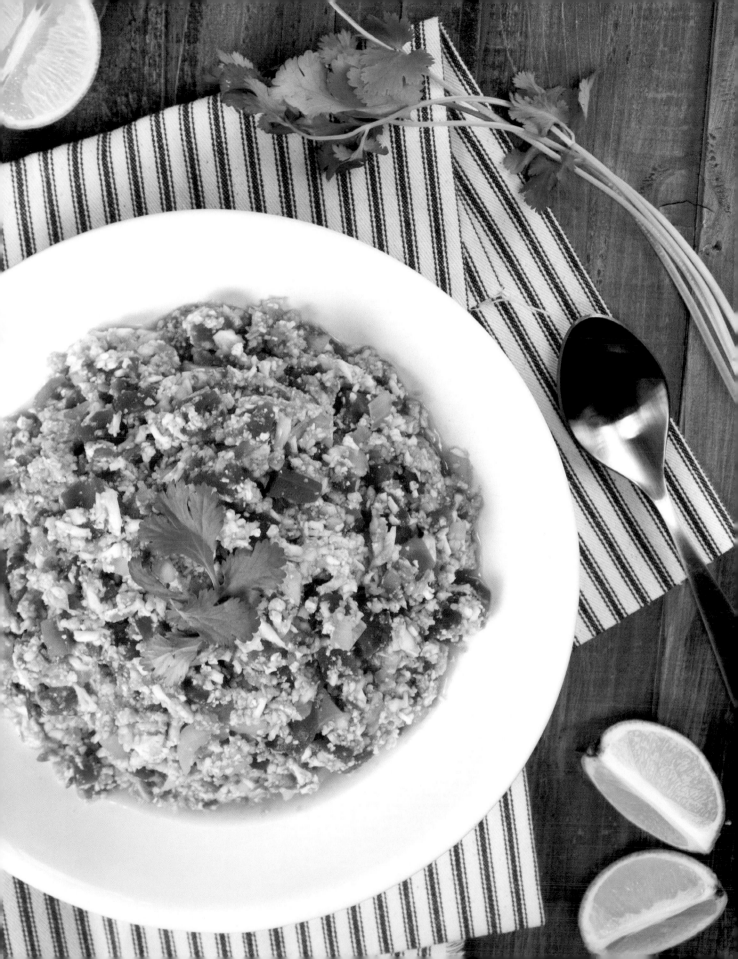

SESAME GINGER
BROCCOLINI

This is yet another recipe that showcases how just a few spices can bring out the natural flavor of a vegetable. Broccolini is almost identical to broccoli but has smaller florets and longer, thinner stalks. If you can't find broccolini, broccoli will work just as well.

Prep Time: 2 minutes   **Cook Time:** 15 minutes   **Yield:** 4 to 6 servings

2 teaspoons sesame seeds, for garnish

1 tablespoon ghee (page 320), lard (page 322), or tallow (page 324)

2 cloves garlic, finely chopped

1 pound broccolini

⅓ cup beef stock (page 310)

1 tablespoon coconut aminos or soy sauce substitute (page 283)

1 teaspoon sesame oil

1 teaspoon ground ginger

¼ teaspoon fine sea salt

⅛ teaspoon ground black pepper

1. In a medium saucepan over medium-high heat, toast the sesame seeds for 30 seconds, or until lightly browned. Remove from the pan and set aside.

2. In the same pan, melt the ghee, then add the garlic and sauté for 1 minute. Add the broccolini and toss to coat, then add the stock. Cover and reduce the heat to low. Simmer for 10 minutes, or until the broccolini is tender.

3. Add the coconut aminos, sesame oil, ginger, salt, and pepper. Toss to coat and cook for 1 more minute, uncovered.

4. Transfer the broccolini and sauce to a serving platter, top with the toasted sesame seeds, and serve.

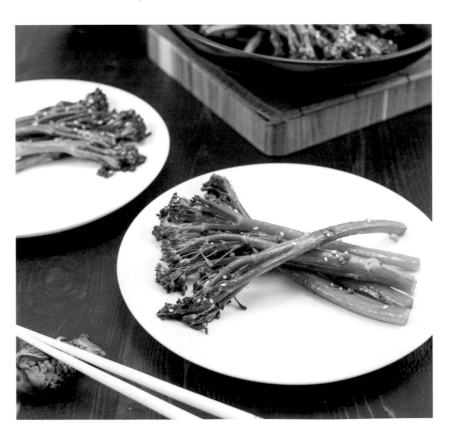

SLOW COOKER APPLESAUCE

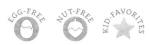

EGG-FREE · NUT-FREE · KID-FAVORITES

Homemade applesauce made with fresh apples is a thousand times better than any store-bought brand. I like to combine different types of apples, such as Golden Delicious and Granny Smith, to give the applesauce a mix of tart and sweet flavors.

Prep Time: 10 minutes   **Cook Time:** 3 hours   **Yield:** 4 to 6 servings

3 pounds apples, peeled, cored, and chopped

¼ cup water

⅓ cup raw honey, warmed if solid

¼ teaspoon ground cinnamon

1. Place the apples in a slow cooker, then add the water, honey, and cinnamon. Cook on high for 2½ to 3 hours, until the apples are tender.

2. Mash the apples with a potato masher or blend with an immersion blender until the desired consistency is reached. Serve warm, or allow to cool to room temperature and then store in the refrigerator in a sealed container for up to 3 days.

TRY THIS!

Try adding a tablespoon of freshly squeezed lemon juice and a dash of nutmeg to the slow cooker.

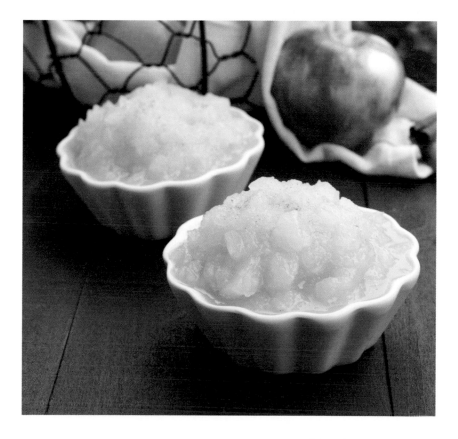

SPICY SMASHED SWEET POTATOES

I meet so many people who are starting out on a Paleo diet and don't know what to cook, and a good number of them end up eating the same thing for dinner every night: a piece of plain grilled steak or chicken and a plain baked sweet potato. Eating the same food every day for a week or two is bound to put you in a rut. Don't get me wrong, plain sweet potatoes are delicious, but sprinkling them with a mixture of sweet and spicy seasoning and letting the edges get crispy in the oven really knocks them out of the park.

Prep Time: 15 minutes   Cook Time: 45 minutes   Yield: 4 to 6 servings

FOR THE SPICE MIXTURE

½ teaspoon chili powder

½ teaspoon ground cumin

½ teaspoon garlic powder

½ teaspoon onion powder

½ teaspoon paprika

½ teaspoon fine sea salt

⅛ teaspoon ground black pepper

3 medium red-skinned sweet potatoes (about 1 pound)

2 tablespoons ghee (page 320) or extra-virgin olive oil

1 tablespoon raw honey, warmed if solid

1 tablespoon chopped fresh parsley, for garnish (optional)

1. Preheat the oven to 400°F. Line a 9-by-13-inch baking sheet with parchment paper or a baking mat.

2. Mix together all the ingredients for the spice mixture in a small bowl and set aside.

3. Poke each sweet potato with a fork 3 or 4 times and place directly on the oven rack. Cook for 25 to 35 minutes, until the sweet potatoes are just tender but not mushy (the cooking time will vary depending on how thick the potatoes are).

4. Take the potatoes out of the oven and turn the oven to broil. Carefully peel the potatoes, cut into 1½-inch-thick slices, and place the slices on the prepared baking sheet, spaced a few inches apart. With a cup or a small flat-bottomed pan, gently press down on each sweet potato circle until the sides split open slightly. This will allow the edges to get nice and crispy in the oven.

5. Whisk together the ghee and honey in a small bowl, then drizzle half of the sauce over the sweet potatoes. Sprinkle half of the spice mixture over the sweet potatoes.

6. Return the potatoes to the oven and broil for 3 minutes, or until the edges start to caramelize and turn a dark brown color, checking them often so they do not burn. Take the pan out and carefully flip each potato slice over. Drizzle the remaining sauce over the sweet potatoes and then sprinkle the remaining spice mixture on top. Return to the oven and broil for another 3 to 4 minutes, until the edges are crispy and browned. Serve garnished with the parsley, if desired.

KITCHEN TIP

Recipes are guidelines; they're not carved in stone. If it's not a main ingredient, you can usually omit it or substitute something else and the dish will still turn out fine. If you change something and it works, always write it down! That way you will be reminded how to re-create it next time.

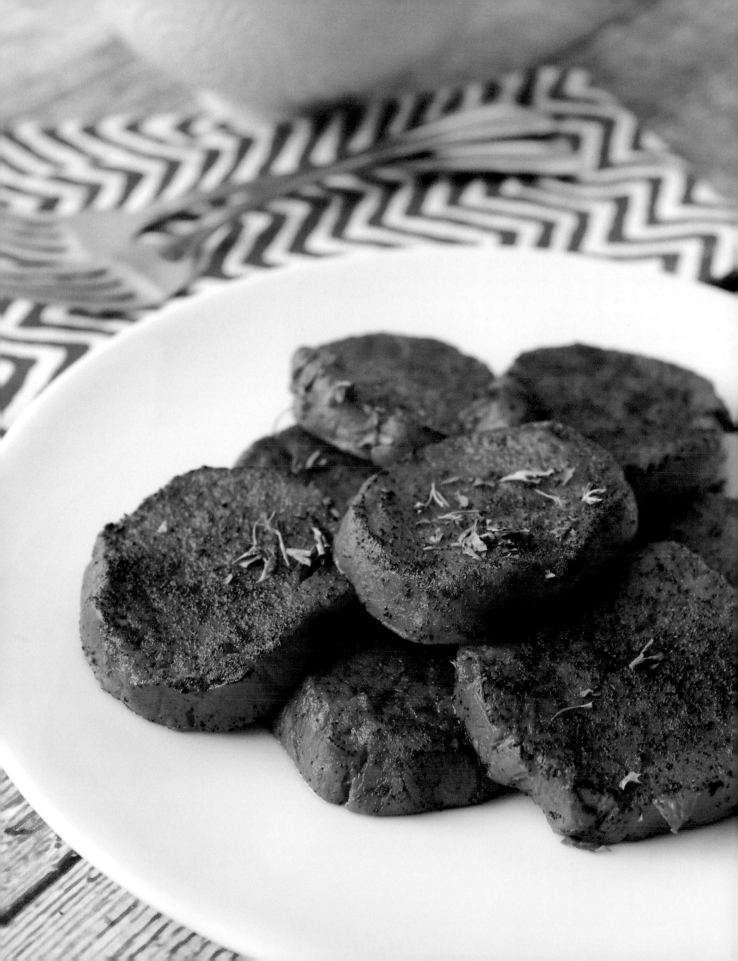

TORTILLAS

EGG-FREE · KID-FAVORITES · 40 MINUTES OR LESS

Since I was born and raised in southern California, tortillas have always been a staple in my life. I never really liked bread that much growing up (I know, I'm weird), but living a life without an occasional tortilla was just not an option. These tortillas mimic a traditional flour tortilla, and they will stay flexible if kept warm.

Make sure to measure your flours by dipping the measuring cup into the flour and scraping the top with a knife. Pouring the flour from the bag into the cup will result in much less flour in the dish.

Prep Time: 10 minutes   **Cook Time:** 15 minutes   **Yield:** 8 tortillas

1 cup almond flour (page 316) or sunflower seed flour

1 cup tapioca flour, plus more for dusting the work surface

½ teaspoon fine sea salt

¼ cup light olive oil

¼ cup warm water

1. In a medium-sized mixing bowl, whisk together the almond flour, tapioca flour, and salt until well combined.

2. Slowly drizzle the olive oil into the flour mixture while stirring with a fork until it's incorporated into the flour (the dough will be chunky). Add the warm water to the bowl and stir until well combined.

3. Sprinkle a cutting board lightly with tapioca flour and transfer the dough to the cutting board. Knead the dough for about 1 minute, or until it's slightly moist but not sticky. If the dough is too wet, add more almond flour, a tablespoon at a time. If it's too dry, add a little more water, ½ teaspoon at a time.

4. Place a large skillet over medium-high heat to heat while you make the tortillas. Separate the dough into 8 equal pieces and knead each piece with your hands for about 30 seconds, then roll it into a ball and place back in the mixing bowl. Keep the bowl covered with a dish towel or plastic wrap so the dough does not dry out.

5. One at a time, flatten each ball in the palm of your hand to a thick disk, then place it between two pieces of parchment paper and flatten using a tortilla press or a rolling pin. The tortillas should be about 6 inches in diameter.

6. Place the tortilla into the hot skillet and cook until bubbly, about 30 seconds. Flip the tortilla over and cook the other side for 30 seconds to 1 minute. Do not overcook: you want the tortilla to be soft with small golden brown spots on the surface.

7. Transfer the cooked tortilla to a tortilla warmer or lay it between two clean kitchen towels. Repeat steps 5 and 6 with the remaining dough balls. Serve right away.

KITCHEN TIP

If you're having trouble peeling the tortillas from the parchment paper, try this: Take the edge of the top piece of paper and gently peel it off. Hold the bottom piece of paper with both hands, flip it over, and place the tortilla side onto the hot pan. Allow the tortilla to cook for about 20 seconds, then take the edge of the parchment paper and gently peel it away. Continue to cook as directed.

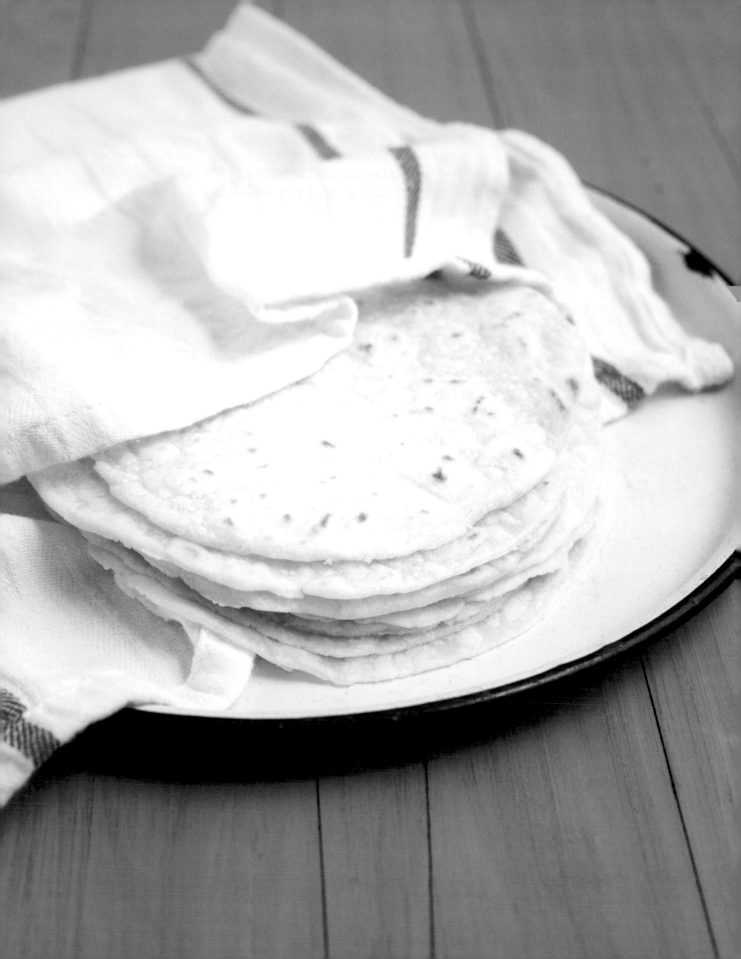

SUMMER VEGETABLE CASSEROLE

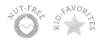

I really hate naming recipes, mostly because people get so worked up over names. Especially names that aren't even that helpful when you're deciding whether you want to make the recipe. If you call a strata a "gratin" or a casserole a "quiche," some folks go into a tailspin. If I had it my way, all recipes would have descriptive and helpful titles like "Super Delicious Way to Get a Lot of Fresh Vegetables into One Dish." That's a lot more useful than "casserole," if you ask me. And speaking of useful, make sure to salt the zucchini ahead of time, as instructed—that's key for this recipe because it draws out the excess water; otherwise, you will have a small swimming pool at the bottom of the dish.

Prep Time: 20 minutes, plus 20 minutes to salt the vegetables   **Cook Time:** 40 minutes   **Yield:** 6 servings

1 large red-skinned sweet potato (about ¾ pound), peeled and grated

1½ teaspoons fine sea salt, divided

1 large zucchini (about ⅓ pound), cut into ¼-inch slices

3 tablespoons ghee (page 320), lard (page 322), or tallow (page 324), divided

½ cup chopped onion (about 1 small)

1 clove garlic, minced

4 cups broccoli florets (about 2 medium heads)

2 large carrots, peeled and thinly sliced

1 cup sliced cremini or white mushrooms (about 4 ounces whole)

4 large eggs, beaten

¾ cup coconut milk (page 314)

¾ teaspoon ground black pepper, divided

1. In a medium-sized mixing bowl, toss the grated sweet potato with ½ teaspoon of the salt and set aside. Place the zucchini slices in a colander, sprinkle with ¼ teaspoon of the salt, and toss to coat. Place the colander over a larger bowl and allow the zucchini to drain for 20 minutes to remove any excess moisture. Line a cutting board with paper towels or a clean kitchen towel and layer the zucchini slices on top. Press them gently with additional paper towels to remove as much liquid as possible.

2. Preheat the oven to 350°F.

3. Melt 2 tablespoons of the ghee in a large skillet over medium-high heat. Add the onion and sauté for 3 minutes, then add the garlic, broccoli, carrots, mushrooms, and zucchini and cook for 1 more minute, tossing to combine. Transfer the vegetables to a 9-inch square baking dish or 2-quart casserole dish.

4. In a medium-sized mixing bowl, whisk together the eggs, coconut milk, ½ teaspoon of the salt, and ½ teaspoon of the pepper. Pour the mixture evenly over the vegetables.

5. Use a few paper towels or a clean kitchen towel to squeeze any excess liquid from the grated sweet potato. Drain the bowl of any liquid, then return the potatoes to the bowl. Melt the remaining 1 tablespoon of ghee, then drizzle it over the potato. Add the remaining ¼ teaspoon of salt and remaining ¼ teaspoon of pepper, tossing to coat. Sprinkle the grated sweet potato evenly over the top of the vegetable mixture, then gently pat down to create a flat surface.

6. Bake for 30 minutes, then turn the oven to broil and cook for another 2 to 4 minutes, until the egg mixture is fully set and the sweet potatoes are lightly browned. Remove from the oven and let cool for at least 5 minutes, then slice into squares and serve.

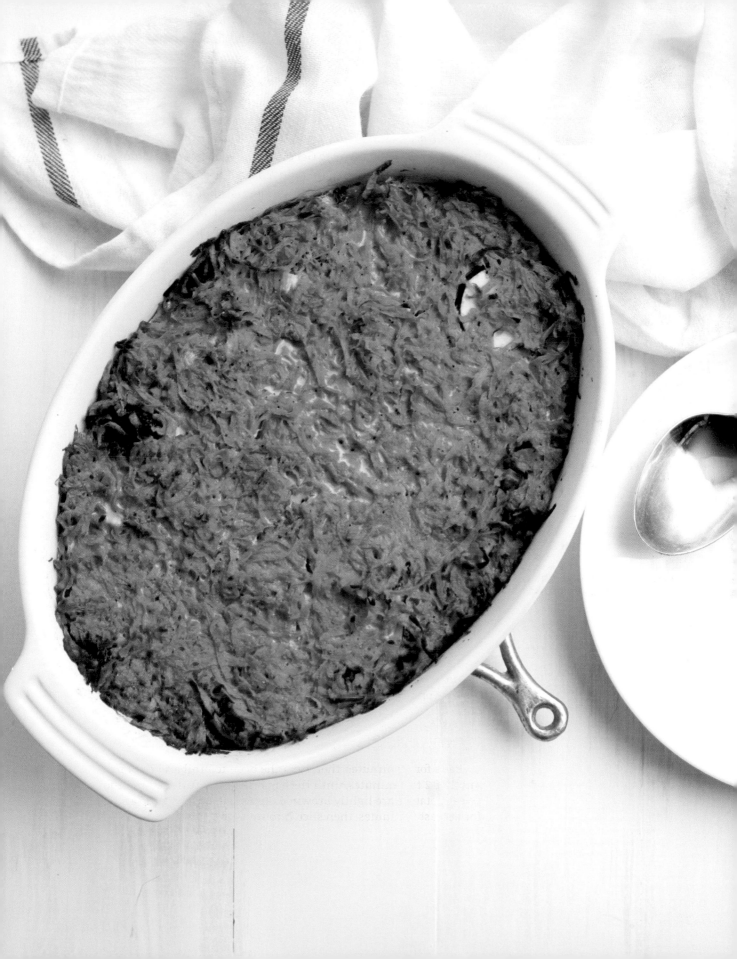

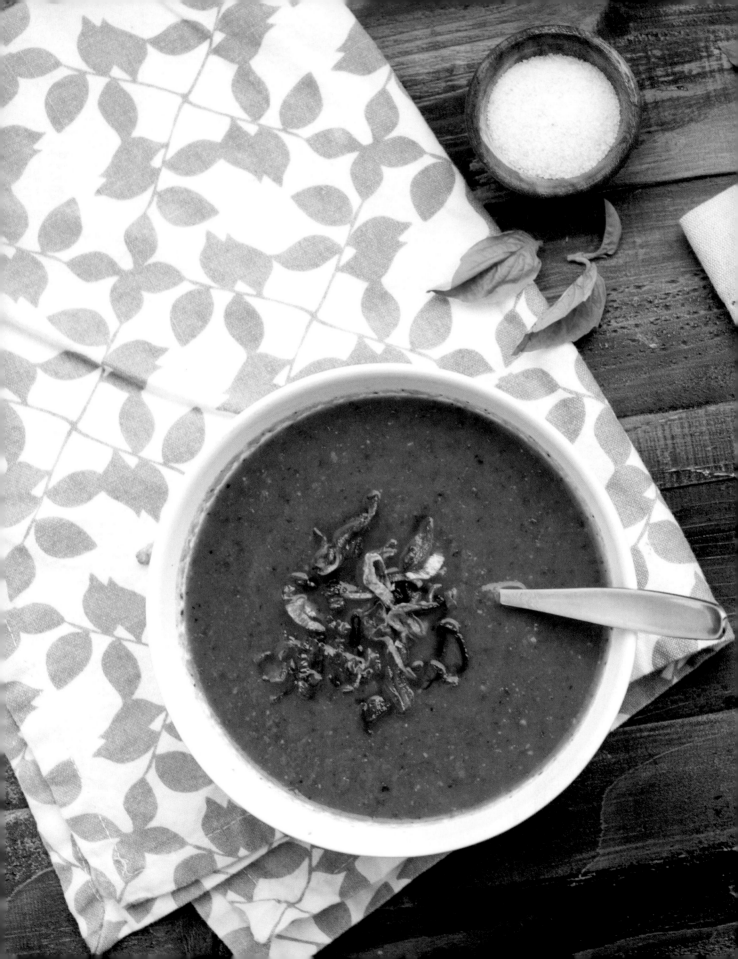

soups, stews, and salads

ASIAN SESAME CHICKEN SALAD

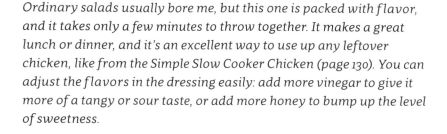

EGG-FREE · KID-FAVORITES · 40 MINUTES OR LESS

Ordinary salads usually bore me, but this one is packed with flavor, and it takes only a few minutes to throw together. It makes a great lunch or dinner, and it's an excellent way to use up any leftover chicken, like from the Simple Slow Cooker Chicken (page 130). You can adjust the flavors in the dressing easily: add more vinegar to give it more of a tangy or sour taste, or add more honey to bump up the level of sweetness.

Prep Time: 15 minutes   **Cook Time:** 5 minutes   **Yield:** 4 servings

FOR THE DRESSING

⅓ cup plus 1 tablespoon apple cider vinegar

3 tablespoons raw honey

⅓ cup extra-virgin olive oil

1½ teaspoons sesame oil

½ teaspoon fine sea salt

¼ teaspoon ground black pepper

¼ teaspoon ground ginger

1 (18-ounce) bag broccoli slaw, or 4½ cups julienned broccoli stems and 1½ cups julienned carrots

1 medium red onion, finely chopped (about 1 cup)

⅓ cup chopped fresh cilantro, plus more for garnish

1 pound boneless skinless chicken breasts, grilled and chopped into bite-sized pieces

⅓ cup sliced almonds

¼ cup sesame seeds, for garnish

1. Make the dressing: Place the vinegar and honey in a small saucepan over medium heat. Stir until the honey dissolves, about 2 minutes, then reduce the heat to low. Very slowly drizzle the olive oil into the pan, whisking constantly until the oil and vinegar mixture are well combined. Next drizzle in the sesame oil, whisking constantly until well combined. Add the salt, pepper, and ginger and stir, then remove from the heat and set aside.

2. In a large mixing bowl, combine the broccoli slaw, red onion, cilantro, chicken pieces, and almonds and toss. Drizzle the dressing over the top and toss again until well coated. Add additional salt and pepper to taste.

3. Sprinkle with chopped cilantro and sesame seeds before serving.

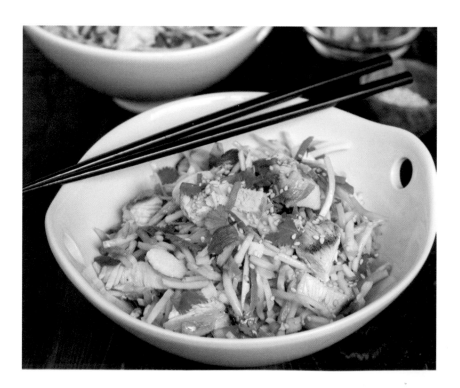

BROCCOLI RAISIN SALAD

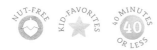

This is a good recipe to keep around for when you need to bring a dish to a picnic or potluck. You just need to do a bit of chopping, and then you have a tasty salad that everyone can enjoy. If I'm making it a day ahead, I like to hold off on adding the bacon until the day it is served, so the bacon stays extra crispy.

Prep Time: 15 minutes   **Yield:** 6 servings

FOR THE DRESSING

1 cup mayonnaise (page 278)

3 tablespoons apple cider vinegar

3 tablespoons raw honey

2 teaspoons freshly squeezed lemon juice

1 teaspoon fine sea salt

1 teaspoon ground black pepper

2 large heads broccoli, chopped into bite-sized pieces (about 5½ cups)

½ pound thick-cut bacon, cooked and crumbled

½ cup raw shelled sunflower seeds

½ cup finely chopped red onion (about 1 small)

½ cup raisins

1. Combine all the ingredients for the dressing in a blender or food processor and blend until smooth.

2. Mix together the broccoli, bacon, sunflower seeds, red onion, and raisins in a large bowl. Pour the dressing on top and toss until well coated. Serve right away or cover and place in the refrigerator until ready to serve.

TRY THIS!

For extra crunch and a nutty flavor, try adding ¼ cup of coarsely chopped toasted walnuts.

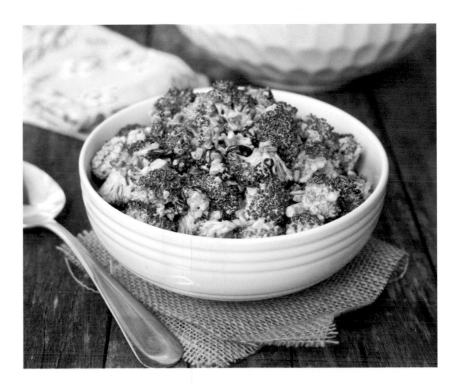

BRUSSELS SPROUTS *and* BACON SALAD

If you're tired of having coleslaw at every picnic and barbecue, these thinly sliced Brussels sprouts with tangy dressing are a great alternative. If you're making this dish ahead of time, prep the salad and dressing and wait until right before serving to combine them.

Prep Time: 20 minutes   **Cook Time:** 5 minutes   **Yield:** 4 servings

1 pound Brussels sprouts

6 slices thick-cut bacon

FOR THE DRESSING

1 small shallot, minced

2 tablespoons freshly squeezed lemon juice

2 tablespoons apple cider vinegar

1½ tablespoons raw honey

1 tablespoon extra-virgin olive oil

2 teaspoons prepared Dijon mustard

¼ teaspoon ground black pepper

½ cup slivered almonds

½ cup dried blueberries

1. Thinly slice the Brussels sprouts crosswise to just above the stem, which you can discard. Toss out any tough pieces, and break apart the chopped layers so that you have mostly thin ribbons. Set aside.

2. In a large skillet over medium-high heat, cook the bacon until crispy. Transfer the bacon to a paper towel–lined plate to drain, then crumble and set aside. Transfer 2 tablespoons of the bacon drippings from the pan to a medium-sized mixing bowl.

3. Make the dressing: To the bacon drippings, add the shallot, lemon juice, vinegar, honey, olive oil, mustard, and pepper, and whisk to combine. Taste and adjust the seasonings as desired (remember that the bacon will add some saltiness and the blueberries will add some sweetness to the finished dish). Set the dressing aside.

4. Combine the sliced Brussels sprouts, almonds, and dried blueberries in a large serving bowl. Pour the dressing over the salad and toss to coat. Crumble the cooked bacon and sprinkle over the top to serve.

TRY THIS!

If you like tart flavors, substitute dried cranberries for the blueberries. Dress up your salad even more by adding 2 chopped hard-boiled eggs or 1 small avocado, halved, pitted, and chopped.

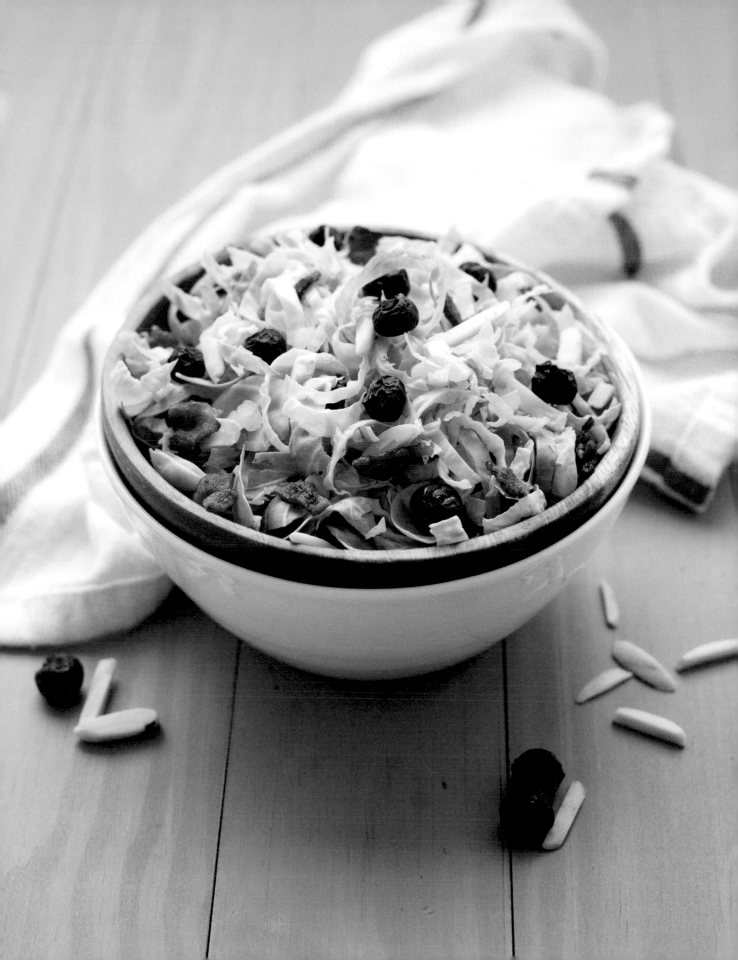

SPINACH *and* BACON SALAD

I have to confess, I am a big fan of bacon, especially the thick-cut variety. This spinach and bacon salad is simple enough to make a nice side dish, but with the addition of some grilled chicken or salmon, it makes a hearty meal. The tanginess of the vinegar combined with the sweetness of the honey and saltiness of the bacon hit a flavor home run.

Prep Time: 10 minutes   **Cook Time:** 20 minutes   **Yield:** 6 servings

4 large eggs

¾ teaspoon fine sea salt, divided

10 ounces fresh baby spinach, rinsed and dried

8 ounces grape tomatoes

8 large white mushrooms, sliced

1 small red onion, thinly sliced (about ½ cup)

4 slices thick-cut bacon

3 tablespoons apple cider vinegar

1 tablespoon raw honey

1 teaspoon prepared Dijon mustard

¼ teaspoon ground black pepper

1. To hard-boil the eggs, place the eggs and ½ teaspoon of the salt in a medium-sized saucepan and fill with enough cold water to cover by 1 inch. Bring to a rolling boil over medium-high heat. Turn off the stove, keeping the pan on the burner. Cover the pan and allow to sit for 12 minutes. Transfer the eggs to a bowl of ice water to stop the cooking process. Allow the eggs to cool for 5 minutes, then peel them under a gentle stream of running water. Slice in half lengthwise and set aside.

2. While the eggs cook, toss together the spinach, tomatoes, mushrooms, and onion in a large mixing bowl and set aside.

3. In a large skillet over medium-high heat, cook the bacon until crispy. Transfer to a paper towel–lined plate to drain, leaving the bacon drippings in the pan, then crumble and set aside.

4. Transfer ¼ cup of the bacon drippings to a small saucepan over medium-high heat. Add the vinegar, honey, mustard, pepper, and the remaining ¼ teaspoon of salt to the pan and whisk until well combined. Cook for 1 to 2 minutes, until the sauce is warm.

5. Pour the sauce over the spinach mixture and toss to combine. Divide the salad evenly on 6 serving plates and top with the crumbled bacon and sliced eggs before serving.

TRY THIS!
For extra crunch, try sprinkling ½ cup of toasted sliced almonds over the finished salad.

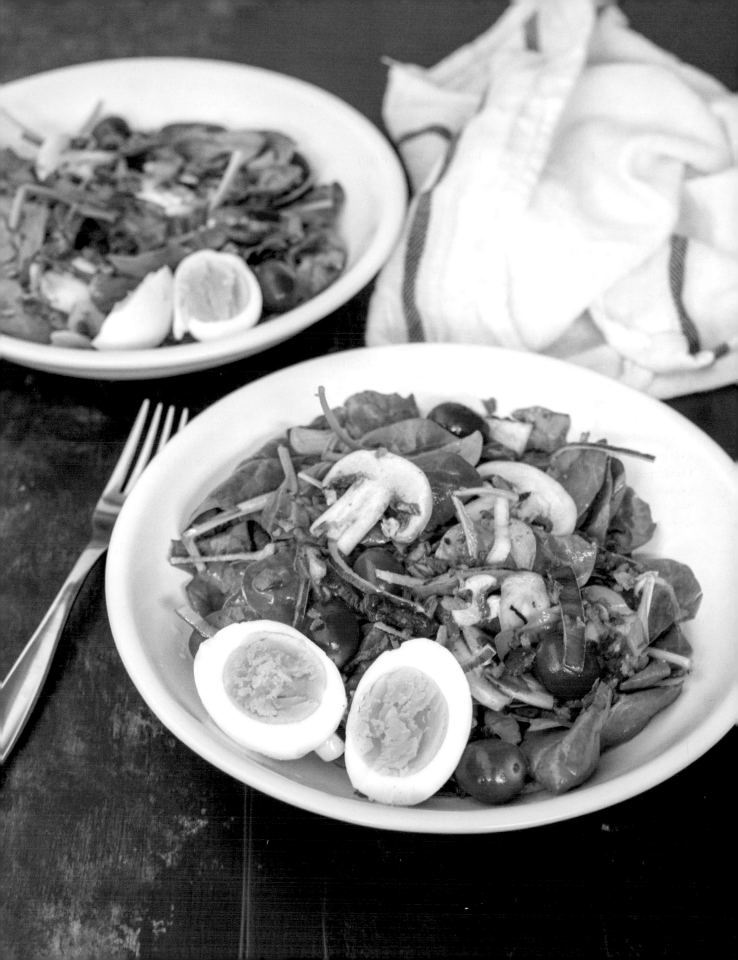

TOMATO
AVOCADO STACK
with CRISPY
PROSCIUTTO

This recipe is a Paleo-friendly spin on caprese salad that uses creamy avocado in place of cheese. The addition of crispy prosciutto gives it a salty crunch, and a drizzle of balsamic vinegar adds a sweet and tangy flavor.

Prep Time: 15 minutes   **Cook Time:** 5 minutes   **Yield:** 4 servings

1 teaspoon ghee (page 320), lard (page 322), or tallow (page 324)

2 ounces prosciutto, thinly sliced

2 large tomatoes (about 1 pound)

½ teaspoon fine sea salt

¼ teaspoon ground black pepper

2 large avocados (about ¾ pound), halved, pitted, and peeled

4 tablespoons extra-virgin olive oil

4 tablespoons balsamic vinegar

½ packed cup fresh basil, thinly sliced

1. Melt the ghee in a medium skillet over medium-high heat. Add the prosciutto slices and cook for 2 minutes, or just until crispy, stirring frequently. Transfer to a paper towel–lined plate and set aside.

2. Remove the stems from the tops of the tomatoes. Core each tomato by inserting the tip of a small knife into the top, with the knife pointed at an angle toward the center of the tomato. Hold the tomato and cut in a circular motion all the way around the top middle of the fruit. Remove the tomato core and discard it. Cut each tomato into 6 to 8 slices and sprinkle the salt and pepper over the slices.

3. Cut each avocado half into 6 to 8 slices. Create 4 stacks by layering the tomato and avocado slices (3 or 4 slices per stack). Drizzle each stack with 1 tablespoon olive oil and 1 tablespoon balsamic vinegar. Sprinkle each stack with the crispy prosciutto and sliced basil and serve.

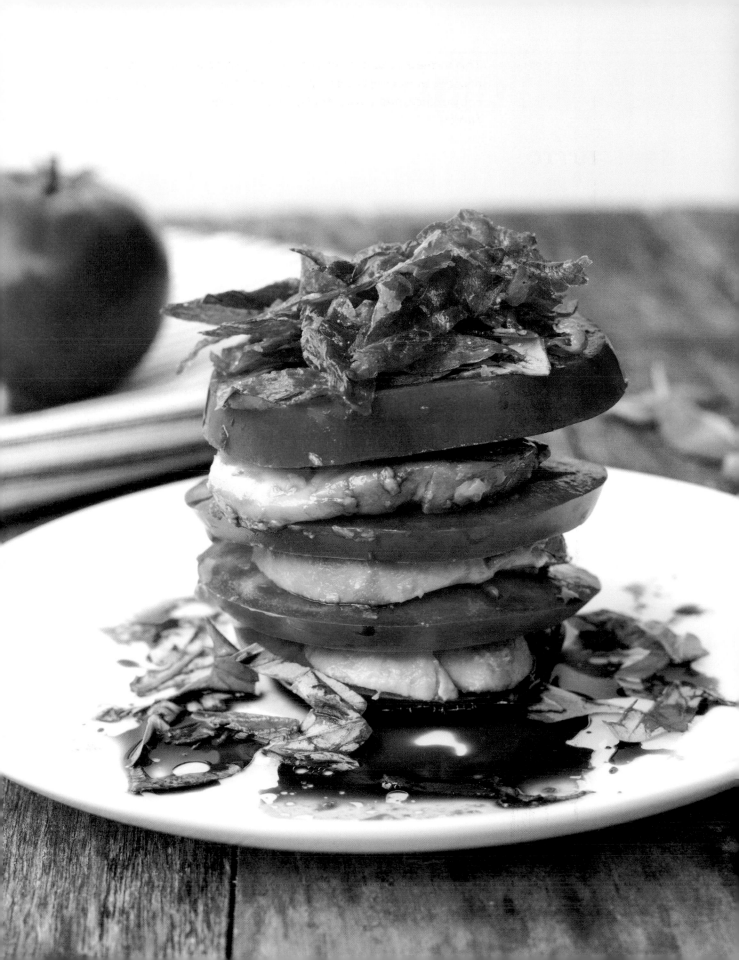

CIOPPINO

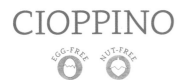

EGG-FREE NUT-FREE

Cioppino is a stew made from a variety of seafood, such as fish, mussels, clams, shrimp, crab, and scallops. The seafood is cooked in a savory tomato stock seasoned with herbs and spices. This was a dish I grew up eating frequently, and my family still enjoys it to this day. You can tailor this recipe based on whatever seafood you like or is in season. Don't like mussels? Add some more shrimp. Don't like clams? Add some more fish.

Prep Time: 15 minutes   Cook Time: 40 minutes   Yield: 6 servings

2 tablespoons ghee (page 320), lard (page 322), or tallow (page 324)

1 small onion, chopped (about ½ cup)

3 cloves garlic, minced

¾ cup tomato paste

2 large tomatoes (about 1 pound), chopped (about 1½ cups)

6 cups fish stock (page 312) or chicken stock (page 310)

2 teaspoons dried basil

1 teaspoon dried thyme

½ teaspoon crushed red pepper

2 teaspoons fine sea salt

½ teaspoon ground black pepper

2 bay leaves

1½ pounds fish fillets (cod, halibut, or mahi mahi), cut into 1½-inch pieces

1 pound clams

1 pound mussels, cleaned and debearded

½ pound medium shrimp, peeled and deveined, tails removed

⅓ cup chopped fresh parsley, for garnish (optional)

1 lemon, quartered, for serving

1. Melt the ghee in a large stockpot over medium-high heat. Add the onion and garlic and sauté for 4 to 5 minutes, until the onion is tender. Add the tomato paste and stir to combine. Add the chopped tomatoes, stock, basil, thyme, crushed red pepper, salt, black pepper, and bay leaves and stir. Bring to a boil, then reduce the heat to low. Cover and simmer for 20 minutes.

2. Add the fish, clams, mussels, and shrimp to the pot and simmer for another 5 to 8 minutes, until the clams are open and the rest of the seafood is cooked through. Taste and add additional salt and pepper if desired. Remove the bay leaves, ladle the stew into bowls, sprinkle with parsley, if desired, and serve with lemon wedges.

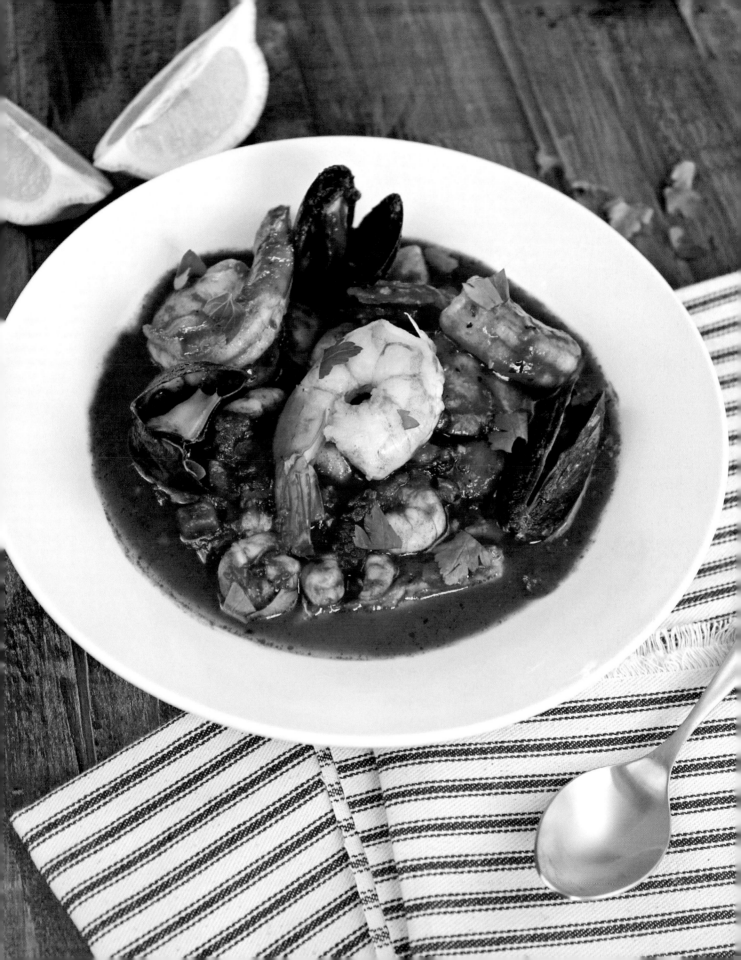

CREAMY
MUSHROOM
SOUP

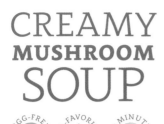

Mushroom soup is a classic comfort food. This recipe makes the perfect light meal, or you can pair it with a salad for a heartier lunch or dinner. Feel free to mix and match your favorite type of mushrooms, and consider sprinkling some crumbled bacon on top for added protein.

Prep Time: 10 minutes   Cook Time: 30 minutes   Yield: 4 servings

16 ounces white mushrooms

5 tablespoons ghee (page 320), lard (page 322), or tallow (page 324), divided

1 medium onion, finely chopped (about ¾ cup)

2 cloves garlic, minced

1 teaspoon dried thyme

1 teaspoon fine sea salt

½ teaspoon ground black pepper

4 cups chicken stock (page 310)

2 cups almond milk (page 318)

¼ cup plus 2 tablespoons tapioca flour or arrowroot flour

3 tablespoons chopped fresh flat-leaf parsley, for garnish (optional)

1. Wipe the mushrooms clean with a slightly damp paper towel, then slice. Melt 2 tablespoons of the ghee in a large saucepan over medium-high heat. Add the mushrooms and sauté for 5 to 7 minutes, until the mushrooms have released their liquid. Transfer the contents of the pan to a bowl, then return the pan to the heat.

2. In the same saucepan, melt the remaining 3 tablespoons of ghee. Add the chopped onion and sauté for 3 minutes, then add the garlic and sauté for 1 more minute. Add the thyme, salt, and pepper, stir to coat the onion mixture, and sauté for 1 more minute. Slowly add the chicken stock to the pan, whisking to combine.

3. Whisk the almond milk and tapioca flour together in a small bowl, then add to the pan and whisk quickly. Bring just to a boil, then stir in the mushrooms and reduce the heat to low. Cover and simmer for 10 minutes, or until the mushrooms are tender and the soup has thickened.

4. Taste and add more salt and pepper if desired. Ladle into bowls, top with a sprinkle of fresh parsley, if desired, and serve.

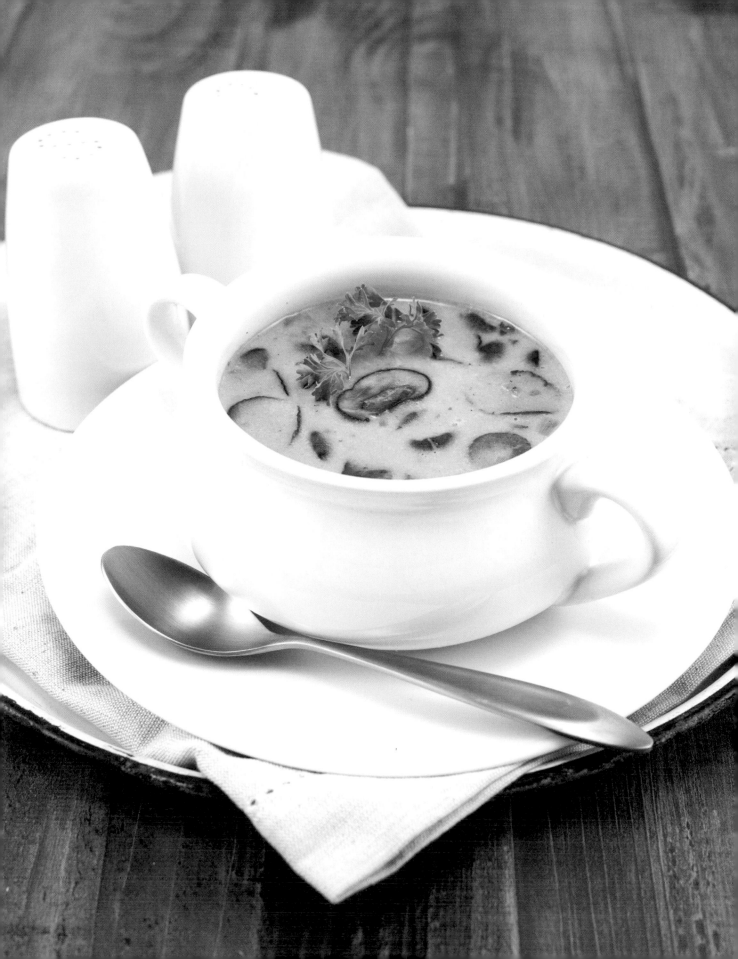

GUMBO

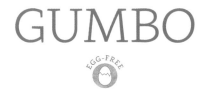

Gumbo is the type of dish that everyone makes a little differently, which is one of the reasons I love it. Some people add okra or crab, some have a very specific spice blend that they believe is the one and only blend, and others have top-secret ingredients that they will never divulge to another soul. But no matter how you make it, gumbo is a comforting and flavorful meal that is sure to be loved by all. Serve it as is or over Seasoned Cauliflower Rice (page 200).

Prep Time: 20 minutes   Cook Time: 1 hour 45 minutes   Yield: 4 servings

1 cup plus 1 tablespoon lard (page 322) or tallow (page 324), divided

1 pound boneless skinless chicken thighs, cut into 1-inch pieces

1 pound andouille or other sausage, cut into 1-inch pieces

¾ cup almond flour (page 316)

½ cup tapioca flour

1½ cups chopped onion

1 cup chopped celery

1 cup chopped red bell pepper

5 cloves garlic, chopped

1½ teaspoons fine sea salt

½ teaspoon ground black pepper

¼ teaspoon cayenne pepper

1 teaspoon paprika

1 teaspoon dried oregano

1 teaspoon dried thyme

5 cups chicken stock (page 310), or more if desired

2 bay leaves

1 pound medium shrimp, peeled and deveined, tails removed

3 tablespoons chopped fresh flat-leaf parsley, for garnish (optional)

1. Melt 1 tablespoon of the lard in a large Dutch oven over medium heat. Add the chicken and sausage and cook for 8 minutes, or until browned, stirring frequently. Transfer the chicken and sausage to a bowl and return the pan to the stove.

2. Melt the remaining 1 cup of lard in the pan, then add the almond flour and tapioca flour and stir to combine. The mixture should resemble a thin pancake batter. Cook for 20 minutes, or until a dark, chocolate-brown roux forms, stirring frequently so it does not burn. Add the onion, celery, bell pepper, garlic, salt, pepper, cayenne, paprika, oregano, and thyme and cook for 2 more minutes, stirring frequently.

3. Slowly add the chicken stock to the pan, whisking to combine. Add the bay leaves and return the chicken and sausage to the pan. Bring just to a boil, then reduce the heat to medium-low and simmer, uncovered, for 1 hour, stirring occasionally. Check the gumbo about halfway through and add an additional cup of stock if a thinner consistency is desired.

4. Add the shrimp and simmer for another 15 minutes, or until the shrimp are cooked through. Remove the bay leaves, ladle the gumbo into bowls, and top with fresh parsley, if desired. Serve with your favorite hot sauce.

KITCHEN TIP

A roux is a thickening and flavoring agent made by combining heated flours and fat, and it is the foundation of a good gumbo. A quality gumbo roux takes time to cook, and that is what gives the flavor its richness, so don't rush the process.

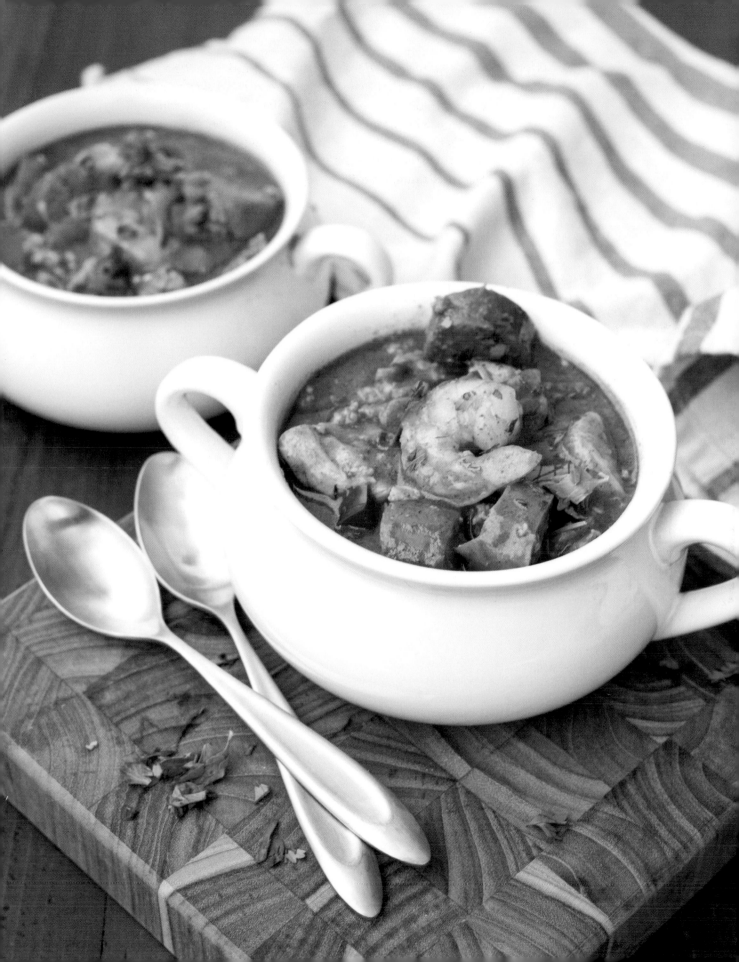

COMFORTING
BEEF
STEW

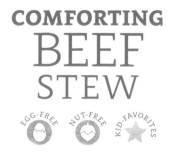

There's something about having a big pot of soup or stew simmering on the stove that makes me feel all warm and fuzzy, and for a few brief moments I forget about things like laundry, a dirty house, and that report I owe my boss on Tuesday. And for that reason alone I eat it year-round, no matter what the weather is like. Most soups and stews also freeze remarkably well, which makes them easy meals to defrost and warm up when you don't have time to cook. This beef stew is great on its own and also tastes great served over Mashed Sweet Potatoes (page 189).

Prep Time: 10 minutes   Cook Time: 1 hour 30 minutes   Yield: 4 servings

3 tablespoons lard (page 322) or tallow (page 324)

2 pounds boneless beef round roast, cut into 2-inch pieces

½ teaspoon fine sea salt

¼ teaspoon ground black pepper

1 large onion, chopped (about 1 cup)

3 cloves garlic, minced

3 tablespoons tomato paste

3 cups beef stock (page 310)

2 teaspoons paprika

1 teaspoon dried thyme

1 teaspoon dried oregano

2 bay leaves

3 tablespoons tapioca flour or arrowroot flour

3 tablespoons water

2 medium carrots, peeled and chopped (about 1½ cups)

8 ounces white mushrooms, sliced

¼ cup chopped fresh parsley, for garnish (optional)

1. Melt the lard in a large Dutch oven over medium-high heat. Season the beef with the salt and pepper and add half of the beef to the pan. Cook for 3 minutes, or until browned on all sides. Remove with a slotted spoon and transfer to a plate. Repeat with the rest of the beef.

2. Add the onion to the pan and sauté for 4 to 5 minutes, until tender. Add the garlic and cook for 1 more minute, stirring frequently. Add the tomato paste and stir to combine.

3. Add the beef stock, paprika, thyme, oregano, and bay leaves to the pan and stir until the sauce is well combined. Return the beef to the pan and bring to a boil. Reduce the heat to low, cover, and simmer for 1 hour, or until the beef is tender.

4. Whisk the tapioca flour and water together in a small bowl and add to the stew, stirring to combine. Raise the heat to medium-high, bring to a boil, add the carrots and mushrooms, and cook, uncovered, for 7 to 10 minutes, until the carrots are tender and the sauce has thickened, stirring occasionally. Taste and add more salt and pepper if desired.

5. To serve, ladle into 4 bowls and top each with a tablespoon of chopped fresh parsley, if desired.

> **TRY THIS!**
> Try adding 1 cup of chopped celery and 1 cup of chopped green bell pepper at the same time as the onion.

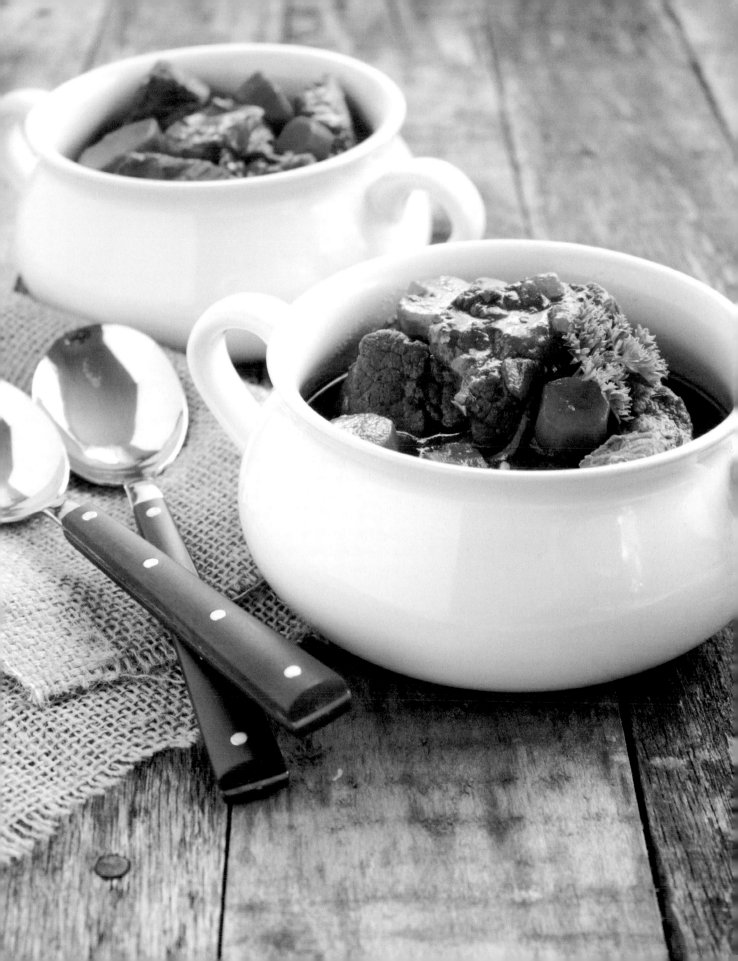

MEXICAN SHRIMP BISQUE

This recipe takes a normal shrimp bisque and gives it a south-of-the-border flair. The creamy coconut milk balances out the zesty chili powder, cumin, and coriander, and a squeeze of fresh lime juice right at the table gives it a burst of freshness. Try adding avocado slices just before serving for even more creamy, buttery flavor. Serve with a crisp green salad for a perfect comforting meal.

Prep Time: 15 minutes   **Cook Time:** 25 minutes   **Yield:** 2 to 4 servings

2 tablespoons ghee (page 320), lard (page 322), or tallow (page 324)

1 large onion, chopped (about 1 cup)

4 cloves garlic, minced

3 tablespoons tapioca flour

2 tablespoons tomato paste

3 cups chicken stock (page 310) or fish stock (page 312)

2 teaspoons chili powder

1 teaspoon ground cumin

1 teaspoon ground coriander

½ teaspoon paprika

½ teaspoon fine sea salt

1 pound medium shrimp, peeled and deveined, tails removed, and chopped, plus more whole cooked shrimp for garnish (optional)

1 cup coconut milk (page 314)

½ cup chopped fresh cilantro, for garnish (optional)

2 limes, quartered, for serving

1. Melt the ghee in a medium-sized saucepan over medium-high heat. Add the onion and sauté for 4 minutes, or until tender. Add the garlic and sauté for another minute. Add the tapioca flour and stir until blended, then add the tomato paste and stir again. Pour in the chicken stock, then add the chili powder, cumin, coriander, paprika, and salt and stir until well incorporated. Bring to a boil, then reduce the heat to low and simmer for 5 minutes, or until the sauce is slightly thickened.

2. Add the shrimp and coconut milk to the soup and simmer for another 10 minutes, or until the shrimp are cooked through.

3. Taste and add more salt and pepper if desired. Ladle the soup into bowls, top with the cilantro and additional whole cooked shrimp, if desired, and serve with lime wedges.

> TRY THIS!
> For an extra boost of creaminess, try topping the bisque with a dollop of sour cream (page 281).

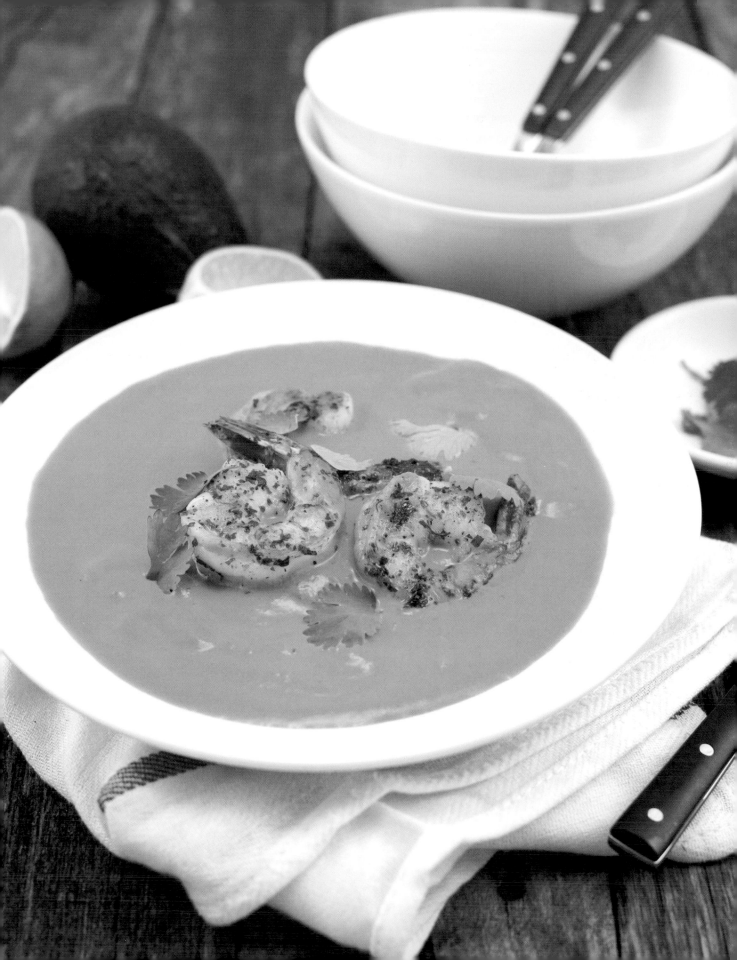

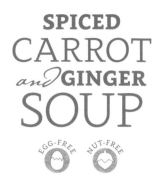

SPICED CARROT *and* GINGER SOUP

EGG-FREE · NUT-FREE

I have a good friend who loves to try unusual recipes, and one day she asked me to come over and make nettle soup with some nettles that she had just picked from her yard. I found out the hard way why they're often referred to as "stinging nettles"—when you touch them, they sting the heck out of you. In the end, the soup was delicious and full of flavor, but after looking at my poor arms covered in red bumps, I decided that I prefer to make soups that are a little more on the safe side. This carrot and ginger soup is both comforting and savory, and best of all, it's made with ingredients that don't fight back.

Prep Time: 10 minutes   Cook Time: 40 minutes   Yield: 4 to 6 servings

3 tablespoons ghee (page 320), lard (page 322), or tallow (page 324)

1 teaspoon ground coriander

½ teaspoon dry yellow mustard

½ teaspoon curry powder

1 teaspoon ground ginger

2 large onions, chopped (about 2 cups)

4 cups peeled and chopped carrots (about 4 large)

1 small red-skinned sweet potato (about ¼ pound), peeled and chopped into 1-inch pieces

4 cloves garlic, minced

3½ cups chicken stock (page 310), plus more if desired

1½ cups coconut milk (page 314)

2 teaspoons freshly squeezed lime juice

1 teaspoon fine sea salt

½ teaspoon ground black pepper

¼ pound thick-cut bacon, cooked and crumbled, for garnish (optional)

¼ cup chopped fresh cilantro, for garnish (optional)

¼ cup sour cream (page 281), for garnish (optional)

1. Melt the ghee in a large stockpot over medium-high heat. Add the coriander, mustard, curry powder, and ginger and cook for 1 minute, stirring constantly. Add the onions, carrots, and sweet potato and stir to combine. Cook for 3 minutes, then add the garlic and cook for 1 more minute.

2. Add the stock and coconut milk and bring to a boil. Reduce the heat to medium-low and simmer, uncovered, for 30 minutes, or until the carrots and sweet potato are tender.

3. Add the lime juice, salt, and pepper. Use an immersion blender to puree the soup until smooth, or carefully transfer the soup to a blender, working in batches if needed, and blend until smooth. If you want the soup to be a little thinner, add ¼ to ½ cup stock and blend again. Taste and add additional salt and pepper if desired.

4. To serve, ladle into bowls and garnish with the crumbled bacon, cilantro, and sour cream, if desired.

KITCHEN TIP

Bacon drippings are a great fat for cooking savory foods, and whenever you cook bacon you can easily save the drippings for later use. Strain the hot drippings through a fine-mesh sieve and store in an airtight container in your refrigerator for up to 6 months. Use them anytime you would use lard or tallow and you want to add a hint of bacon flavor to your recipes. Bacon drippings also freeze well and will melt when added to a hot pan. Pour the drippings into ice cube trays and place in the freezer for 4 hours, or until solid. Transfer to a sealed container and store in the freezer for up to 9 months.

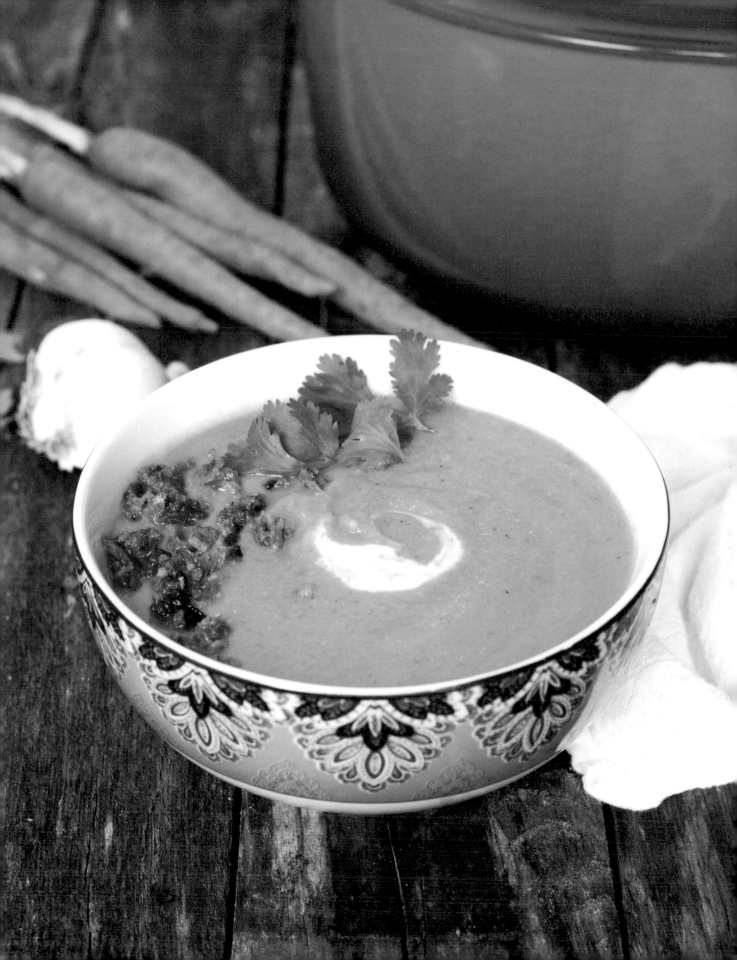

TACO SOUP

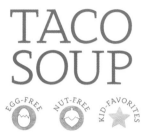

Cooking this soup slow and low allows the flavors of the vegetables, meat, and seasonings to softly blend together, and adding a fresh squeeze of lime juice at the table takes it to a whole new level. Feel free to make it a day ahead, because an overnight visit with your refrigerator will give the soup even more flavor. If you want to add a hint of creaminess, serve it with a dollop of chilled sour cream (page 281) on top.

Prep Time: 10 minutes   Cook Time: 1 hour 15 minutes   Yield: 4 to 6 servings

1 tablespoon ghee (page 320), lard (page 322), or tallow (page 324)

2 pounds ground beef

1 small onion, chopped (about ½ cup)

3 cloves garlic, minced

3 medium carrots, peeled and chopped (about 2 cups)

1 medium red bell pepper, chopped (about ¾ cup)

1 medium green bell pepper, chopped (about ¾ cup)

1 cup beef stock (page 310)

1 (15-ounce) can tomato sauce

1 (4-ounce) can roasted green chiles

2 large tomatoes (about 1 pound), chopped (about 1½ cups)

1 teaspoon fine sea salt

½ teaspoon ground black pepper

½ teaspoon chili powder

½ teaspoon ground cumin

½ teaspoon paprika

1 large ripe avocado, sliced, for serving

¼ cup chopped fresh cilantro, for garnish (optional)

2 limes, quartered, for serving

1. Melt the ghee in a large stockpot over medium-high heat. Add the ground beef, onion, and garlic and cook for 7 minutes, or until the meat is browned. Add the carrots and bell peppers and cook for 2 more minutes, stirring to combine.

2. Add the stock, tomato sauce, green chiles, and tomatoes to the pot. The mixture will be thick, but the tomatoes will release their liquids while cooking. Bring the soup to a boil, then reduce the heat to low. Add the salt, pepper, chili powder, cumin, and paprika and stir to combine. Cover and simmer for 1 hour, stirring occasionally.

3. Ladle into bowls and top with the avocado slices and a sprinkle of fresh cilantro, if desired. Serve with the lime wedges.

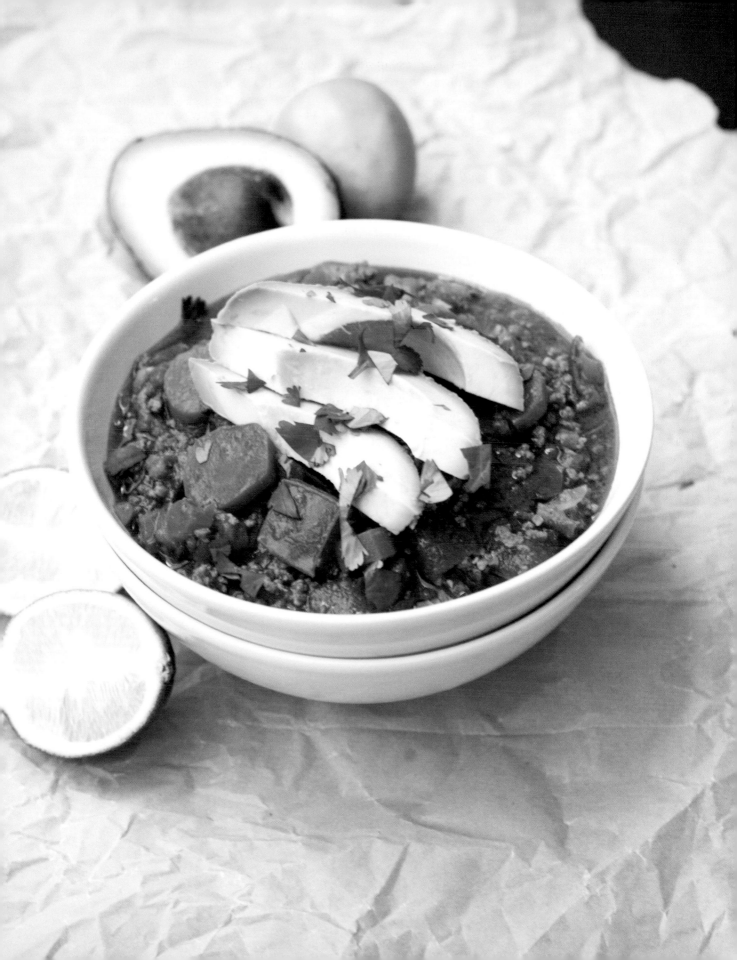

THAI COCONUT SOUP

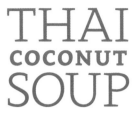

This Thai-inspired soup is rich and creamy, full of chunks of tender chicken, peppers, and mushrooms, and brimming with fragrant ginger and basil.

Prep Time: 10 minutes   Cook Time: 15 minutes   Yield: 4 servings

2 (13.5-ounce) cans full-fat coconut milk or 3⅓ cups homemade coconut milk (page 314)

3 cups chicken stock (page 310)

3 tablespoons freshly squeezed lime juice

1 teaspoon raw honey

1½ tablespoons fish sauce

½ teaspoon ground ginger

1 pound boneless skinless chicken thighs, cut into 1-inch pieces

⅓ cup thinly sliced red bell pepper (about 1 medium)

1½ cups sliced white mushrooms

2 tablespoons fresh basil leaves, thinly sliced, for garnish (optional)

2 tablespoons chopped fresh cilantro, for garnish (optional)

2 limes, quartered, for serving

1. In a medium saucepan over medium-high heat, combine the coconut milk, stock, lime juice, honey, fish sauce, and ginger. Bring to a boil, then add the chicken pieces, bell pepper, and mushrooms and reduce the heat to low. Simmer for 7 to 10 minutes, until the chicken is cooked through.

2. To serve, ladle into bowls, garnish with the fresh basil and cilantro, if desired, and serve with the lime wedges.

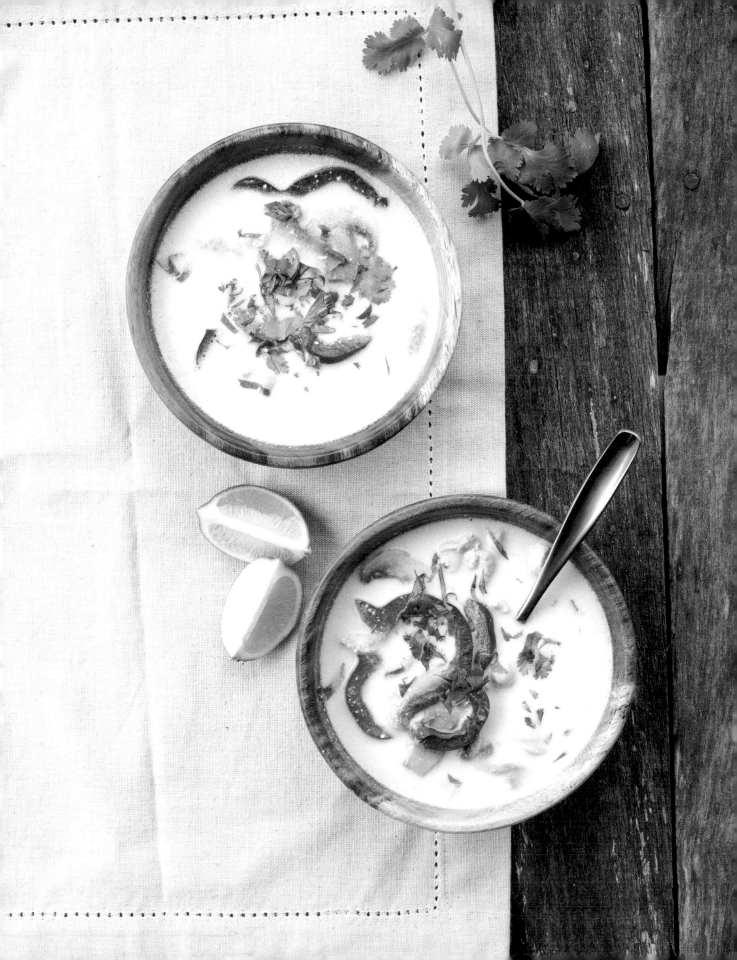

TOMATO BASIL SOUP with CRISPY SHALLOTS

Roasting the tomatoes for this soup brings out a warm and earthy taste, and the fresh herbs make sure this recipe is packed full of rich Italian flavors. Crispy shallots are a nice substitute for croutons and also make a great topping for Mashed Sweet Potatoes (page 189).

EGG-FREE   NUT-FREE

Prep Time: 20 minutes   Cook Time: 1 hour 30 minutes   Yield: 4 servings

FOR THE SOUP

8 large Roma tomatoes (about 2 pounds), cut in half lengthwise

2 tablespoons extra-virgin olive oil

1 teaspoon fine sea salt

½ teaspoon ground black pepper

2 tablespoons ghee (page 320), lard (page 322), or tallow (page 324)

2 large onions, chopped (about 2 cups)

¼ teaspoon crushed red pepper

5 cloves garlic, minced

1½ cups tomato sauce

3½ cups chicken stock (page 310)

1 teaspoon raw honey

2 packed cups fresh basil leaves, chopped

1 tablespoon chopped fresh thyme

1 tablespoon chopped fresh oregano

FOR THE SHALLOTS

½ cup ghee (page 320), lard (page 322), or tallow (page 324)

2 large shallots, peeled and sliced into thin rings (about 1½ cups)

1. Preheat the oven to 400°F. Line a 9-by-13-inch baking sheet with parchment paper or a baking mat.

2. In a large mixing bowl, toss together the tomatoes, olive oil, salt, and pepper. Transfer the tomatoes to the prepared baking sheet, skin side up, and roast for 40 minutes. Remove from the oven and let cool for 5 minutes, then peel the tomatoes.

3. While the tomatoes are roasting, cook the shallots: Melt the ghee in a large skillet over medium-low heat. Add the sliced shallots and cook for 15 minutes, or until golden brown and crispy, stirring occasionally. Reduce the heat to low if the shallots start to cook too quickly. Remove the shallots from the pan with a slotted spoon and transfer to a paper towel–lined plate to drain.

4. Once the tomatoes are done, melt the 2 tablespoons of ghee in a large saucepan over medium heat. Add the onions and crushed red pepper and sauté for 4 minutes, or until the onions begin to soften. Add the garlic and sauté for another minute. Add the peeled tomatoes, tomato sauce, chicken stock, and honey and stir to combine. Bring just to a boil, then reduce the heat to low and simmer, uncovered, for 30 minutes.

5. Add the basil, thyme, and oregano and stir to combine. Cook for another 5 minutes, then remove from the heat. Use an immersion blender to puree the soup until smooth, or carefully transfer the soup to a blender, working in batches if needed, and blend until smooth. Taste and add more salt and pepper if desired. To serve, ladle the soup into serving bowls and sprinkle with the sliced shallots.

TRY THIS!
For extra creaminess, add ½ cup of almond or coconut milk to the soup right before serving.

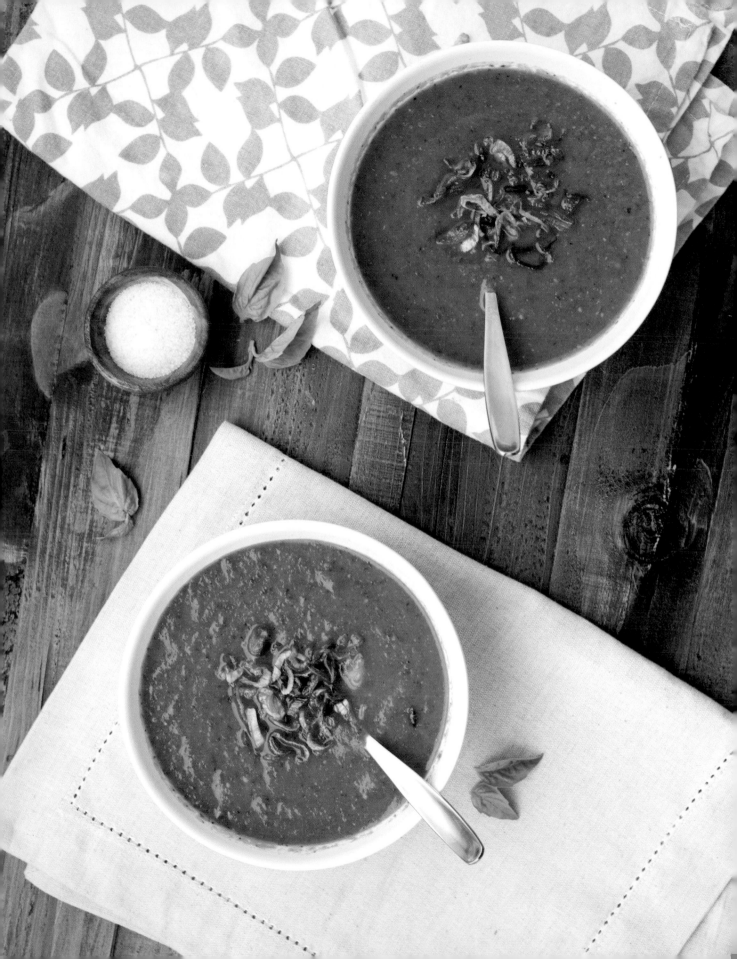

ZUPPA TOSCANA

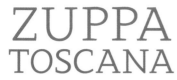
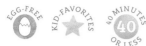

If you want a comforting soup that is both creamy and savory, this is the one for you. It's the food equivalent of a warm hug, and whenever I'm not feeling well or I just need something tasty to pick me up, this is what I turn to. For some folks, myself included, the bitterness of raw kale can be hard to swallow. But when it's allowed to simmer in a savory broth, the bitter flavor disappears, and even picky eaters will fall in love and ask for seconds.

Prep Time: 15 minutes   **Cook Time:** 25 minutes   **Yield:** 4 to 6 servings

2 tablespoons ghee (page 320), lard (page 322), or tallow (page 324)

1 pound ground Italian sausage

1 medium onion, chopped (about ¾ cup)

3 cloves garlic, chopped

1 teaspoon crushed red pepper (optional)

8 cups chicken stock (page 310)

4 medium turnips, peeled and chopped into 1-inch cubes

4 cups chopped kale leaves, center ribs and stems removed

1 cup almond milk (page 318)

Fine sea salt and ground black pepper

1. Melt the ghee in a large stockpot over medium-high heat. Add the Italian sausage and cook for 5 minutes, or until the sausage has browned, breaking the sausage apart into chunks as it cooks. Add the chopped onion, garlic, and crushed red pepper (if using) to the pan. Sauté for 3 minutes, or until the onion begins to soften.

2. Add the chicken stock and turnips to the pot and stir to combine. Bring just to a boil, then reduce the heat to low and simmer for 10 minutes.

3. Add the kale and almond milk, stir, and simmer for another 5 minutes, or until heated through and the turnips and kale are tender. Add salt and pepper to taste, ladle into bowls, and serve.

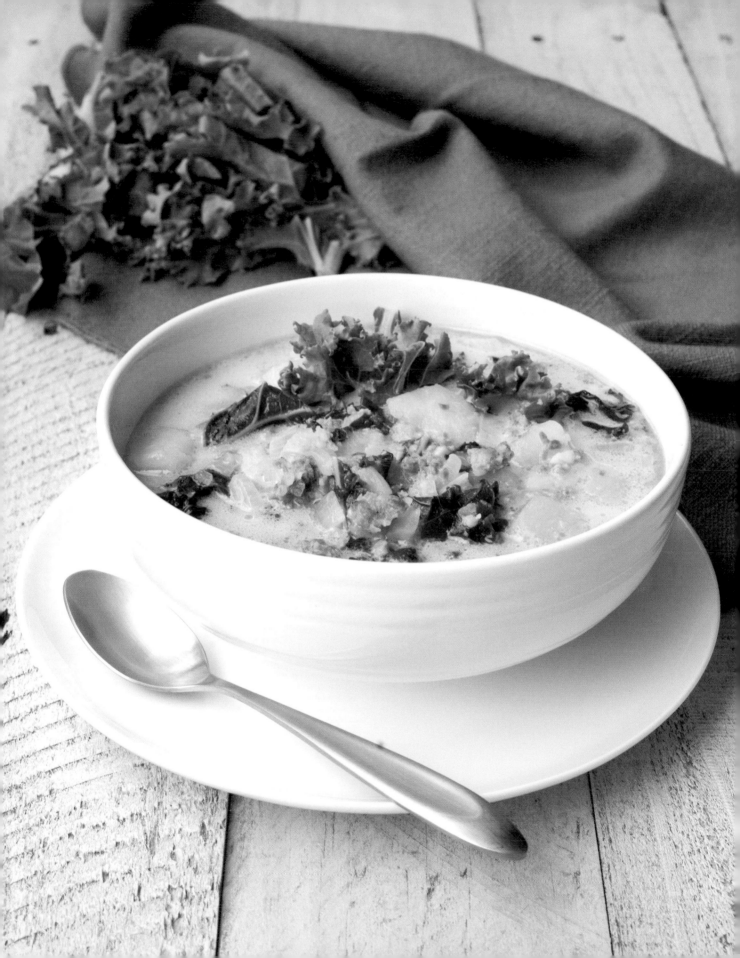

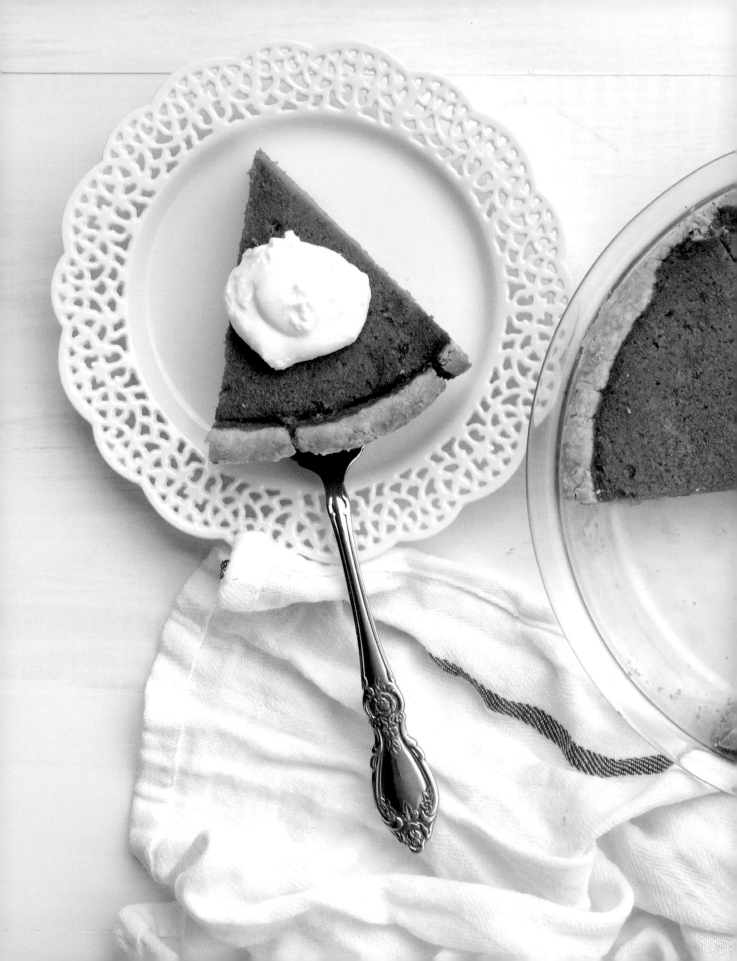

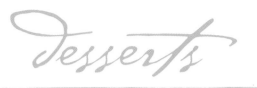

desserts

BLACKBERRY PEACH UPSIDE-DOWN CAKE

KID-FAVORITES

I used to steer clear of upside-down cakes because they reminded me of fruitcakes, those horrible, hard, nasty-looking cakes that some people serve around Christmastime. My grandmother insisted on having one, and every Christmas it sat on the table for a week or so on display, showing off all of its ugliness. It very well could have been the same fruitcake year after year, because nobody would eat a single bite, not even her.

Luckily I eventually realized that an upside-down cake is nothing like a fruitcake, and thus was born this tasty treat. This cake has a moist texture similar to that of bread pudding, which highlights the flavors of the fresh fruit. Nectarines or plums also work instead of the peaches, and raspberries can be substituted for the blackberries.

Prep Time: 10 minutes   **Cook Time:** 55 minutes   **Yield:** One 9-inch round cake (8 to 10 servings)

FOR THE TOPPING

¼ cup raw honey

3 tablespoons ghee (page 320) or coconut oil

2 large peaches (about 1 pound), pitted and sliced into ½-inch-thick wedges

1 cup fresh blackberries

FOR THE CAKE

1½ cups almond flour (page 316), sifted

½ cup tapioca flour

½ teaspoon baking soda

½ teaspoon fine sea salt

⅓ cup raw honey, warmed if solid

¼ cup ghee (page 320) or coconut oil, warmed if solid

½ cup coconut milk (page 314)

1 teaspoon pure vanilla extract

2 large eggs

1. Preheat the oven to 350°F. Grease the inside of a 9-inch round springform pan with ghee or coconut oil.

2. Make the caramel topping: In a small saucepan over medium-high heat, bring the ¼ cup raw honey and 3 tablespoons ghee to a boil. Allow to boil without stirring for 3 to 4 minutes, until the foam is medium brown in color. Remove the pan from the heat and whisk for 20 seconds, or until the foam subsides, then pour into the greased pan and quickly swirl to coat the bottom of the pan. Gently press the peach slices and blackberries in a single layer on top of the caramel, making sure the fruit is packed closely together.

3. Make the cake: Combine the almond flour, tapioca flour, baking soda, and salt in a medium-sized mixing bowl and stir with a fork or small whisk for 1 minute, or until no clumps appear. In another medium-sized mixing bowl, combine the honey, ghee, coconut milk, vanilla extract, and eggs and blend with a hand mixer on medium speed for 30 seconds, or until well combined. Slowly pour the wet mixture into the dry mixture, blending with the hand mixer as you pour until the batter is smooth and well combined. Pour the batter over the fruit layer in the pan.

4. Place the pan in the oven and bake for 40 to 45 minutes, until a toothpick inserted into the center comes out clean. Let cool on a wire rack for 20 minutes, or until the pan is cool enough to touch.

5. Gently run a butter knife around the edge of the pan and then unmold the outside of the pan from the cake. Place a serving plate facedown on top of the cake. Holding the bottom of the pan with one hand and the plate with the other, flip the pan over so that the cake is now face up on the plate and gently remove the pan bottom from the top of the cake. Allow the cake to cool completely before serving.

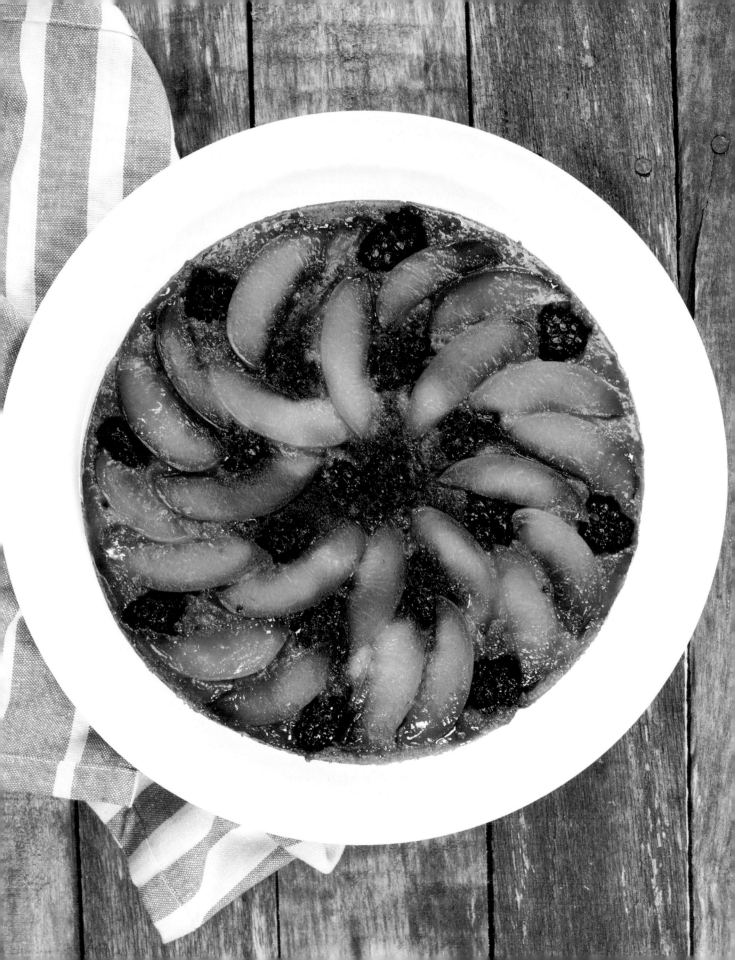

CHOCOLATE SOUFFLÉ *with* STRAWBERRY SAUCE

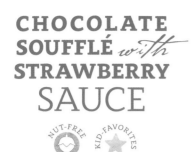

NUT-FREE · KID-FAVORITES

Some people are intimidated by the idea of making a soufflé, but it's actually not that difficult. Don't let a dessert scare you; get in there and show it who's boss! If you are making a soufflé for the first time and want to cut back on the number of steps, make the strawberry sauce first or leave it out entirely. The soufflés will taste just fine without it, and you won't be trying to juggle as many things at once. I try to use 100 percent cacao baking bars for this recipe, but if you have trouble finding them, look for a bar with at least 70 percent cacao.

Prep Time: 15 minutes   Cook Time: 30 minutes   Yield: 4 soufflés (4 servings)

FOR THE SOUFFLÉS

⅓ cup raw honey

3½ ounces dark chocolate (at least 70% cacao), chopped

1 tablespoon cacao powder

3 tablespoons ghee (page 320) or coconut oil

1 teaspoon pure vanilla extract

2 large egg yolks, room temperature

6 large egg whites, room temperature

Pinch of fine sea salt

4 fresh strawberries, for garnish (optional)

FOR THE STRAWBERRY SAUCE

1 cup chopped fresh strawberries

1 tablespoon raw honey

2 tablespoons water

1. Preheat the oven to 400°F. Grease 4 (6-ounce) oven-safe ramekins with ghee or coconut oil and place on a 9-by-13-inch baking sheet.

2. Fill a small saucepan with 1 inch of water and bring to a light simmer. Place a metal bowl over the saucepan and add the honey, chocolate, cacao powder, ghee, and vanilla extract. Heat for 4 minutes, or until all the ingredients are melted, combined, and smooth, stirring occasionally. Remove the bowl from the heat and allow to cool for 3 to 5 minutes. Stir in the egg yolks, whisking quickly until fully combined. Set aside.

3. Place the egg whites and salt in a large mixing bowl. Beat the whites with a hand mixer on medium speed for 1 minute, or until very frothy, then increase the speed to high and beat until stiff peaks form. Fold about 1 cup of the egg whites into the chocolate mixture until combined, then pour the chocolate mixture into the middle of the egg whites. Gently fold the egg whites into the chocolate until fully mixed and no more white is showing. Spoon the mixture into the prepared ramekins and bake for 17 to 19 minutes, until puffy and the tops begin to slightly brown.

4. While the soufflés are cooking, make the strawberry sauce: Place the strawberries, honey, and water in a small saucepan over medium heat. Bring to a simmer and then reduce the heat to low. Cook for 10 to 12 minutes, until the sauce has thickened slightly, breaking up the strawberries with a wooden spoon as they soften.

5. Remove the soufflés from the oven, top with the strawberry sauce, and garnish with the fresh strawberries, if desired. Serve right away.

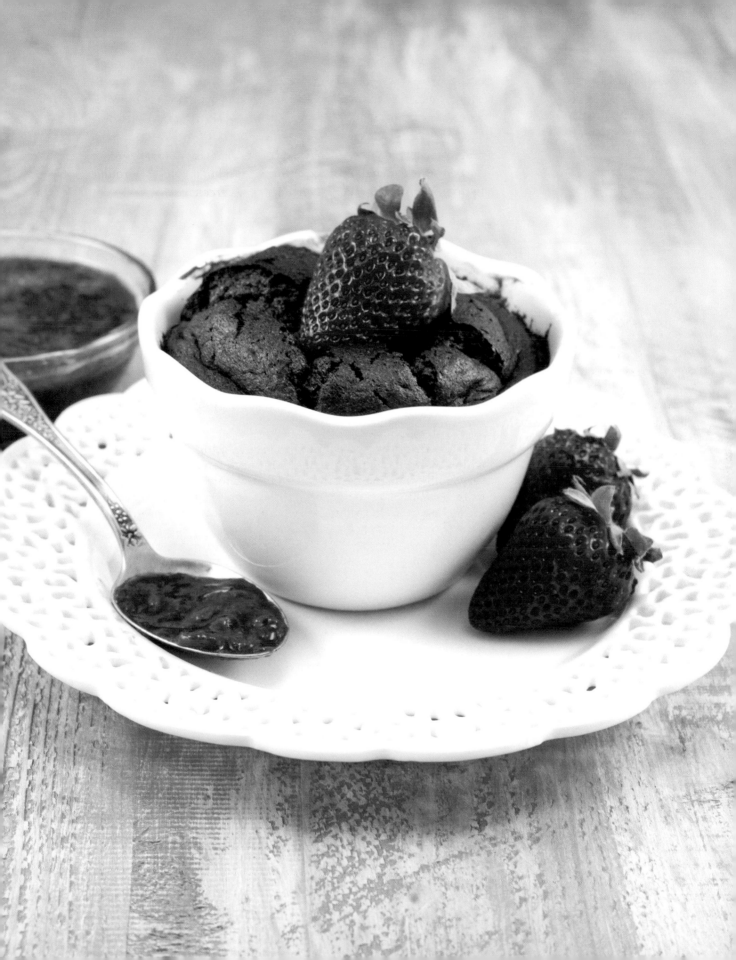

COCONUT
CREAM
TARTS

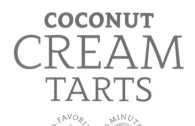

Everyone has a bit of a different opinion on the difference between a pie and a tart. Tarts generally do not have a top crust, but some pies do and some pies don't. Tarts have straight sides while pies have sloped sides. Tarts usually have a firmer crust and pies have a flakier crust, but sometimes tarts can have flaky crusts. It can be a bit overwhelming, really. I like to think of tarts as the chicer, smaller cousins of pies. Feel free to disagree with me, but who has time to argue about these things when there are delicious tart-pie-thingies that need to be eaten?

Prep Time: 10 minutes, plus 4 hours to chill   **Cook Time:** 25 minutes
Yield: Four 4½-inch tarts (4 servings)

FOR THE FILLING

1 (13.5-ounce) can full-fat coconut milk or 1⅔ cups homemade coconut milk (page 314)

2 tablespoons tapioca flour or arrowroot flour

3 large egg yolks

¼ cup raw honey

1 teaspoon pure vanilla extract

⅓ cup unsweetened shredded coconut (optional)

2 tablespoons unsweetened shredded coconut, for serving

FOR THE CRUST

1½ cups almond flour (page 316)

½ cup tapioca flour or arrowroot flour

¼ cup raw honey, warmed if solid

¼ cup ghee (page 320) or coconut oil, warmed if solid

1 teaspoon pure vanilla extract

1 batch Whipped Coconut Cream (page 261), for serving (optional)

1. Make the filling: Whisk together the coconut milk and tapioca flour in a medium-sized saucepan. Add the egg yolks, honey, and vanilla extract and whisk to combine. Place the saucepan over medium-low heat and cook for 8 minutes, or until the mixture is the consistency of pudding, whisking frequently.

2. Remove the saucepan from the heat and stir in the shredded coconut (if using). Allow to cool completely, then transfer to a bowl, cover, and refrigerate for 4 hours, or until set. The mixture will have the consistency of a thick pudding.

3. While the filling sets, toast the coconut for the topping: Place the 2 tablespoons shredded coconut in a large skillet and cook over medium heat, stirring frequently, until the flakes are light golden brown. Set aside.

4. Once the filling has set, make the crusts. Preheat the oven to 350°F. Grease 4 (4½-inch) tart pans with a thin layer of ghee.

5. In a medium-sized mixing bowl, combine the almond flour, tapioca flour, honey, ghee, and vanilla extract and stir with a fork until well combined. Press the dough into the bottom of the tart pans and up the sides, forming a thin crust. Poke each tart crust with a fork 5 times. Set the tart pans on a 9-by-13-inch baking sheet, then bake for 13 to 15 minutes, until they are light golden brown. Remove from the oven and set aside to cool fully.

6. Spoon the filling into the tart crusts. Add a dollop of whipped coconut cream on top, if desired, sprinkle each tart with ½ tablespoon of the toasted coconut, and serve.

KITCHEN TIP

Because the filling for this dish needs to set in the refrigerator before you make the crusts, you can make the filling and whipped coconut cream a day ahead of time and store them in the refrigerator until ready to serve.

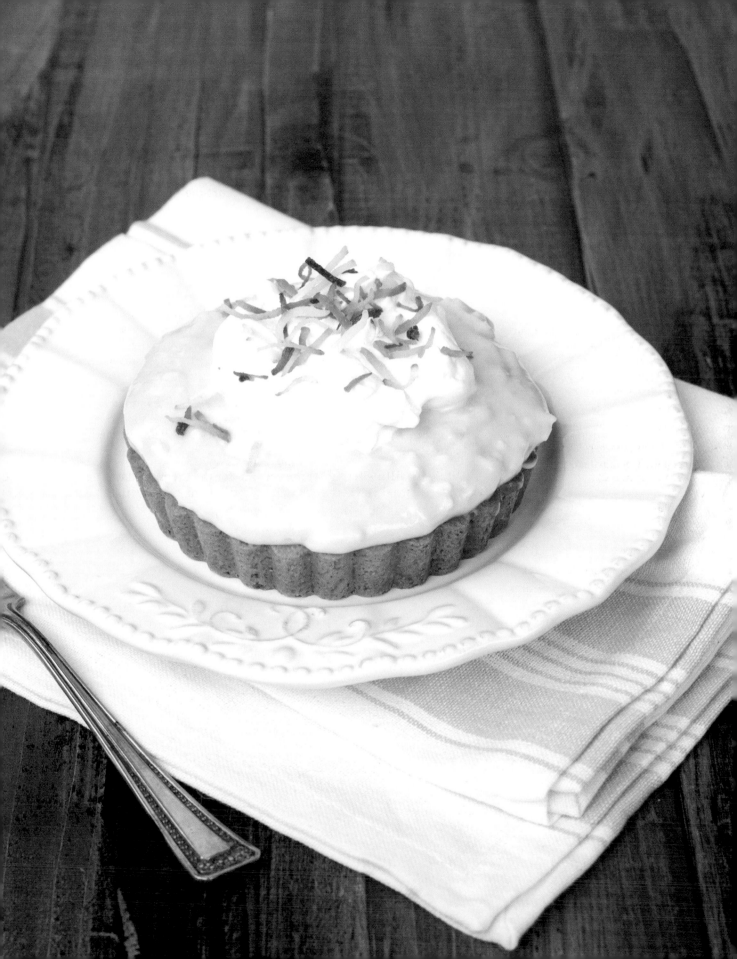

CREAMY **CHOCOLATE** MOUSSE

This is an easy make-ahead dessert that both kids and adults love. You can serve it plain or dress it up a little by garnishing it with Whipped Coconut Cream (page 261) and berries.

Prep Time: 10 minutes, plus 1 hour to chill   **Cook Time:** 5 minutes   **Yield:** 4 to 6 servings

1 tablespoon pure vanilla extract

1 tablespoon water

1 teaspoon grass-fed gelatin

¼ cup raw honey

¼ cup cacao powder or unsweetened cocoa powder, plus more to taste

¼ cup ghee (page 320) or coconut oil

Cream from 2 (13.5-ounce) cans full-fat coconut milk (see page 315) or 2 cups homemade coconut cream (page 315)

Whipped Coconut Cream (page 261), for topping (optional)

Fresh berries, for topping (optional)

1. In a small bowl, whisk together the vanilla extract and water. Sprinkle the gelatin over the top and set aside to bloom for 10 minutes.

2. Combine the honey, cacao powder, and ghee in a small saucepan over medium heat. Bring just to a boil, whisking frequently, then remove from the heat. Stir in the gelatin mixture and whisk again until smooth and well combined. Set aside.

3. In a large mixing bowl, beat the coconut cream with a hand mixer on medium speed for 1 minute. Slowly pour in the chocolate mixture and continue to beat until combined. Taste and add more cacao powder if you want a stronger chocolate taste, blending with the hand mixer until fully combined.

4. Spoon into bowls or glasses, cover, and chill in the refrigerator for 1 hour. Serve with whipped coconut cream and fresh berries if desired.

TRY THIS!

For a version of this recipe with a little extra kick, try adding ¼ teaspoon of ground cinnamon and a pinch of cayenne pepper at the same time you combine the honey, cacao powder, and ghee. It's like Mexican hot chocolate in mousse form!

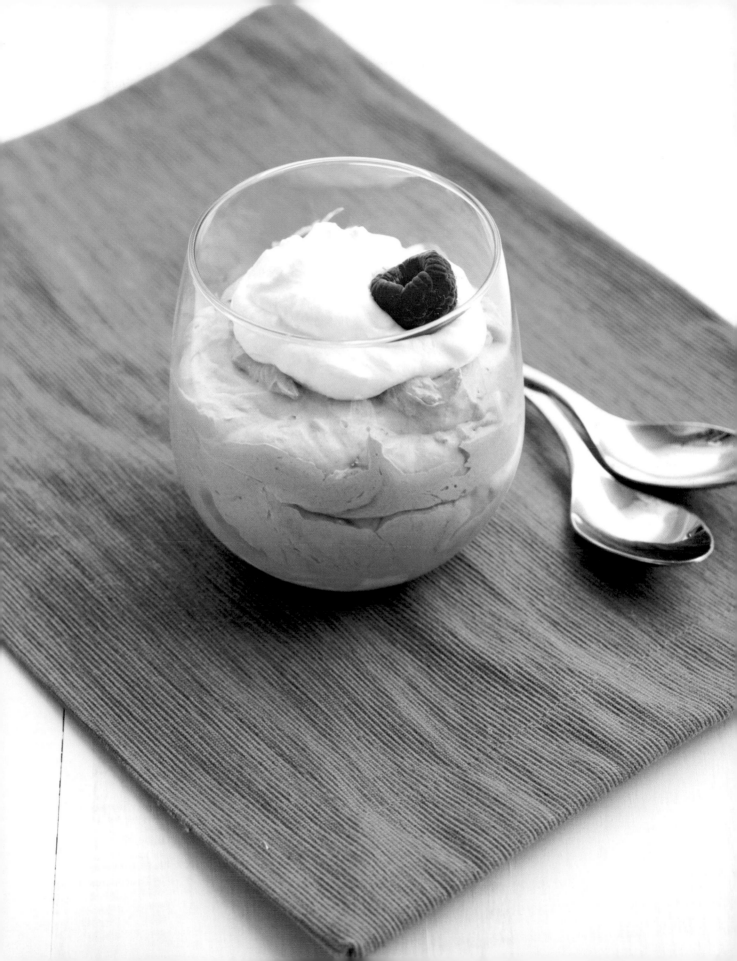

CRÈME BRÛLÉE

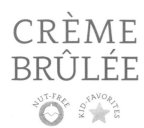

I don't eat dessert often, but crème brûlée is one of my favorite desserts of all time. It's creamy and rich and delicious, and if you put one near me, it is very likely that it will disappear in a matter of seconds. Crème brûlée is elegant enough to serve at a dinner party and yet simple enough to devour while standing at your kitchen counter, and despite what some people think, it is actually very easy to make. So whip out your whisk and let's make this amazing dessert!

Prep Time: 5 minutes, plus 2 hours 15 minutes to chill   Cook Time: 55 minutes   Yield: 4 servings

1 (13.5-ounce) can full-fat coconut milk or 1⅔ cups homemade coconut milk (page 314)

3 large egg yolks

2½ tablespoons raw honey

1 teaspoon pure vanilla extract

1 cup fresh berries or sliced fresh fruit, for topping (optional)

4 sprigs mint, for garnish (optional)

1. Preheat the oven to 325°F.

2. In a small saucepan over medium-high heat, bring the coconut milk just to a boil, then reduce the heat to low and simmer for 5 minutes.

3. Whisk the egg yolks, honey, and vanilla extract together in a medium-sized mixing bowl for 1 minute, or until well blended. Slowly drizzle the heated coconut milk into the egg mixture, whisking constantly. The slow drizzle heats the eggs without cooking them.

4. Pour the mixture into 4 small, shallow oven-safe bowls. Place the bowls into a large baking dish or roasting pan and pour hot water into the pan until it is halfway up the sides of the bowls. Place the baking dish in the oven and bake for 40 to 45 minutes, until the crème brûlée is set around the edges but still wiggles in the center.

5. Allow the custard to cool for 15 minutes, then refrigerate for at least 2 hours, or until fully set. Garnish with your favorite berries or seasonal fresh fruit and mint, if desired, before serving.

KITCHEN TIP

If you happen to have coconut sugar and a baking torch, you can caramelize the sugar on top of the custard to give it a more traditional brittle sugary topping. Remove the crème brûlée from the refrigerator and allow to come to room temperature for at least 30 minutes prior to browning the sugar on top. Sprinkle 2 tablespoons of coconut sugar evenly across the top of the 4 bowls. Using the baking torch, melt the coconut sugar so that it forms a crispy top, being careful not to let it burn. Allow to sit for at least 5 minutes before serving.

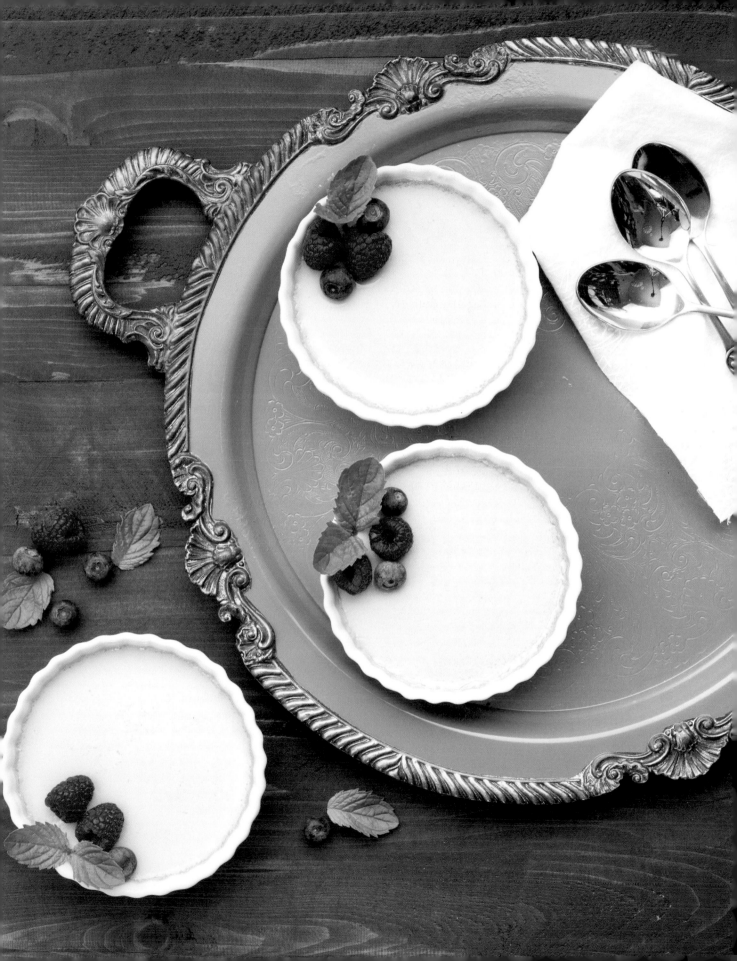

LEMON BARS

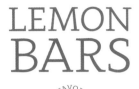
KID-FAVORITES

These lemon bars combine the tart flavor of lemons with the sweetness of raw honey. Using lime juice and zest instead of lemon, or half lime and half lemon, also works well.

Prep Time: 15 minutes, plus 2 hours 30 minutes to chill   Cook Time: 45 minutes   Yield: 12 bars

FOR THE CRUST

½ cup almond flour (page 316)

½ cup tapioca flour or arrowroot flour

3 tablespoons ghee (page 320) or coconut oil, warmed if solid

3 tablespoons raw honey, warmed if solid

Finely grated zest of ½ lemon

FOR THE FILLING

½ cup raw honey

5 large eggs, room temperature

½ cup freshly squeezed lemon juice

1 tablespoon tapioca flour

1. Preheat the oven to 350°F.

2. Make the crust: Mix together the almond flour, tapioca flour, ghee, honey, and zest in a medium-sized mixing bowl. Press the dough into the bottom of an 8-inch square glass baking dish with your fingers. Bake for 15 minutes, or until light golden brown around the edges. Allow the crust and pan to cool for 30 minutes. Reduce the oven temperature to 325°F.

3. When the crust is almost done cooling, make the filling: Place the honey in a small saucepan over medium heat. Bring just to a boil, then turn off the heat.

4. Whisk the eggs in a medium-sized mixing bowl. In a separate bowl, whisk together the lemon juice and tapioca flour until fully combined, and then whisk in the eggs. Very slowly drizzle the hot honey into the egg mixture, a few drops at a time, whisking the entire time.

5. Once fully combined, pour the lemon mixture over the crust and bake for another 22 to 25 minutes, until just set. The edges should be firm but the center should jiggle just slightly. The bars will continue to firm up as they cool.

6. Remove from the oven and allow to cool completely, then refrigerate for 2 hours, or until fully set. Slice into 12 equal-sized bars and serve.

KITCHEN TIP

If you need to measure out both ghee (or another oil) and honey for a recipe, measure the ghee first and then use the same cup or spoon for the honey—it will slide right out instead of sticking to the spoon.

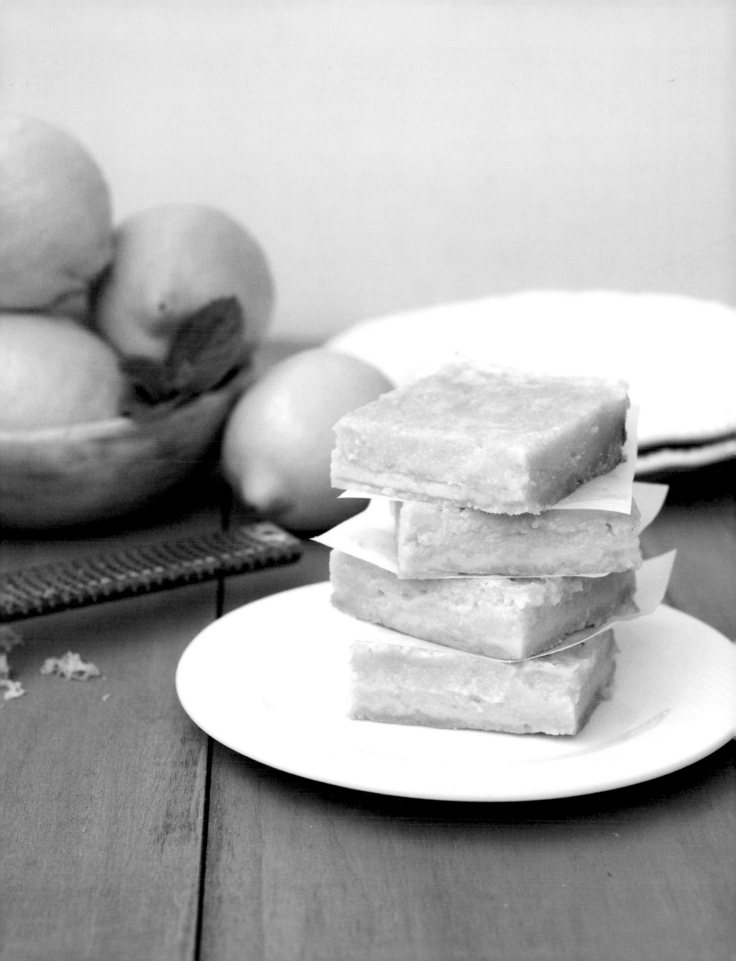

MELON GRANITA

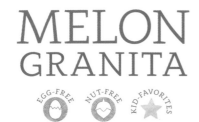

EGG-FREE · NUT-FREE · KID-FAVORITES

This melon granita is an easy way to make a refreshing dessert without using any fancy equipment. The best way to choose a good cantaloupe for this recipe is to give it a sniff test. Yes, that means you will be the person standing at the store smelling produce, and if anyone looks at you funny, just turn away and proceed with sniffing. Remember, you're on a mission and can't be bothered with those folks. If the stem end of the cantaloupe smells sweet and fruity and the shell has no green tint to it, then it is a good choice. If it has no smell at all, most likely it won't have much flavor, either. And if you don't like cantaloupe, you can use your favorite type of melon, such as watermelon or honeydew, instead.

Prep Time: 10 minutes, plus 3 hours to chill   **Yield:** 4 to 6 servings

2 tablespoons raw honey

1 large cantaloupe, chopped (about 5 cups)

1 cup apple juice

Fresh mint leaves, for garnish (optional)

1. Combine the honey, cantaloupe, and apple juice in a blender or food processor and puree until smooth. Pour the mixture into a 9-by-13-inch glass baking dish and place in the freezer, uncovered. Chill for 2½ to 3 hours, until the granita is firm but not frozen, stirring with a fork every 30 minutes to break apart any large lumps.

2. Remove the dish from the freezer and scoop the granita into bowls. Garnish with mint leaves, if desired, and serve.

TRY THIS!

Try adding 2 tablespoons of freshly squeezed lime juice along with the apple juice to give the granita a nice underlying citrus flavor. You can also stick any leftover granita and an extra splash of apple juice in a blender for a few seconds to make a cool summertime drink.

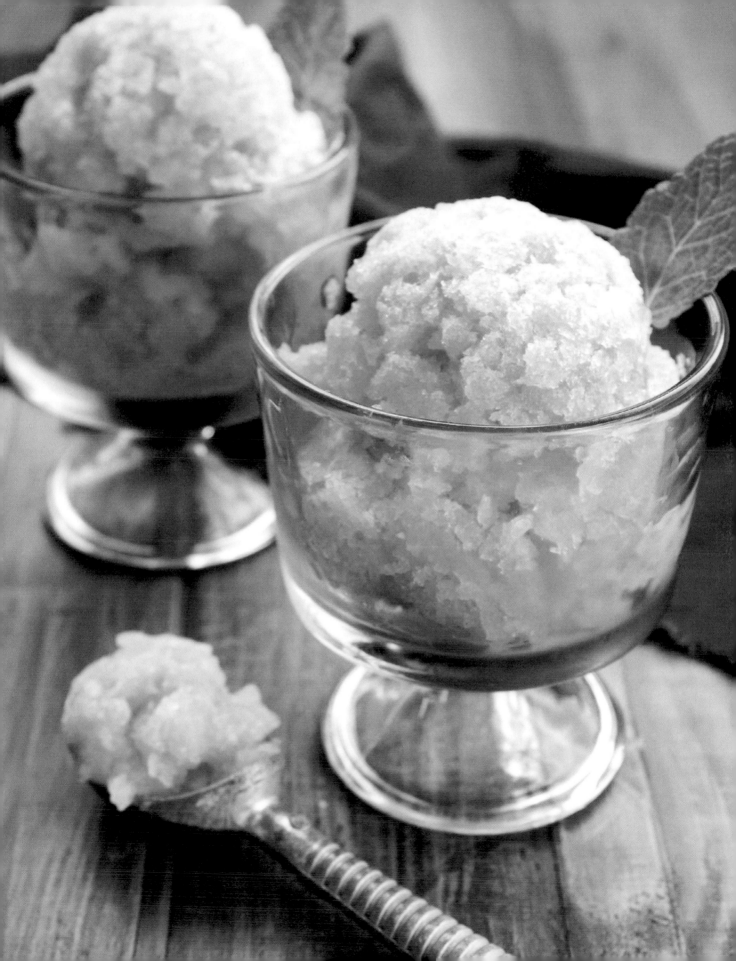

SALTED CARAMEL SAUCE

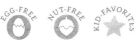

I don't know who came up with the idea of adding salt to caramel sauce, but I want to shake their hand. The combination of salty and sweet in a creamy sauce is pure genius. Drizzle it over apple slices, put a couple teaspoons in a cup of coffee, or eat it with a spoon.

Prep Time: 2 minutes, plus 20 minutes to cool   **Cook Time:** 30 minutes   **Yield:** ½ cup

1 (13.5-ounce) can full-fat coconut milk or 1⅔ cups homemade coconut milk (page 314)

½ cup raw honey

2 tablespoons ghee (page 320) or coconut oil

1 teaspoon pure vanilla extract

½ teaspoon fine sea salt

1. In a medium-sized saucepan over medium heat, bring the coconut milk and honey to a boil, whisking occasionally, then reduce the heat to medium-low and simmer for 25 minutes, stirring occasionally, until the sauce has thickened and turned a golden brown color.

2. Remove from the heat and whisk in the ghee, vanilla extract, and salt. Allow to cool for 20 minutes, stirring every 5 minutes or so. Use right away or store in a sealed container in the refrigerator for up to 1 week.

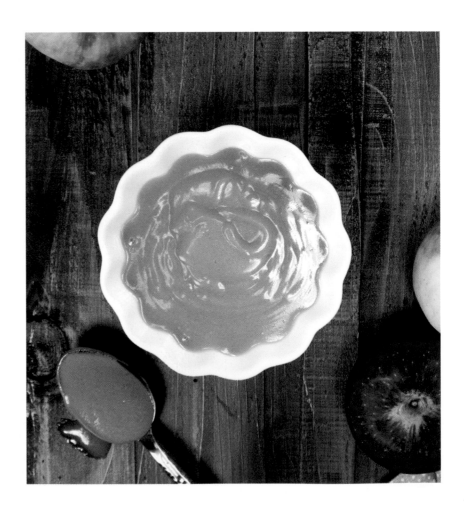

WHIPPED COCONUT CREAM

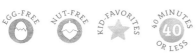

EGG-FREE · NUT-FREE · KID-FAVORITES · 40 MINUTES OR LESS

Whipped coconut cream is perfect served with fruit or as a topping, just like a dairy-based whipped cream. Coconut cream does not whip up like heavy cream does, though, so standing there with a hand mixer for 30 minutes won't get you very far—unless of course you want a good arm workout, in which case, carry on. Fortunately, making whipped coconut cream is even faster and easier.

Prep Time: 5 minutes   Yield: 1¼ cups

Cream from 1 (13.5-ounce) can full-fat coconut milk (see page 315) or 1 cup homemade coconut cream (page 315)

1 teaspoon pure vanilla extract

2 tablespoons raw honey

In a medium-sized mixing bowl, combine the coconut cream, vanilla extract, and honey. Whip with a hand mixer at medium speed for 2 minutes, until smooth and well combined. Serve right away or cover and place in the refrigerator until ready to serve.

TRY THIS!
For a flavorful whipped cream, try adding ¼ teaspoon of cardamom or 1 teaspoon of freshly squeezed lemon juice.

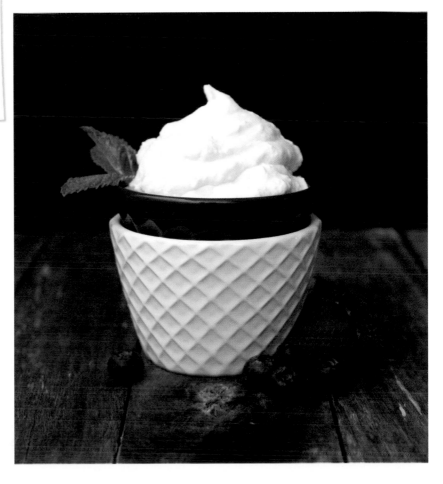

CIDER BAKED APPLES

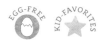

These apples are stuffed with a crunchy nut filling and surrounded by a vanilla-infused cider, then slowly cooked until just tender. You can use any type of apples, from tart to sweet, so experiment with your favorites. Smaller apples will cook faster than larger, so adjust the cooking time as needed. Slightly undercooked apples are better than overcooked, soggy apples.

Prep Time: 15 minutes   **Cook Time:** 45 minutes to 3½ hours, depending on cooking method   **Yield:** 5 servings

5 medium apples (about 2 pounds)

1 cup apple juice

½ teaspoon finely grated lemon zest

2 tablespoons freshly squeezed lemon juice

1 teaspoon pure vanilla extract

¼ teaspoon ground allspice

¼ teaspoon ground nutmeg

⅓ cup finely chopped walnuts

3 tablespoons raisins

3 tablespoons raw honey

2½ teaspoons ghee (page 320; optional)

1 stick cinnamon

1. Slice the top off of each apple and set aside (don't discard), then remove the core of the apple, leaving the bottom intact to create a bowl shape within the apple. A small knife or a melon baller works well to remove the core.

2. In a small bowl, combine the apple juice, lemon zest, lemon juice, vanilla extract, allspice, and nutmeg; set aside.

3. In a separate medium-sized bowl, mix the walnuts, raisins, and honey until well combined. Spoon an equal amount of the mixture into the center of each apple, add ½ teaspoon of ghee (if using), then place the top of each apple back on.

4. **To use a slow cooker:** Pour the apple juice mixture into the slow cooker. Add the cinnamon stick to the liquid, then place the apples in the slow cooker, top side up. Cook on low for 3 to 3½ hours or on high for 1½ to 2 hours, until the apples are slightly tender but not mushy.

   To use an oven: Preheat the oven to 375°F. Pour the apple juice mixture into the bottom of an 8-inch square baking dish, add the cinnamon stick, and place the apples in the pan, top side up. Bake for 30 to 45 minutes, until the apples are slightly tender but not mushy.

5. To serve, pour the cooking liquid into a serving bowl and add the apples.

TRY THIS!

Use cranberries instead of walnuts for a little extra tartness, or drizzle a couple tablespoons of Salted Caramel Sauce (page 260) over the apples right before serving.

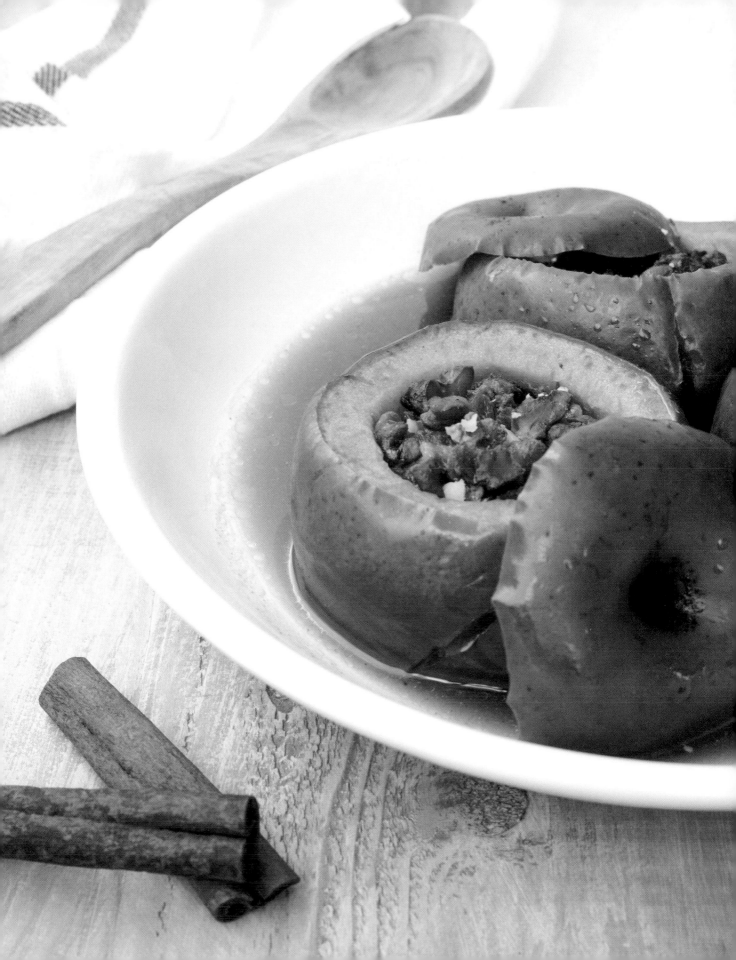

SWEET POTATO PIE

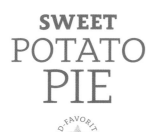

There's a reason that sweet potato pie is so popular in the United States, especially around the holidays. When sweet potato, cinnamon, nutmeg, and vanilla come together, it's like a big warm hug for your mouth. There's no need for a rolling pin with this recipe; just press the dough into the dish with your fingers and your crust is ready to go into the oven. Whipped Coconut Cream (page 261) makes a nice optional topping.

Prep Time: 15 minutes   **Cook Time:** 2 hours   **Yield:** One 9-inch pie (6 servings)

FOR THE FILLING

1 pound red-skinned sweet potatoes

½ cup ghee (page 320) or coconut oil, warmed if solid

½ cup raw honey

½ cup almond milk (page 318) or coconut milk (page 314)

2 large eggs, beaten

¾ teaspoon ground cinnamon

½ teaspoon ground nutmeg

½ teaspoon fine sea salt

1½ teaspoons pure vanilla extract

FOR THE CRUST

1½ cups almond flour (page 316)

½ cup tapioca flour

¼ teaspoon fine sea salt

1 large egg, beaten

1 tablespoon water

2 tablespoons ghee (page 320) or coconut oil, room temperature

1. Preheat the oven to 425°F.

2. Pierce the sweet potatoes a few times with a fork and then bake in the oven for 40 to 50 minutes, until very tender. Remove the potatoes and cool for 5 to 10 minutes, then remove the skin and discard. Turn the oven down to 350°F.

3. Make the crust: Mix the almond flour, tapioca flour, and salt in a large mixing bowl and stir until well combined. Add the beaten egg, water, and ghee and stir with a fork until the dough begins to form large clumps, and then use your hands to knead the dough in the bowl until well combined. The dough should be slightly moist and not crumbly. Press the dough into the bottom of a 9-inch pie pan and up along the edges. Pierce the bottom of the crust a few times with a fork, and then bake at 350°F for 10 minutes. Remove from oven and set aside to cool slightly.

4. While the crust bakes, make the filling: In a large mixing bowl, combine the peeled baked sweet potatoes with the ghee, honey, almond milk, eggs, cinnamon, nutmeg, salt, and vanilla extract. Beat with a hand mixer on medium speed for 1 to 2 minutes, until smooth.

5. Pour the sweet potato filling into the crust. Return the pie to the oven and bake for 55 to 60 minutes, until a toothpick inserted in the center comes out clean. Let cool for at least 20 minutes before slicing.

TRY THIS!
Try adding 1 teaspoon of finely grated orange zest to the filling at the same time as the nutmeg and cinnamon.

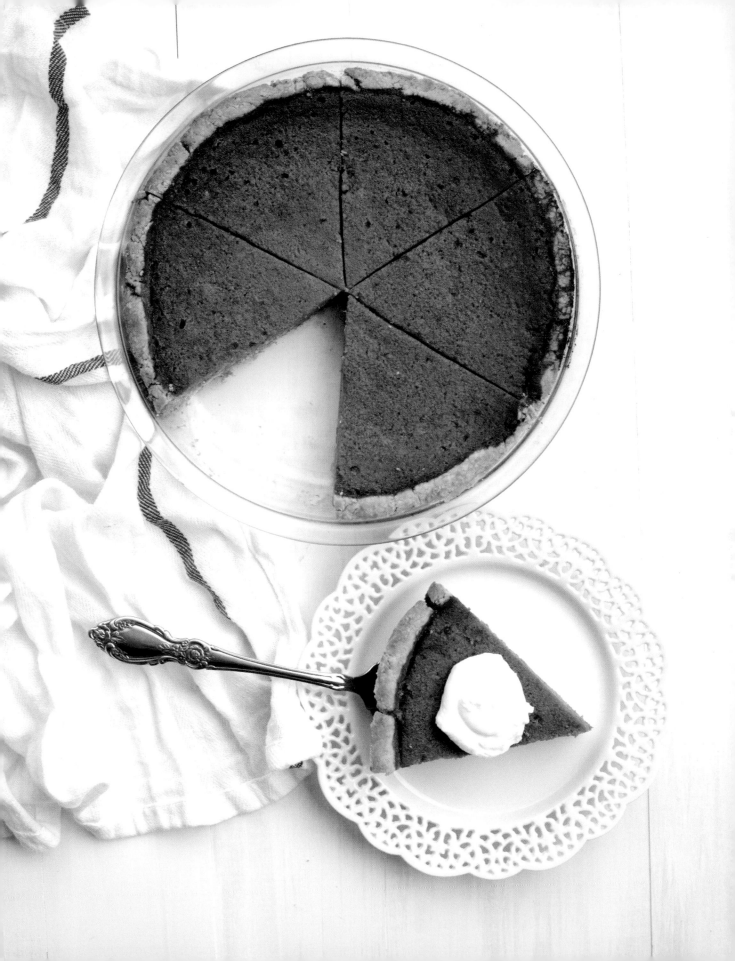

WATERMELON
CAKE

EGG-FREE · NUT-FREE · KID-FAVORITES · 40 MINUTES OR LESS

This watermelon cake was one of the first recipes I posted on my blog, and within a few weeks it had blown up all over social media. The weirdest part for me was that some people were outraged that I had the audacity to call this a "cake." They insisted that cake had to be made from flour and white sugar and covered in icing, and anything else was blasphemy. Many folks were worried that a poor kid might cut into it and have their whole childhood ruined! These were people who took pastries way too seriously.

So for those who can't eat a traditional gluten-filled cake, and for those who just want a healthier option, I present to you this Paleo watermelon CAKE.

Prep Time: 15 minutes   **Yield:** One cake (8 servings)

1 cup sliced almonds or shredded coconut

1 large seedless watermelon (15 to 20 pounds)

2 batches Whipped Coconut Cream (page 261)

Seasonal fresh fruit, such as blackberries, strawberries, and kiwi, for topping

1. Toast the almonds in a large skillet over medium heat for 5 to 10 minutes, until golden brown, stirring frequently. Transfer to a plate to cool.

2. Slice off both ends of the watermelon, then turn it on its side and shave around the edges of the rind, top to bottom, until you're left with a cake-shaped watermelon with no rind. Pat the outside of the watermelon dry with paper towels or a clean kitchen towel to remove any excess moisture, then cut the watermelon cake into 8 wedges.

3. Dip the outside edge of each wedge into the whipped coconut cream and then into the toasted almonds, then reassemble the wedges in the cake shape on a serving platter. Top with more whipped coconut cream and your favorite fresh fruit. Serve right away, or store in the refrigerator until ready to serve.

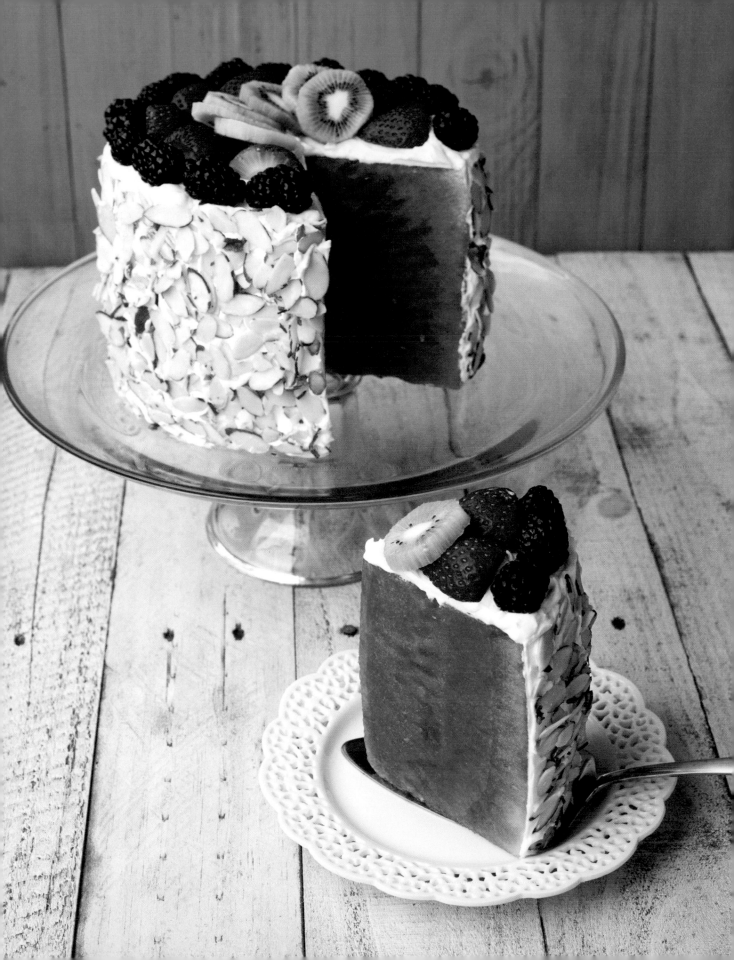

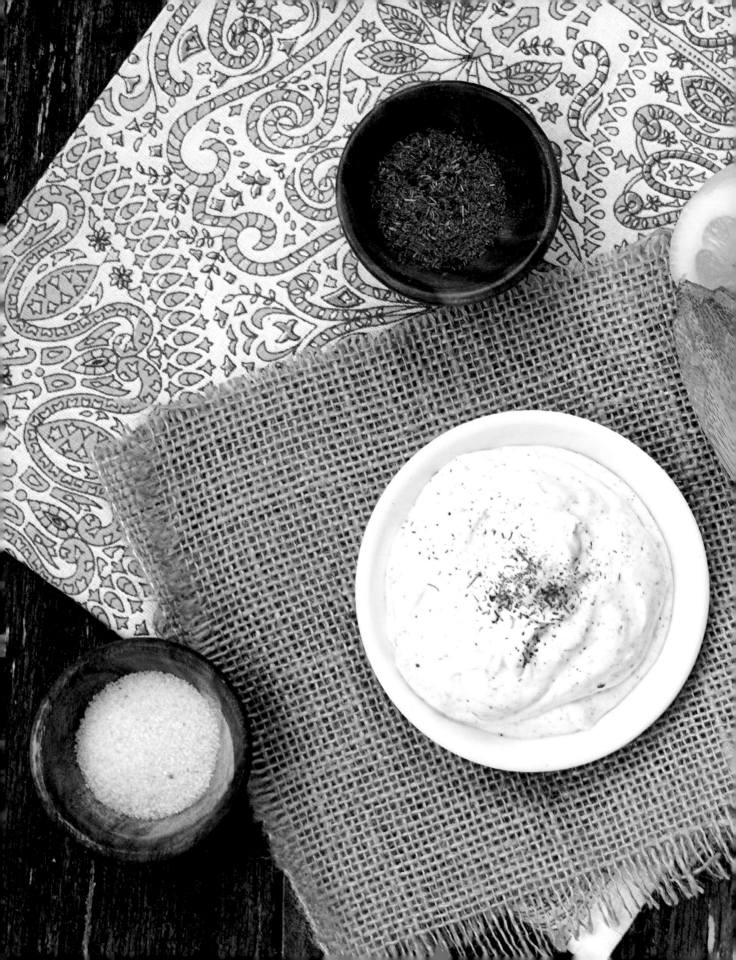

dips and sauces

AVOCADO
BASIL
CREAM SAUCE

EGG-FREE NUT-FREE 40 MINUTES OR LESS

As far as sauces go, it doesn't get much easier than this one. You basically just need to turn on your blender and it's done.

Prep Time: 8 minutes **Yield:** ¾ cup

2 large avocados (about ¾ pound), halved, pitted, and peeled

3 cloves garlic, minced

¼ cup packed fresh basil leaves

2 tablespoons extra-virgin olive oil

1 tablespoon freshly squeezed lemon juice

½ teaspoon fine sea salt

½ teaspoon ground black pepper

Place all of the ingredients in a food processor and blend until smooth.

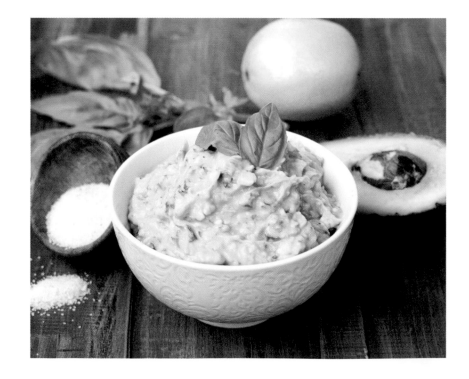

EGGPLANT DIP

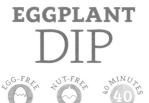

EGG-FREE · NUT-FREE · 40 MINUTES OR LESS

This creamy dip, usually called "baba ghanoush," is similar to hummus, but instead of chickpeas it's made with grilled or roasted eggplant mixed with tahini (ground sesame seed paste), olive oil, and fresh lemon and garlic. Serve with your favorite chopped vegetables or as a topping on grilled chicken, steak, or fish.

Prep Time: 8 minutes   **Cook Time:** 15 or 30 minutes, depending on cooking method   **Yield:** 1½ cups

1 medium eggplant (about 1½ pounds)

2 tablespoons extra-virgin olive oil, divided

¼ cup tahini (see Kitchen Tip, page 276)

¼ cup freshly squeezed lemon juice

2 cloves garlic, minced

¼ teaspoon ground cumin

¼ teaspoon fine sea salt

¼ teaspoon ground black pepper

1 tablespoon chopped fresh flat-leaf parsley, for garnish (optional)

1. Cut the ends off of the eggplant and then slice lengthwise into 4 pieces. Place 1 tablespoon of the olive oil in a bowl and brush each slice lightly with the olive oil.

2. **To use a grill:** Preheat the grill to medium heat. Place the eggplant slices on the grill and cook for 15 minutes, or until tender.

    To use an oven: Preheat the oven to 400°F. Line a 9-by-13-inch baking sheet with parchment paper or a baking mat. Place the eggplant slices on the prepared baking sheet and bake for 30 minutes, or until tender.

3. Peel the skins from the eggplant with a small knife and place the flesh in a blender or food processor. Add the tahini, lemon juice, garlic, cumin, salt, and pepper and blend for 30 seconds, or until the dip is fully combined.

4. Transfer to a serving bowl, drizzle with the remaining 1 tablespoon of olive oil, and sprinkle with parsley, if desired, to serve.

TRY THIS!

For a tasty lunch wrap, spread a tablespoon or two of this dip over a tortilla (page 210) and top with some grilled chicken or steak, romaine lettuce, and sliced tomato.

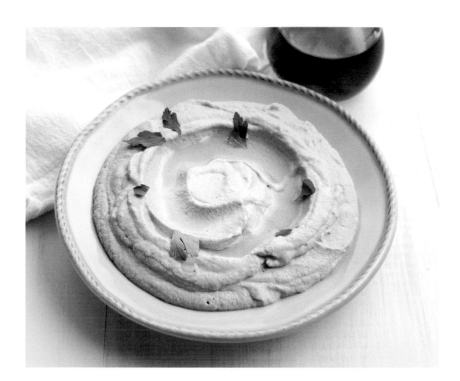

BBQ
SAUCE

EGG-FREE NUT-FREE KID-FAVORITES

Different types of tomatoes have different levels of acidity, and some are sweeter than others. Depending on the type used in the tomato sauce and paste you use, you may need to add a little more raw honey for additional sweetness or a little more apple cider vinegar for tartness. But wait until the sauce is almost done cooking before adjusting the seasonings, as the taste will change as the flavors meld and the sauce reduces.

Prep Time: 5 minutes   Cook Time: 1 hour   Yield: 1½ cups

2 (8-ounce) cans tomato sauce

1 cup water

½ cup apple cider vinegar

5 tablespoons raw honey

2 tablespoons tomato paste

1½ teaspoons ground black pepper

1½ teaspoons onion powder

1½ teaspoons dry yellow mustard

1 teaspoon paprika

Place all ingredients in a medium saucepan over medium-high heat and stir to combine. Bring just to a boil, then reduce the heat to low and simmer for 1 hour, or until thickened to your liking. The longer you leave it on the stove, the more it will reduce and the thicker it will get. Taste and adjust seasonings if desired.

TRY THIS!
Try adding 1 tablespoon of freshly squeezed lemon juice at the same time as the rest of the ingredients.

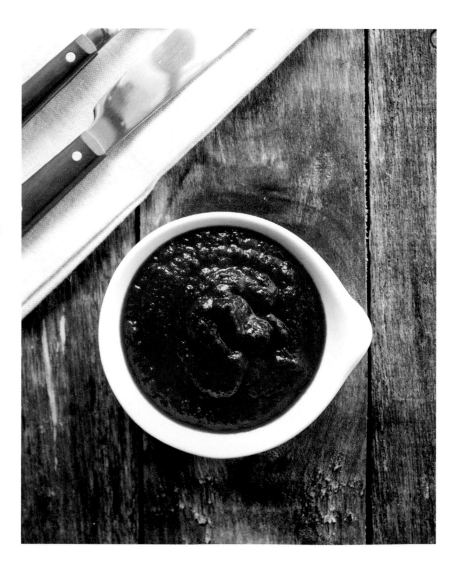

CHIMICHURRI

Chimichurri is made slightly differently in different countries, but almost all versions contain fresh parsley, garlic, and olive oil. I like to use a mixture of half parsley and half cilantro, but you can use 2 full cups of parsley if you dislike cilantro. You will usually find chimichurri served over grilled red meat, but it is also delicious on poultry, fish, and shrimp. I like it best served over a grilled flank steak that has been seasoned with salt and pepper and cut against the grain—simple, fresh, and perfect.

Prep Time: 8 minutes   Yield: 1½ cups

4 cloves garlic, chopped

1 cup tightly packed fresh Italian flat-leaf parsley

1 cup tightly packed fresh cilantro

⅔ cup extra-virgin olive oil

1½ tablespoons freshly squeezed lemon juice or apple cider vinegar

½ teaspoon crushed red pepper

½ teaspoon dried oregano

½ teaspoon fine sea salt

¼ teaspoon ground black pepper

Combine all ingredients in a food processor or blender and blend for 15 seconds, or until well mixed. Taste and adjust seasonings as desired.

TRY THIS!

If you want your sauce to have a little more tang or acidity, add more lemon juice or vinegar. If you like a little more heat, add a few more dashes of crushed red pepper. Add more olive oil to make the sauce thinner, or more parsley to make it thicker.

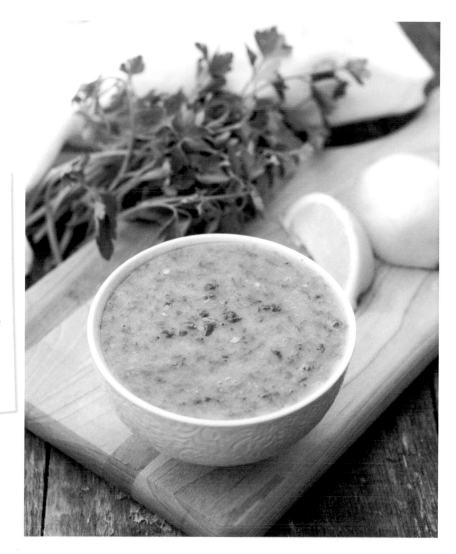

GUACAMOLE

In my house, guacamole is made often, and we love to make it a topping as well as a dip. Guacamole is an easy recipe to tweak, so play around with the amounts and types of seasonings until you get it just the way you like.

Prep Time: 15 minutes   **Yield:** 3 cups

3 large ripe avocados (about 1½ pounds), halved, pitted, and peeled

1 tablespoon freshly squeezed lime juice

½ teaspoon fine sea salt

¼ teaspoon ground black pepper

½ teaspoon garlic powder

½ teaspoon ground cumin

½ teaspoon cayenne pepper

2 cloves garlic, minced

2 medium Roma tomatoes (about ¼ pound), chopped (about ½ cup)

1 small white onion, chopped (about ½ cup)

1 tablespoon chopped fresh cilantro

Place the avocado halves, lime juice, salt, pepper, garlic powder, cumin, and cayenne in a large mixing bowl and mash until the desired consistency is reached. Add the garlic, tomatoes, onion, and cilantro to the mixing bowl and stir until just combined. Taste and season with additional salt and pepper if desired.

TRY THIS!

For extra heat, finely dice and seed 1 small jalapeño and mix it in with the rest of the ingredients.

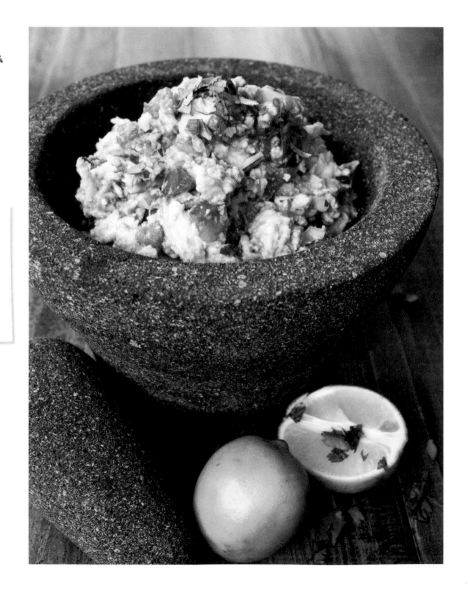

KETCHUP

Like many of my recipes in this book, this one is easy to tailor to suit your personal taste. If you like it a little sweeter, add a little more honey. Like it tangier? Add some more vinegar. Like it a little thinner? Don't cook it as long. Like it with a little kick? Throw in some extra black pepper. I think you're following me: taste and adjust as you go and make it the way YOU like it.

Prep Time: 5 minutes   **Cook Time:** 25 minutes   **Yield:** ¾ cup

½ cup tomato paste

¼ cup raw honey

¼ cup water

¼ cup apple cider vinegar

¾ teaspoon fine sea salt

¾ teaspoon onion powder

¾ teaspoon ground black pepper

½ teaspoon garlic powder

Place all the ingredients in a medium saucepan over medium-high heat. Bring just to a boil, stirring frequently. Reduce the heat to low and gently simmer for 15 to 20 minutes, stirring every couple minutes. Once the sauce has thickened to your liking, remove from the heat and allow to cool completely. Transfer to a sealed container and store in the refrigerator for up to 2 weeks.

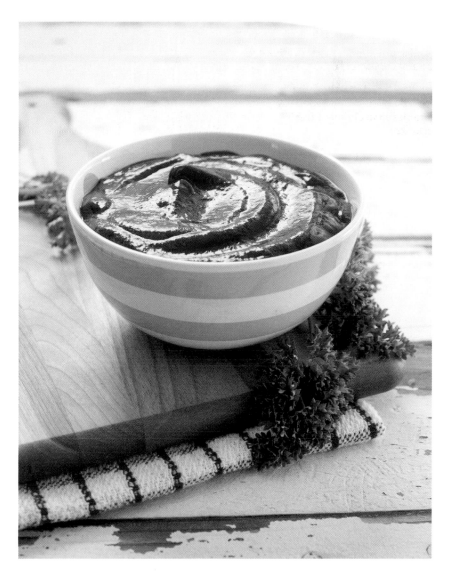

HUMMUS

Hummus is traditionally made with chickpeas, which are not Paleo-friendly, but this tasty dip uses avocado and zucchini to get the same creamy texture. It's perfect with your favorite vegetables.

Prep Time: 10 minutes   Yield: 1½ cups

1 small ripe avocado, halved, pitted, and peeled

1 large zucchini, peeled and chopped (about 1 cup)

1 clove garlic, finely chopped

⅓ cup chopped fresh cilantro, plus more for garnish (optional)

3 tablespoons freshly squeezed lemon juice

3 tablespoons tahini (see Kitchen Tip)

1 tablespoon extra-virgin olive oil, plus more for garnish

½ teaspoon ground cumin

½ teaspoon fine sea salt

¼ teaspoon ground black pepper

Paprika, for garnish (optional)

1. Place all the ingredients but the paprika in a food processor. Blend for 1 minute, or until smooth.

2. Transfer the hummus to a serving bowl. Drizzle with olive oil and add a few dashes of paprika and a sprinkle of chopped cilantro, if desired, before serving.

KITCHEN TIP

If you can't find tahini, almond butter works as a good substitute in this recipe. You can also make your own tahini at home. Place ½ cup of sesame seeds in a large skillet over medium heat and stir until they are toasted and just golden brown. Transfer to a blender or food processor, add 1½ tablespoons of extra-virgin olive oil, and blend until smooth. Store in a sealed container in the refrigerator for up to 2 months.

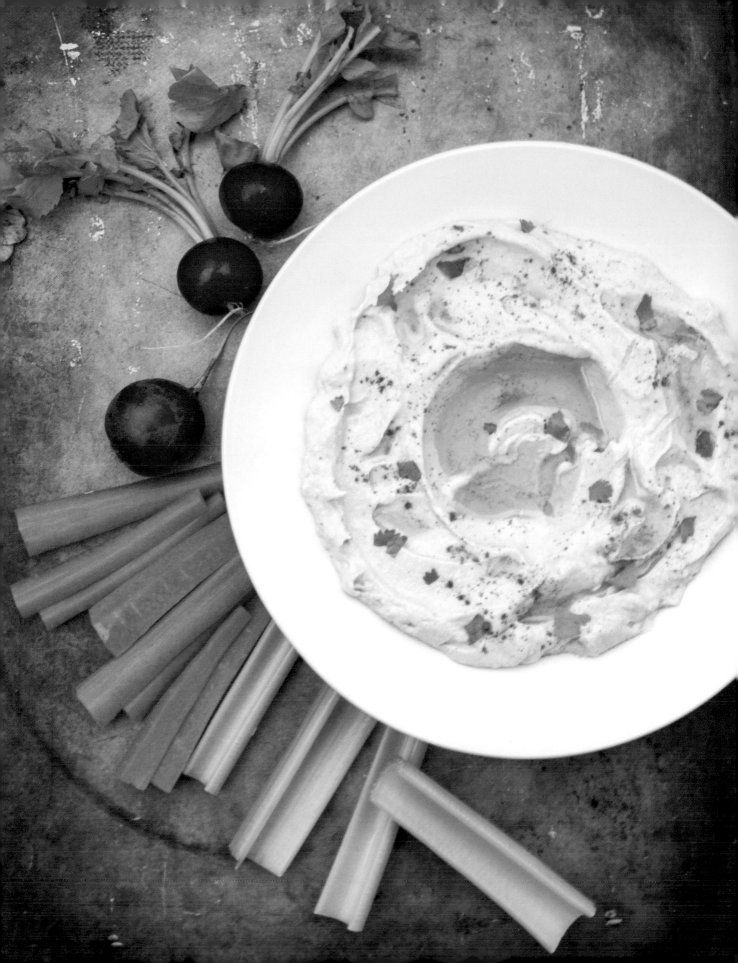

MAYONNAISE

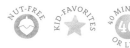

While there are a few brands of Paleo-friendly mayonnaise now, making your own at home is fairly easy. There's some science involved here, so you can't just slap it in a blender and hope for the best, but once you get it down you will be a mayo expert. To make mayonnaise we have to combine ingredients that really don't want to be together under normal conditions, but running a fast blender and very slowly adding the oil drop by drop makes the liquids break apart into tiny droplets, which are then forced to get along and form our creamy mayonnaise.

Prep Time: 10 minutes   **Yield:** 1 cup

1 egg yolk from a large pasteurized egg, room temperature

1 tablespoon freshly squeezed lemon juice

1 cup light olive oil or avocado oil

½ teaspoon fine sea salt

1. **To use a food processor or blender:** Blend the egg yolk and lemon juice in the food processor for 20 seconds. Keeping the food processor running, slowly add the olive oil drop by drop. Do not rush this part; it must be one drop at a time. The mixture will start to thicken and get creamy. Once you have added about ¼ cup of the olive oil and you have a nice thick mixture, you can begin to add the oil a little faster. Once all of the olive oil is added, add the salt and blend once more to fully combine.

    To use an immersion blender: Add all ingredients to a mason jar or wide-mouthed container and allow to settle for about 5 minutes. Place the immersion blender into the jar, all the way to the bottom. Turn the blender on and hold it in place for 30 seconds. Slowly lift the blender up to the top of the mayonnaise and then slowly push it back down again. Once the mayonnaise has turned creamy, you can move the blender around the sides and up and down to make sure everything gets incorporated.

2. Store in a sealed container in the refrigerator for up to 1 week.

KITCHEN TIP
Ripe avocado also works great as a mayonnaise substitute, especially in cold dishes like deviled eggs or chicken salad.

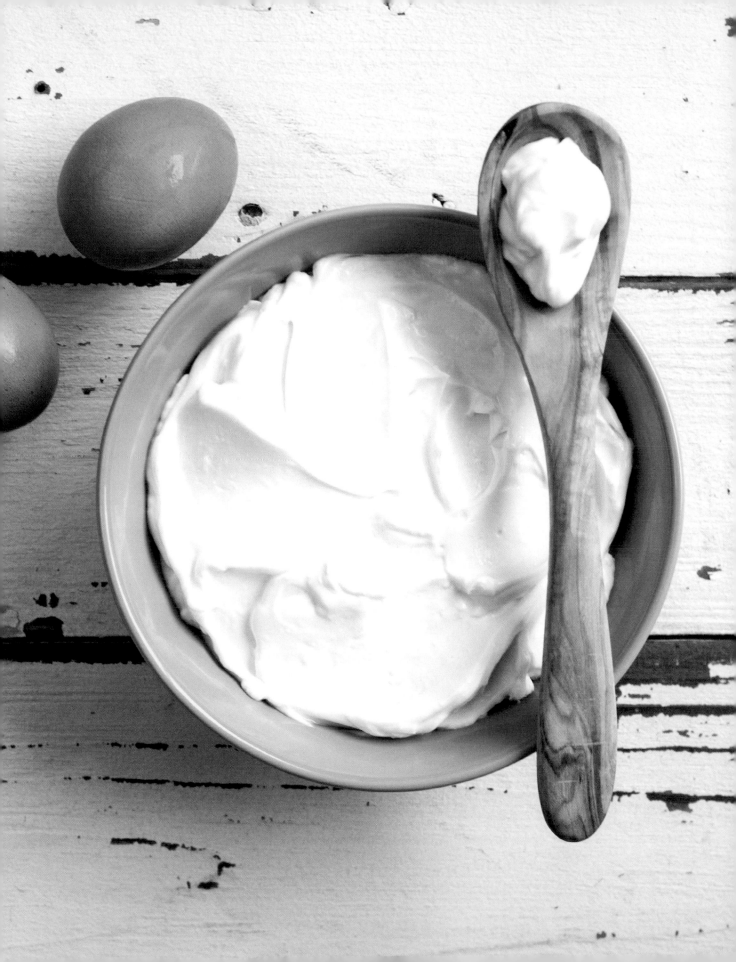

PESTO

EGG-FREE *40 MINUTES OR LESS* **40**

Pesto is a ridiculously simple sauce that is jam-packed with flavor, and just like chimichurri (page 273) it tastes great on all sorts of vegetables, meats, and seafood. For a thicker pesto, increase the amount of basil and pine nuts. For a thinner pesto, increase the amount of olive oil.

Prep Time: 10 minutes   **Cook Time:** 3 minutes   **Yield:** ¾ cup

⅓ cup pine nuts

2 cups packed fresh basil leaves

⅓ cup extra-virgin olive oil

3 cloves garlic, chopped

¼ teaspoon fine sea salt

¼ teaspoon ground black pepper

1. In a small skillet, toast the pine nuts over medium heat for 3 minutes, or until lightly browned.

2. Place the toasted pine nuts, basil, olive oil, garlic, salt, and pepper in a blender and puree until smooth. Store in the refrigerator until ready to use, or freeze in ice cube trays and reheat when needed.

TRY THIS!
Try adding 2 tablespoons freshly squeezed lemon juice and ⅛ teaspoon crushed red pepper.

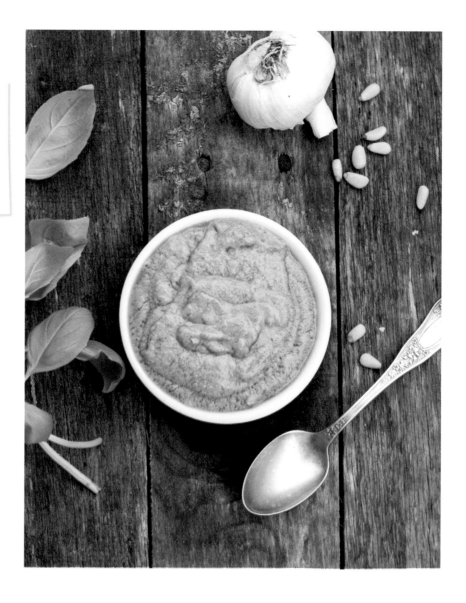

SOUR CREAM

This thick and creamy dairy-free sour cream substitute is great as a topping, or you can mix in your favorite fresh herbs and spices to make a tasty dip for chopped vegetables.

Prep Time: 5 minutes   Yield: 1 cup

Cream from 1 (13.5-ounce) can full-fat coconut milk (see page 315) or 1 cup homemade coconut cream (page 315)

1 tablespoon freshly squeezed lemon juice, or more to taste

⅛ teaspoon fine sea salt

Place the coconut cream in a medium-sized mixing bowl and whisk in the lemon juice and salt until well combined. Taste and add more lemon juice or salt if needed. Store in a sealed container in the refrigerator for up to 1 week.

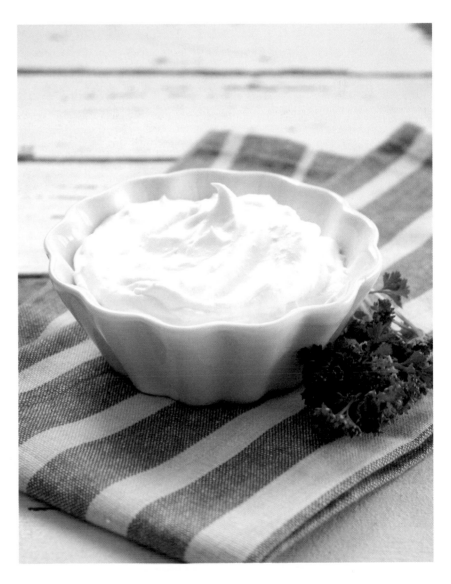

PICO
DE GALLO

EGG-FREE NUT-FREE 40 MINUTES OR LESS

Pico de gallo is a simple dish that is bursting with flavor. The fresh lime juice gives it a little acidity, and the jalapeño adds just a touch of heat. Together they make it far more interesting than just a bowl of chopped onion and tomato. I try to find tomatoes that are ripe but still firm, which hold up best when chopped.

Prep Time: 10 minutes, plus 30 minutes to rest   **Yield:** 2½ cups

3 large tomatoes (about 1½ pounds), seeded and finely chopped (about 1¾ cups)

1 medium onion, chopped (about ¾ cup)

1 jalapeño, seeded and minced

1 clove garlic, minced

¼ cup chopped cilantro

1 tablespoon freshly squeezed lime juice

½ teaspoon fine sea salt

¼ teaspoon ground black pepper

Place all the ingredients in a medium-sized mixing bowl and stir well to combine. Cover and allow to rest at room temperature for 30 minutes for the flavors to combine, or store in the refrigerator until ready to serve.

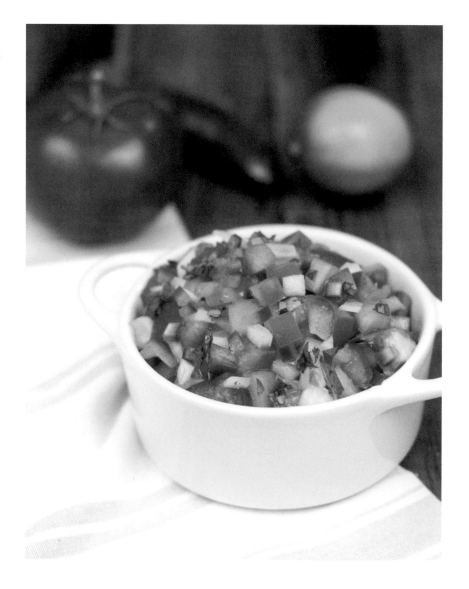

SOY SAUCE
SUBSTITUTE

Since soy is best avoided on a Paleo diet, soy sauce is not an option. Coconut aminos are a great substitute, but if you can't find them or want to make your own replacement, then this recipe also works well. You can use it one-for-one for soy sauce in any recipe.

Prep Time: 5 minutes   **Cook Time:** 20 minutes   **Yield:** ½ cup

1½ cups beef stock (page 310)

1 teaspoon fine sea salt

1 teaspoon apple cider vinegar

1 teaspoon raw honey

¼ teaspoon ground ginger

⅛ teaspoon garlic powder

⅛ teaspoon ground black pepper

Whisk together all the ingredients in a small saucepan over medium-high heat. Bring to a boil, then reduce the heat to low and simmer for 10 to 15 minutes, until the liquid measures about ½ cup. Store in a sealed container in the refrigerator for up to 2 weeks.

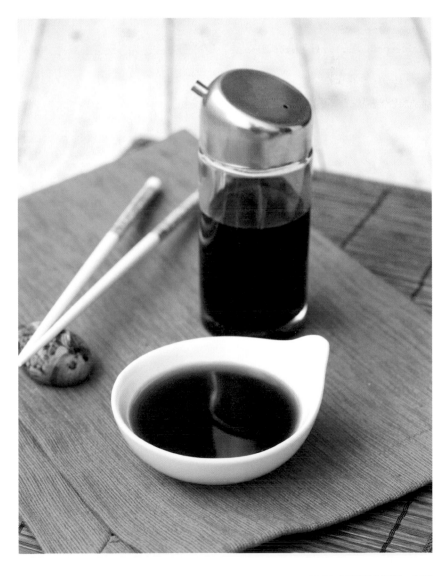

TARTAR
SAUCE

Homemade tartar sauce is easy to make and tastes much better than the store-bought variety. Once you have the mayonnaise base made, it only takes a couple minutes to throw together.

Prep Time: 7 minutes   Yield: 1 cup

1 cup mayonnaise (page 278)

1 tablespoon minced onion

1½ teaspoons freshly squeezed lemon juice or apple cider vinegar

¼ teaspoon fine sea salt

¼ teaspoon garlic powder

¼ teaspoon fresh dill

Mix all the ingredients together in a small bowl until well combined. Taste and adjust the seasonings as desired. Store in a sealed container in the refrigerator for up to 1 week.

TRY THIS!
Try mixing in 2 tablespoons of chopped capers for extra flavor and texture.

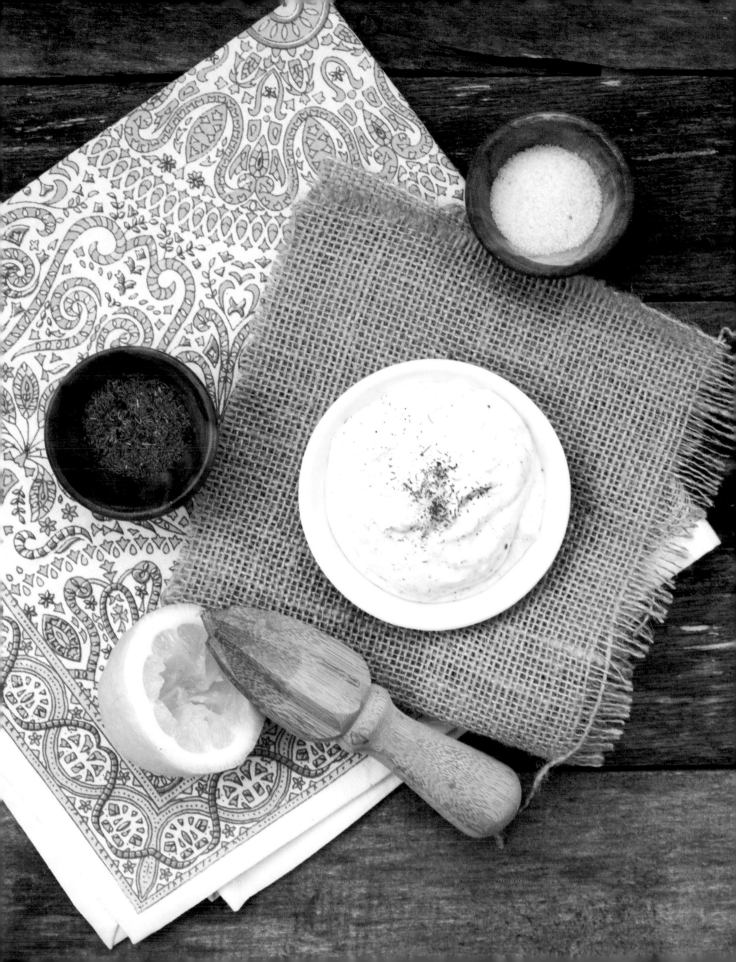

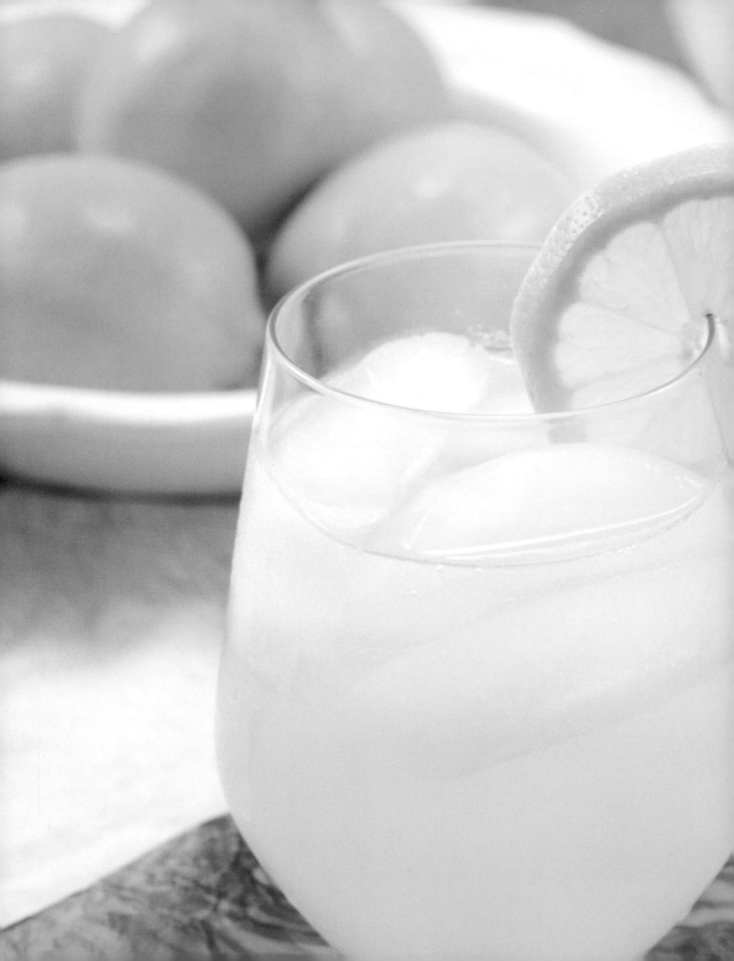

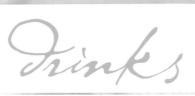

Drinks

APPLE CIDER

This recipe can be made on the stovetop or in a slow cooker, but I love the slow cooker method because on a cold day I get to come home to a house that smells of cinnamon and apples. Having a mug of apple cider is the perfect way to warm up and relax.

Prep Time: 5 minutes   Cook Time: 20 minutes to 8 hours, depending on cooking method   Yield: 4 servings

6 whole cloves

3 sticks cinnamon

6 cups apple juice

Dash of nutmeg (optional)

1. **To use the stove:** Place all the ingredients in a medium-sized saucepan over medium-high heat. Bring to a boil, then reduce the heat to low and simmer for 20 minutes, stirring occasionally. Remove from the heat and cool for about 5 minutes.

   To use the slow cooker: Place all the ingredients in the slow cooker and cook for 3 to 4 hours on high or 6 to 8 hours on low.

2. Ladle into mugs and serve.

TRY THIS!

Try adding a strip or two of orange rind (about 3 inches each) to the pot or slow cooker at the same time as the rest of the ingredients.

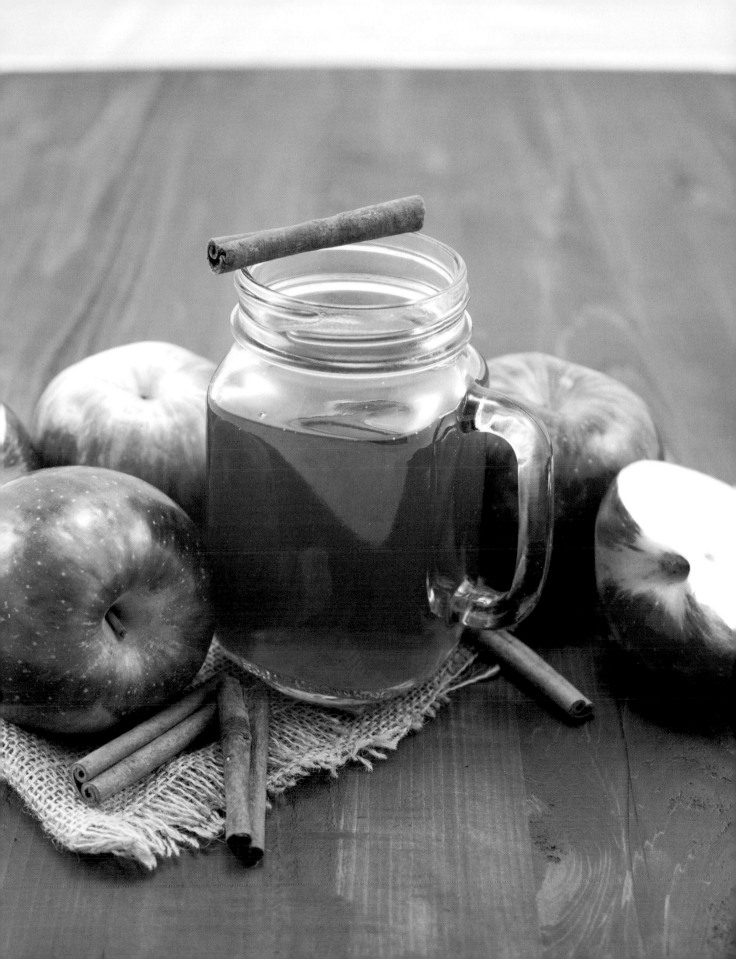

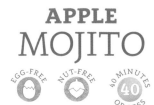

APPLE
MOJITO

EGG-FREE · NUT-FREE · 40 MINUTES OR LESS

This is a fun, nonalcoholic twist on a traditional mojito, and it's especially refreshing on a hot day. Reducing the apple juice makes it more concentrated, so you get more flavor in your glass without having too much liquid. Try to resist the urge to add a splash of rum, but if you do, make me a drink, too.

Prep Time: 5 minutes, plus 10 minutes to cool   Cook Time: 10 minutes   Yield: 2 servings

2 cups apple juice

8 fresh mint leaves

½ teaspoon raw honey

¼ cup freshly squeezed lime juice

½ cup soda water

2 apple slices, for garnish

1. Place 2 glasses in the refrigerator to chill. In a medium saucepan over medium-high heat, bring the apple juice to a boil. Boil for 5 minutes, or until the juice has reduced down to 1 cup. Set aside to cool for 10 minutes.

2. Muddle the mint leaves and honey in the chilled glasses until the mint is crushed. Add the lime juice and the reduced apple juice and stir. Fill with ice almost to the top of the glass, then top off with the soda water. Garnish with an apple slice and serve.

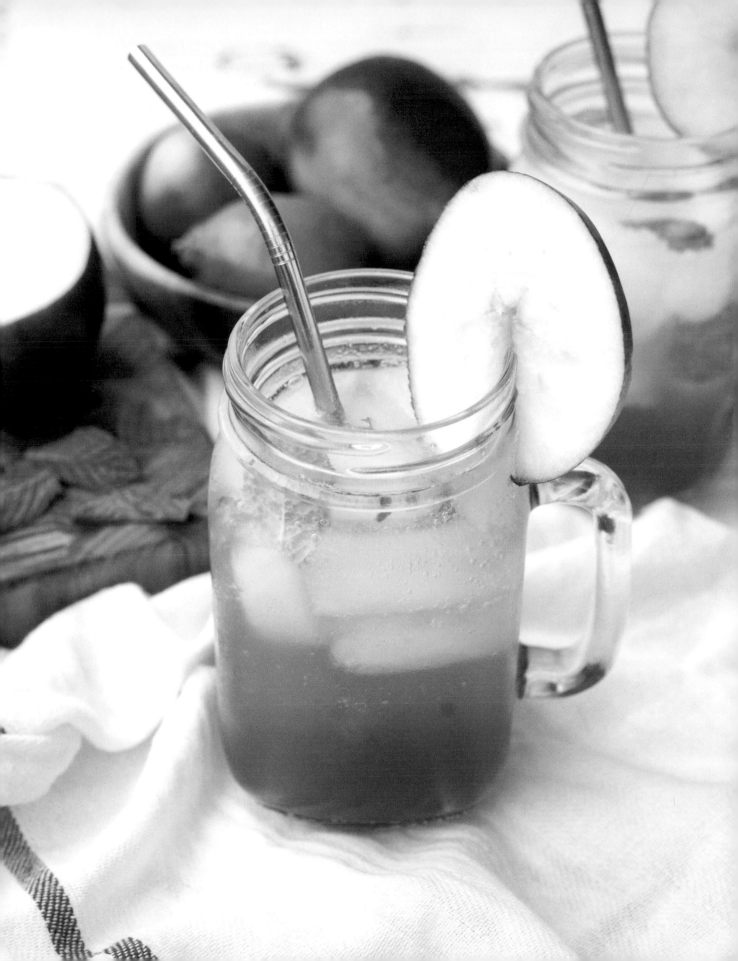

HORCHATA

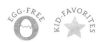

If you have never heard of horchata, then sit back and get ready to be excited. It's a creamy, refreshing, perfectly chilled drink with a hint of cinnamon and sweetness. Sounds good, doesn't it? I like to use a mixture of almond and coconut milk, but you can use either one alone and it will still taste great.

Prep Time: 5 minutes, plus 2 hours to chill   **Cook Time:** 5 minutes   **Yield:** 2 servings

2 cups almond milk (page 318)

1 cup coconut milk (page 314)

¼ cup raw honey

1½ teaspoons ground cinnamon

1½ teaspoons pure vanilla extract

2 sticks cinnamon, for garnish (optional)

1. Place the almond milk and coconut milk in a large pitcher and whisk to combine.

2. In a small saucepan over medium-high heat, bring the honey, cinnamon, and vanilla extract just to a light boil, then pour into the pitcher. Stir until the honey mixture is well combined with the milk.

3. Chill the pitcher in the refrigerator for at least 2 hours. To serve, stir well and then pour over ice. Garnish with a cinnamon stick if desired.

TRY THIS!
Try adding a couple dashes of nutmeg at the same time as the ground cinnamon.

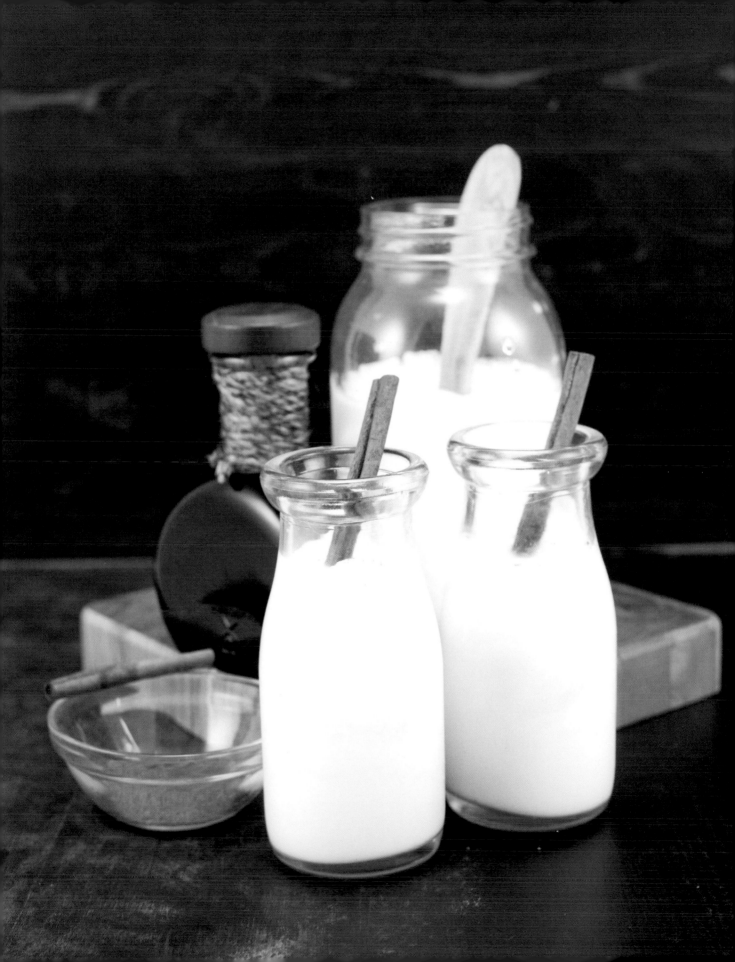

HOT
DULCE DE
LECHE

This recipe is a nice treat for kids who want a sweet warm drink. You can use either coconut milk or almond milk, depending on your taste preferences. Make sure to allow time to make the Salted Caramel Sauce (page 260) and the Whipped Coconut Cream (page 261), if using, before you start.

Prep Time: 5 minutes, plus 30 minutes for the Salted Caramel Sauce   **Cook Time:** 5 minutes   **Yield:** 2 servings

2 cups coconut milk (page 314) or almond milk (page 318)

¼ cup Salted Caramel Sauce (page 260)

½ teaspoon pure vanilla extract

Whipped Coconut Cream (page 261), for topping (optional)

¼ teaspoon ground cinnamon, for topping (optional)

1. In a small saucepan over medium-high heat, combine the coconut milk, caramel sauce, and vanilla extract. Cook for 4 to 5 minutes, until the caramel sauce is fully dissolved, stirring occasionally.

2. Pour into serving mugs and top with whipped coconut cream and a sprinkle of cinnamon, if desired.

TRY THIS!

For a hot chocolate dulce de leche, add 2 tablespoons of cacao powder or unsweetened cocoa powder at the same time as the caramel sauce.

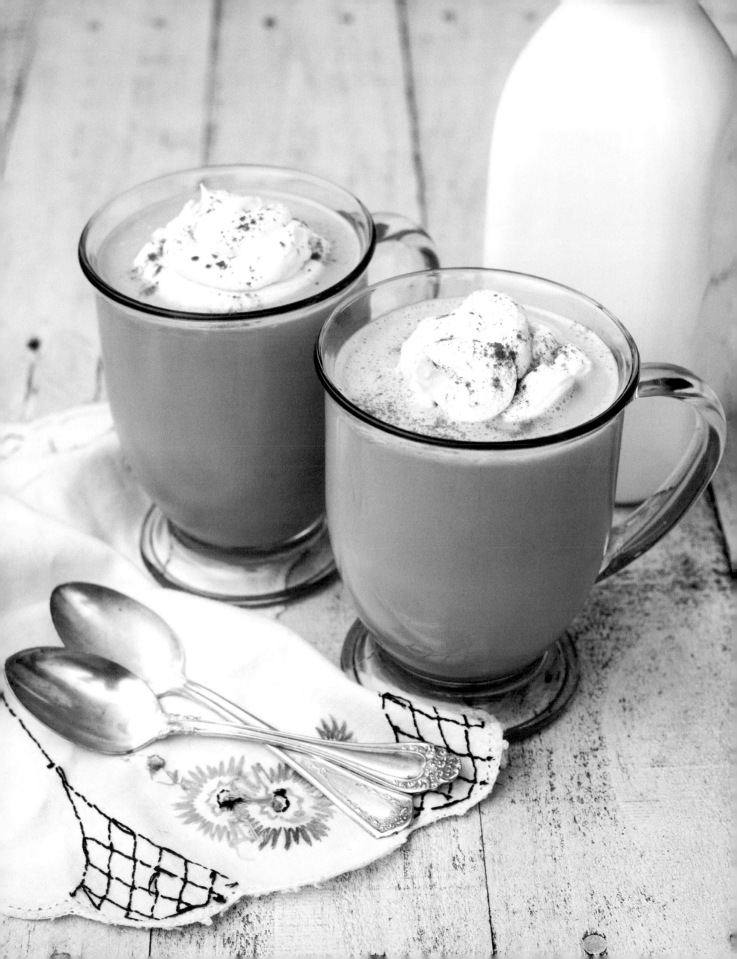

HONEYDEW MINT AGUA FRESCA

Agua fresca is a refreshing and light fruit drink that is great on a hot day. This recipe calls for honeydew melon, but you can use seedless watermelon instead. If you want an extra minty flavor, you can muddle the mint in the glass before adding the ice.

Prep Time: 5 minutes   **Yield:** 4 servings

1 (5-pound) ripe honeydew melon, rind and seeds removed, chopped

3 cups cold water

⅓ cup raw honey

¼ cup freshly squeezed lemon juice

1 lemon, sliced, for garnish

8 sprigs fresh mint, for garnish

1. Puree the chopped melon in a blender until smooth. Strain through a sieve placed over a pitcher and discard any excess pulp.

2. Return the melon juice to the blender and add the water, honey, and lemon juice. Blend for 30 seconds, or until fully combined. Place in the refrigerator until ready to serve.

3. To serve, fill 4 glasses with ice and pour the agua fresca over the ice. Garnish with the lemon slices and mint.

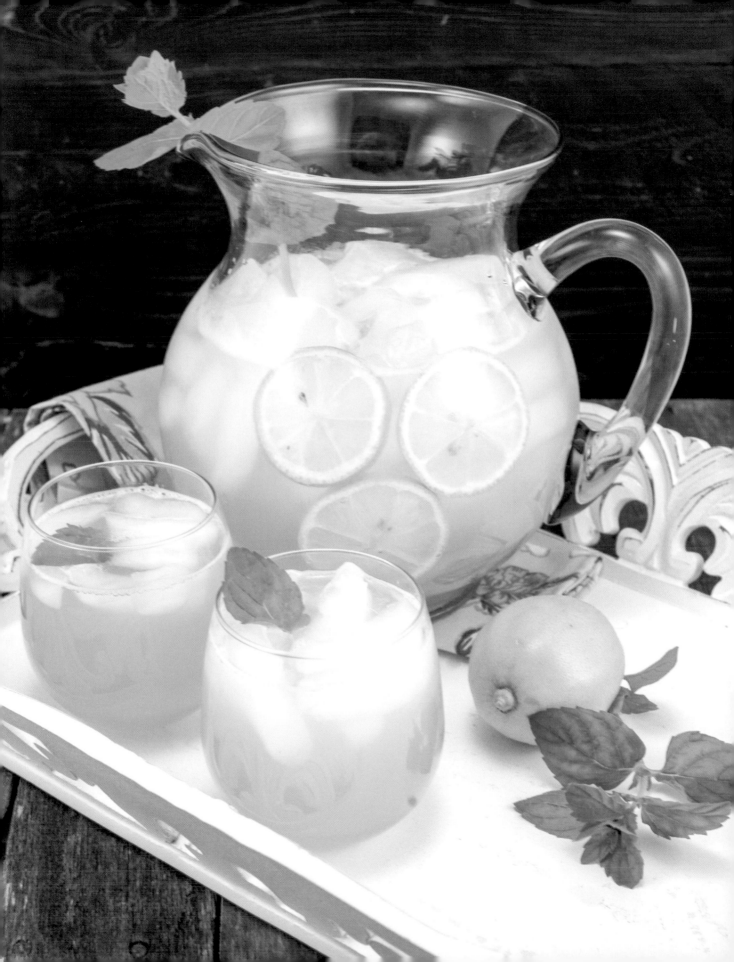

LEMONADE

EGG-FREE NUT-FREE KID-FAVORITES

Lemonade is a classic American beverage, and no picnic or barbecue would be complete without it. The lemon and honey in this recipe create a refreshing combination of sweet and tart. You can adjust the levels to suit your tastes so you can have the perfect glass of lemonade.

Prep Time: 10 minutes, plus 2 hours 15 minutes to chill   **Cook Time:** 5 minutes   **Yield:** 6 servings

1½ cups freshly squeezed lemon juice (8 to 10 large lemons)

8 cups water, divided

1 cup raw honey

1 lemon, sliced, for garnish (optional)

1. In a medium-sized saucepan over medium-high heat, bring the lemon juice, 1 cup of the water, and the honey just to a boil, stirring to make sure it is well combined. Remove from the heat and let cool for 15 minutes.

2. Pour the remaining 7 cups of water into a large pitcher. Add the lemon mixture and stir to combine. Taste to see if it needs any modifications. If too sweet, add a little more water and lemon juice. If too sour, add a little more water and raw honey. Refrigerate for 2 hours, or until chilled. Serve over ice with a lemon garnish if desired.

KITCHEN TIP

Wondering what to do with those leftover lemon rinds? Place a couple in the dishwasher for a clean-smelling load of dishes, or simmer them in a saucepan filled with water for a few hours to create a fresh-smelling house.

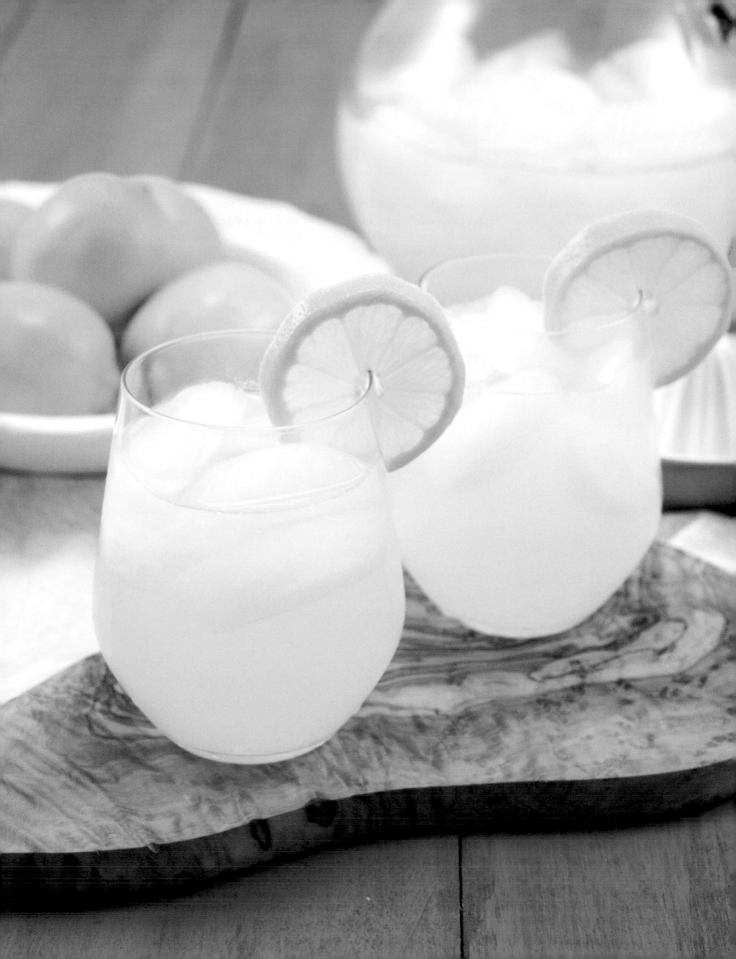

THAI
ICED TEA

EGG-FREE   NUT-FREE   40 MINUTES OR LESS

I am a big fan of Thai tea; it's an occasional treat that I truly enjoy, especially with spicy food. Many Thai tea mixes found online or in stores contain artificial food dyes, which are what give it the bright orange color. Because of that, I usually stick to black tea bags and add vanilla extract and occasionally some additional spices (see the "Try This!" tip below for suggestions).

Prep Time: 5 minutes, plus 1 hour to steep   **Cook Time:** 5 minutes   **Yield:** 4 servings

4 cups water

⅓ cup raw honey

1 teaspoon pure vanilla extract

4 black tea bags

1 cup coconut milk (page 314)

1. In a medium saucepan over medium-high heat, bring the water, honey, and vanilla extract just to a boil, then remove the pan from the heat.

2. Add the tea bags to the saucepan and allow to sit for 1 hour, or until the tea has come to room temperature. Remove the tea bags and discard. Store the tea in the refrigerator until ready to serve.

3. Fill 4 glasses with ice and pour an equal amount of tea into each glass. Slowly pour ¼ cup of coconut milk into each glass and serve.

TRY THIS!

Try adding 6 whole cloves, a dash of cardamom, and/or a cinnamon stick to the honey mixture before you place it on the stove, then discard the spices along with the tea bags before serving.

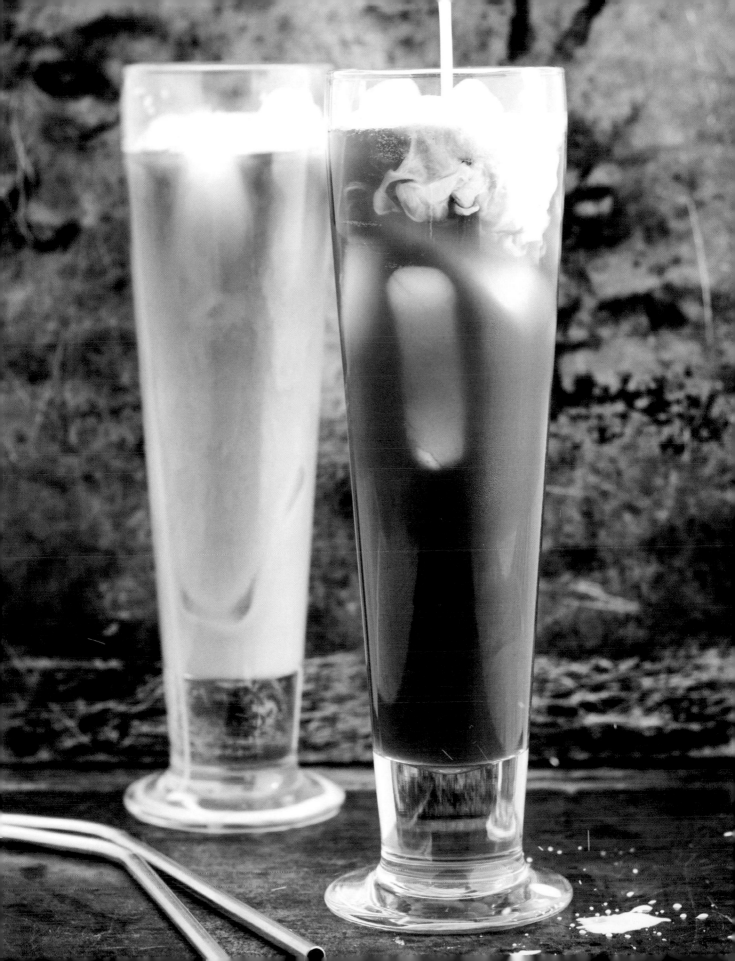

CREAMSICLE SMOOTHIE

This smoothie combines the slight tanginess of fresh orange juice with the creaminess of almond milk and bananas.

Prep Time: 7 minutes   Yield: 2 to 4 servings

1 large orange, peeled and sliced

1 large banana, sliced and frozen (see Kitchen Tip)

1½ cups almond milk (page 318) or coconut milk (page 314)

1½ cups freshly squeezed orange juice

1 teaspoon raw honey

1 teaspoon pure vanilla extract

Place all the ingredients in a blender or food processor and blend for 30 seconds, or until smooth. Pour into glasses and serve right away.

KITCHEN TIP

The best way to freeze a banana is to peel and slice it, place it on a baking sheet lined with parchment paper, and stick it in the freezer for a couple hours until frozen solid. Transfer the banana slices to a sealed container and store in the freezer until ready to use.

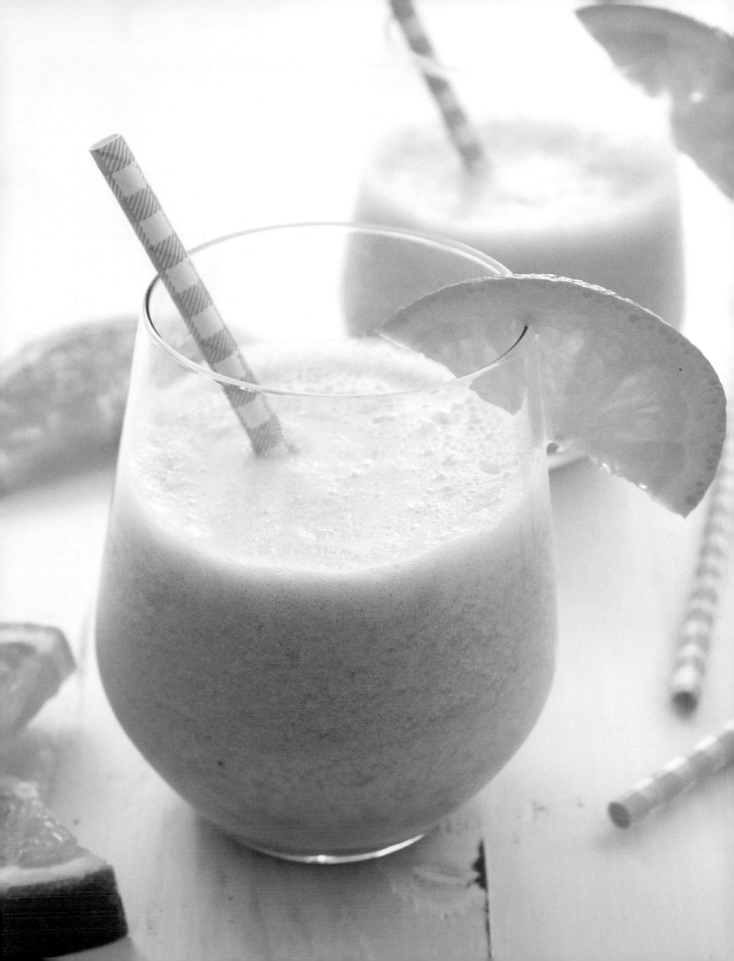

PIÑA COLADA
SMOOTHIE

This smoothie takes just a few minutes to throw together, and it's satisfying no matter what the weather is outside. Just close your eyes, take a big sip, and picture yourself in the middle of summer on a lovely beach surrounded by golden sand.

Prep Time: 5 minutes   **Yield:** 2 servings

1 cup pineapple chunks, frozen

1 medium banana, sliced and frozen (see Kitchen Tip, page 302)

1 cup coconut milk (page 314)

1 tablespoon raw honey

2 tablespoons freshly squeezed lime juice

½ cup Whipped Coconut Cream (page 261), for topping (optional)

In a blender, blend the frozen pineapple, frozen banana, coconut milk, honey, and lime juice for 1 minute, or until smooth. Pour into 2 glasses and top with whipped coconut cream, if desired.

TRY THIS!

Try topping each glass with a sprinkle of toasted shredded coconut (see page 250 for toasting instructions) to give your smoothie some extra texture and flavor.

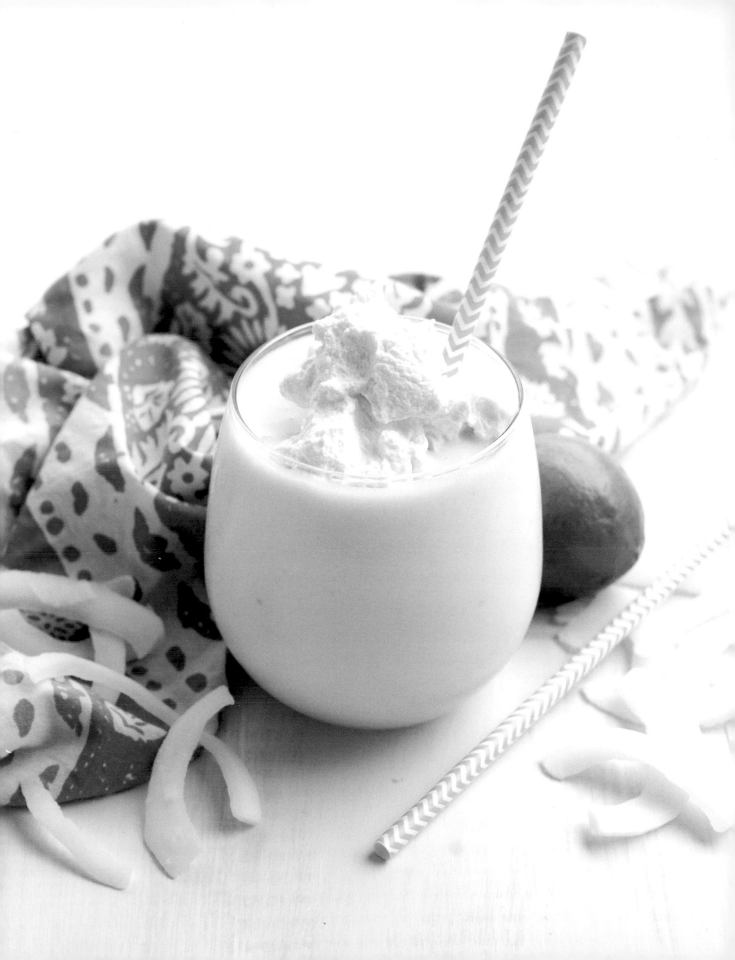

STRAWBERRY
AVOCADO
SMOOTHIE

I have been feeding this smoothie to my kids for at least a year now, and they have no idea they're drinking avocado. All they know is that they get a drink with fun colors that tastes great. The sweetness of the strawberries perfectly complements the creaminess of the avocado, and the two combined make a velvety smooth drink.

Prep Time: 7 minutes   Yield: 2 servings

FOR THE STRAWBERRY LAYER

10 strawberries, plus 2 more for garnish

1 tablespoon raw honey

FOR THE AVOCADO LAYER

1 large avocado (about ½ pound), halved, pitted, and peeled

½ cup pineapple juice

1 cup coconut milk (page 314)

3 tablespoons raw honey

1. First, make the strawberry layer: Place the strawberries and honey in a blender or food processor and blend for 30 seconds, or until smooth. Pour into 2 glasses.

2. Next, make the avocado layer: Place the avocado halves, pineapple juice, coconut milk, and honey in a blender or food processor and blend for 30 seconds, or until smooth. Gently spoon on top of the strawberry layer, then garnish each glass with a strawberry and serve.

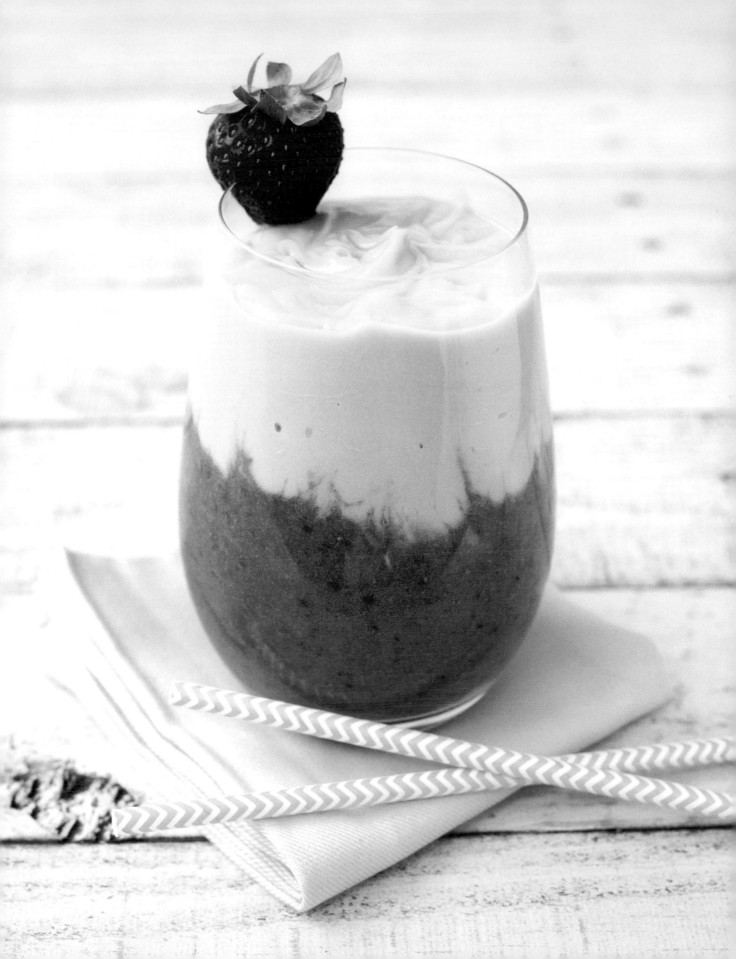

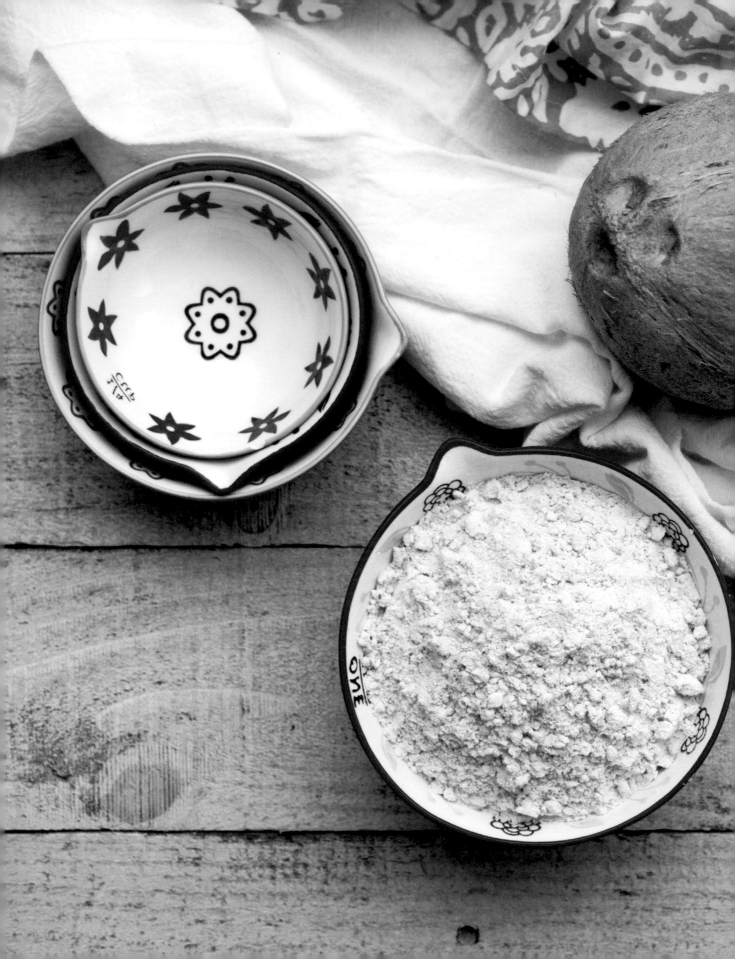

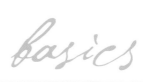

basics

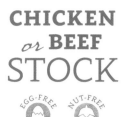

CHICKEN or BEEF STOCK

EGG-FREE   NUT-FREE

Making your own stock at home is easy, and it tastes much better than the canned version, plus you know there are no weird additives or ingredients. This recipe doesn't include salt; it's usually best to add it when you're using the stock in a recipe instead, so that you can use the right amount for that particular dish.

Prep Time: 10 minutes   Cook Time: 5 or 15 hours, depending on the cooking method   Yield: 10 cups

2 pounds chicken or beef bones, and any remaining meat

1 medium onion, quartered

2 medium carrots, cut into 4 pieces each

3 stalks celery, cut into 4 pieces each

5 sprigs fresh thyme

2 bay leaves

5 black peppercorns

2 cloves garlic, peeled

16 cups (1 gallon) water

1. **To use a stovetop:** In a large stockpot over high heat, bring all the ingredients to a boil. Reduce the heat to low and simmer, uncovered, for 5 hours.

   To use a slow cooker: Place all ingredients in the slow cooker and cook on low for 12 to 15 hours.

2. Strain through a fine-mesh sieve into a large container and discard the solids. Use right away, or cool to room temperature for 1 hour, then pour into sealable containers and store in the refrigerator for up to 3 days or freezer for up to 3 months.

KITCHEN TIP

Having a stash of homemade stock in your freezer is a huge time-saver, especially if you freeze the stock in ice cube trays. Knowing how much your ice cube tray holds means that you will know how many cubes you need to grab for a recipe. For me, it's usually 2 tablespoons per cube. I just pour the stock in the tray, leave it to freeze for a few hours, then transfer the frozen cubes of stock to a sealed container that I store in my freezer.

TRY THIS!

If you're using clean bones with no meat on them, you can roast the bones before making the stock to help give it an even richer flavor: just place the bones in a roasting pan and roast in a 400°F oven for 1 hour.

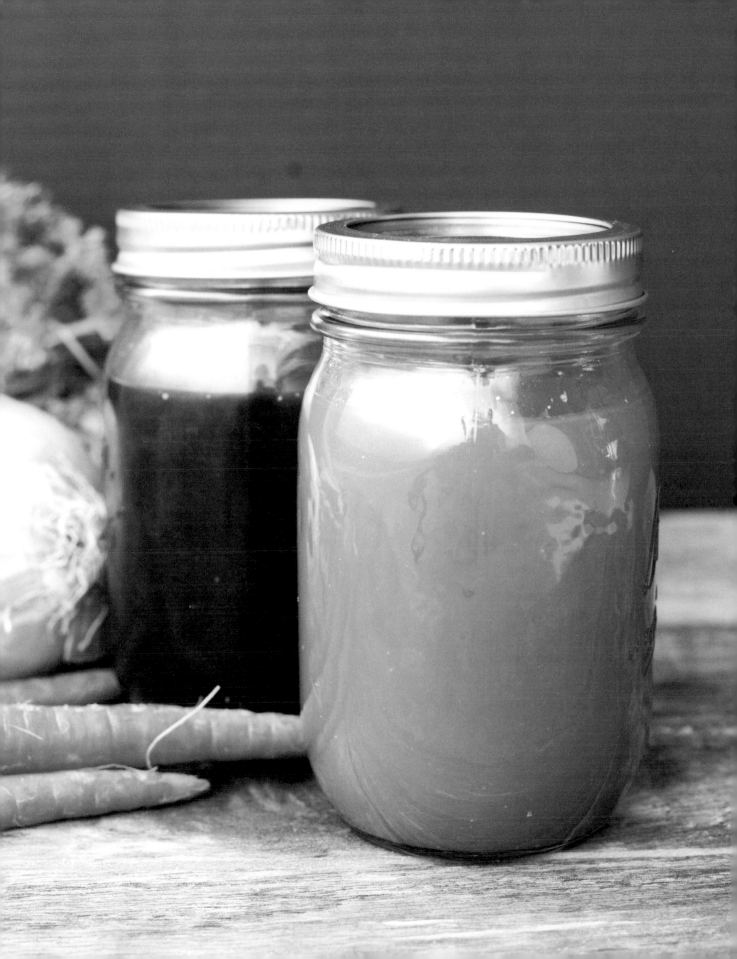

FISH STOCK

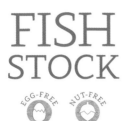

EGG-FREE   NUT-FREE

Unlike chicken and beef stock, which cook for a long period of time, most fish stocks are cooked for 30 minutes or less to prevent the bitter flavor that can result from overcooking some types of fish. This shorter cooking time means the vegetables need to be chopped small, so you can get maximum flavor in minimum time. Less-oily fish, such as snapper, bass, or cod, are good choices. Ask the nice folks at your local seafood counter if they have any fish heads and bones in the back (they tend to not leave those out on the display).

Prep Time: 10 minutes   **Cook Time:** 40 minutes   **Yield:** 10 cups

2 tablespoons ghee (page 320), lard (page 322), or tallow (page 324)

1 large shallot, chopped

2 cloves garlic, chopped

2 medium carrots, chopped (about 1½ cups)

3 stalks celery, chopped

4 pounds fish heads (gills removed) and fish bones

5 sprigs fresh thyme

2 bay leaves

5 black peppercorns

11 cups water

1. Melt the ghee in a large saucepan over medium heat. Add the shallot and garlic to the pan and sauté for 3 minutes. Add the carrots, celery, and fish bones and sauté for another 5 minutes, stirring occasionally. Add the thyme, bay leaves, and peppercorns and cook for 1 more minute.

2. Add the water to the pan and bring to a boil. Use a spoon to skim off any froth and scum from the surface, then reduce the heat to low and simmer, uncovered, for 25 minutes.

3. Strain the stock through a fine-mesh sieve into a large container and discard the solids. Use right away, or cool to room temperature for 1 hour, then pour into sealable containers and store in the refrigerator for up to 3 days or freezer for up to 3 months.

TRY THIS!
To make a shellfish stock, replace the fish bones with shrimp, crab, and/or lobster shells. Shellfish stock can be used in place of fish stock in most recipes.

COCONUT FLOUR

EGG-FREE · NUT-FREE · 40 MINUTES OR LESS

While I don't use coconut flour often and I don't have any recipes that use it in this cookbook, it is an ingredient you will find used in many Paleo baking recipes. Making coconut flour at home is as easy as taking shredded coconut and grinding it into a powder. I recommend making coconut milk (page 314) first and then using the pulp to make coconut flour, so you can get the most out of the coconut (see the Kitchen Tip).

Prep Time: 3 minutes   **Yield:** 1 cup

1 cup unsweetened shredded coconut

Place the shredded coconut in a blender or food processor and pulse until it forms a fine powder, then transfer to an airtight container. Store in a dark, dry place for up to 2 months.

KITCHEN TIP

If you've made coconut milk and are using the leftover coconut pulp, you'll need to dry the pulp before making coconut flour. Preheat the oven to 200°F. Evenly spread the coconut pulp on an unlined 9-by-13-inch baking sheet and bake for 2 to 3 hours, until completely dry, stirring occasionally. Then just follow the instructions above to make the flour.

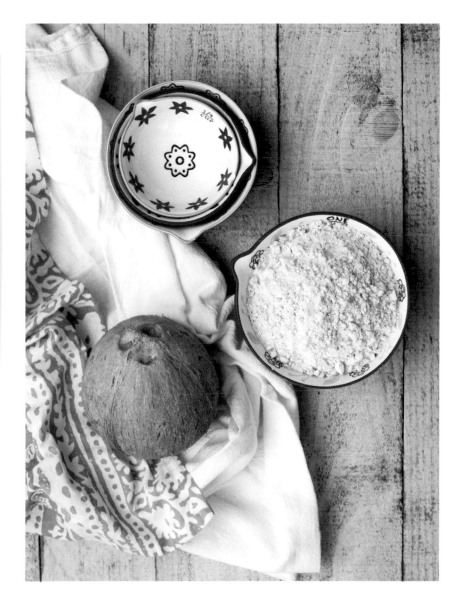

COCONUT MILK

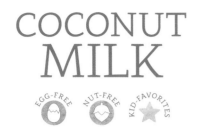

EGG-FREE · NUT-FREE · KID-FAVORITES

It's easy to make your own coconut milk and cream at home using freshly grated coconut or dried shredded coconut, which is more readily available. This recipe will give you coconut milk that is the same consistency as the full-fat store-bought kind, so that you can make coconut cream (page 315). If you do not need coconut cream and want a thinner coconut milk that is similar to almond milk, use 6 cups of water instead of 3. If you use store-bought coconut milk for any of the recipes in this book, make sure you use the full-fat kind.

Prep Time: 5 minutes, plus 1 hour to soak   **Yield:** 2 cups

3 cups unsweetened shredded coconut

3 cups hot water

1. In a blender or food processor, blend the coconut and hot water for 30 seconds. Transfer to a large container, cover, and set aside for at least 1 hour.

2. After an hour, strain the coconut mixture through a nut milk bag or 2 layers of cheesecloth. Squeeze the coconut mixture until all of the liquid has been removed, then set aside the shredded coconut (you can use this to make coconut flour; see page 313).

3. Use the milk right away or store in a sealable container in the refrigerator for up to 4 days or in the freezer for up to 3 months. The milk will separate into water and cream as it sits; to return it to the original consistency, seal and shake the container vigorously or throw the milk in a blender or food processor and blend for a few seconds.

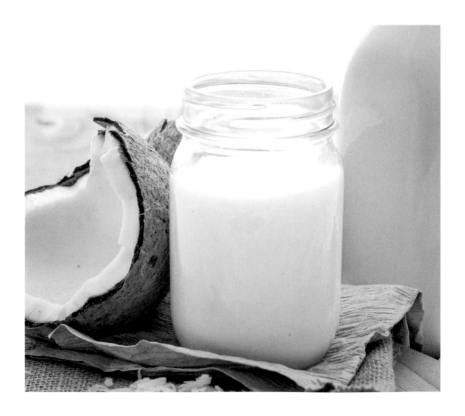

COCONUT CREAM

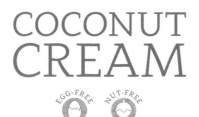

EGG-FREE NUT-FREE

After a few hours in the refrigerator, coconut milk separates into water and cream, and the cream can be skimmed off and used in many recipes—including Whipped Coconut Cream (page 261), a tasty dessert topping. (If you plan to use store-bought coconut milk to make coconut cream, see the Kitchen Tips below for instructions.)

Prep Time: 5 minutes, plus 6 hours to chill   Yield: ¾ cup

1 batch Coconut Milk (page 314)

Place the coconut milk in a sealed container and store upside-down in the refrigerator for about 6 hours to separate the coconut water and cream. Once the water and cream have separated, open the container, pour off the water (you can save it to use later if you like), and scoop the cream out from the bottom.

KITCHEN TIPS

If you want to use canned coconut milk instead of homemade for coconut cream, the process is basically the same: Chill a 13.5-ounce can of full-fat coconut milk upside-down in the refrigerator for 6 hours or longer. Open the can and pour the water into a container to save for later (it's great for smoothies), then scrape out the thick coconut cream into a separate bowl. This will give you about 1 cup of coconut cream.

Many coconut milk companies add preservatives so that the coconut milk will not separate, so look for a brand with very few additives. If you shake the can gently and don't hear any sloshing sounds, that is probably a good brand to use. I always keep an extra can in my refrigerator in case one doesn't fully separate (it happens).

There are a few brands of canned or boxed coconut cream that have very few additives, but I still put these in the refrigerator and allow them to separate just like coconut milk. There is much less liquid to pour out, but it gives you an extra-thick cream.

ALMOND FLOUR

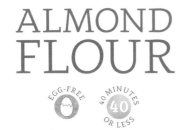

While almond flour is becoming more readily available in grocery stores and online, it is also very easy to make your own at home. Buying almonds in bulk is a great way to keep the cost reasonable, and you can get even more bang for your buck by making almond milk first and then turning the leftover pulp into almond flour (see the Kitchen Tip). If you do use store-bought almond flour for any of the recipes in this book, make sure you use finely ground, blanched almond flour.

Cashews, macadamia nuts, and pistachios also make great nut flours. And the instructions here are the same for sunflower seed flour, which can be used as a one-for-one replacement for almond flour in almost all Paleo recipes and is a good option for people who are allergic to nuts.

Prep Time: 1 minute   **Yield:** 2 cups

2 cups raw blanched almonds (or raw cashews, raw macadamia nuts, raw pistachios, or raw sunflower seeds), divided

1. Place 1 cup of the almonds in a blender or food processor and blend on high speed for 15 seconds, then stir the mixture and blend for another 5 to 10 seconds, until the mixture is finely ground. Overblending the mixture can cause it to start to turn into nut butter, so make sure you check the texture every few seconds. (If you're using sunflower seeds, keep in mind that they will blend faster than the larger almonds.)

2. Transfer the flour to an airtight container, then repeat the process with the remaining cup of almonds. Store in a dark, dry place for up to 3 months.

KITCHEN TIPS

If you've made almond milk and are using the leftover pulp, you'll need to dry the pulp before making almond flour: Preheat the oven to 200°F. Evenly spread the almond pulp on an unlined 9-by-13-inch baking sheet and bake for 2 to 3 hours, until completely dry. Place in a food processor or blender and pulse 7 to 10 times, until very finely ground, then transfer to an airtight container.

I recommend using blanched almonds (skin removed) for almond flour. If you can't find blanched raw almonds at the store, you can remove the almond skins yourself at home. Fill a medium saucepan halfway full with water and bring to a boil. Add the almonds to the water and boil for 1 minute. Transfer the almonds to a colander or sieve to drain and then lay them out on paper towels or a kitchen towel and pat dry. Squeeze each almond gently between your fingers and the skin should slide right off. Discard the skins and allow the almonds to dry completely before using.

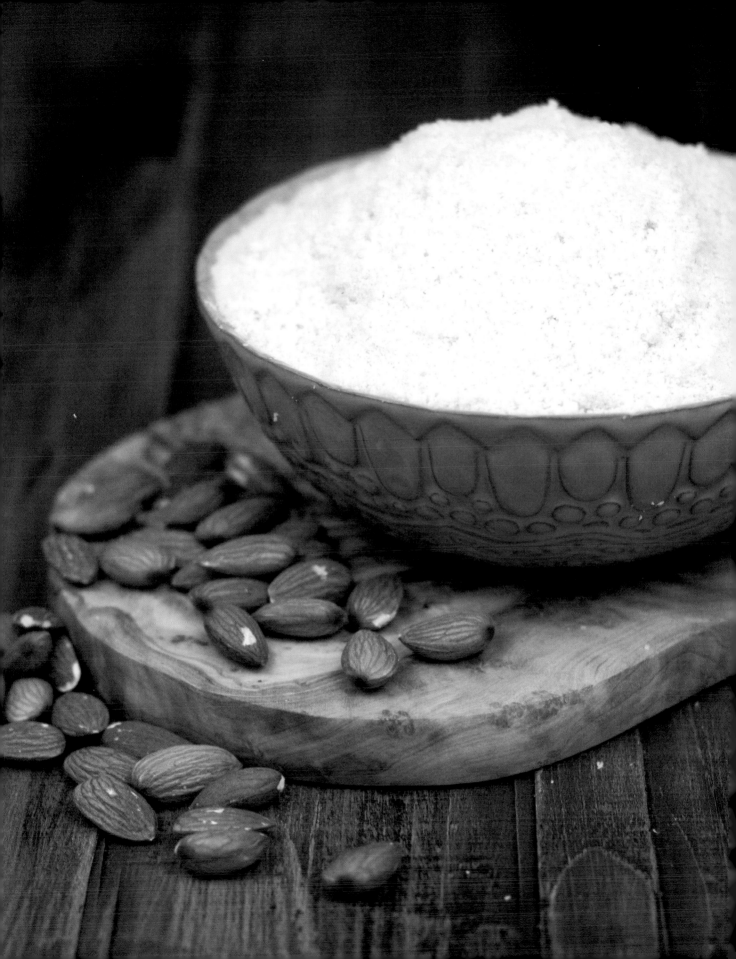

ALMOND MILK

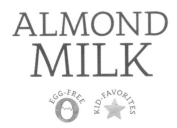

EGG-FREE · KID-FAVORITES

Almond milk is commonly used as a dairy-free milk substitute in Paleo recipes. While coconut milk has a strong coconut flavor to it, almond milk has a mild flavor and is not as thick as coconut milk. The store-bought versions usually have quite a few additives or even sweeteners, but luckily making your own at home is very easy. You don't have to make just almond milk, either; you can use any type of raw nuts or seeds to make a Paleo-friendly milk. As an added bonus, the leftover pulp can be dried and used to make flour (see page 316).

Prep Time: 10 minutes, plus 6 hours to soak   Yield: 3 cups

1 cup raw almonds (or raw cashews, raw macadamia nuts, raw pistachios, or raw sunflower seeds)

3½ cups water, plus more for soaking

1. Place the almonds in a bowl, cover with water, and soak for at least 6 hours or overnight.

2. Drain the water and transfer the almonds to a blender or large food processor. Add the 3½ cups of water and blend on high for 1 minute.

3. Strain the almond mixture through a nut milk bag or 2 layers of cheesecloth into a resealable container. Squeeze the nut milk bag until all of the almond milk has been removed. The almond milk will keep, covered, in the refrigerator for up to 4 days.

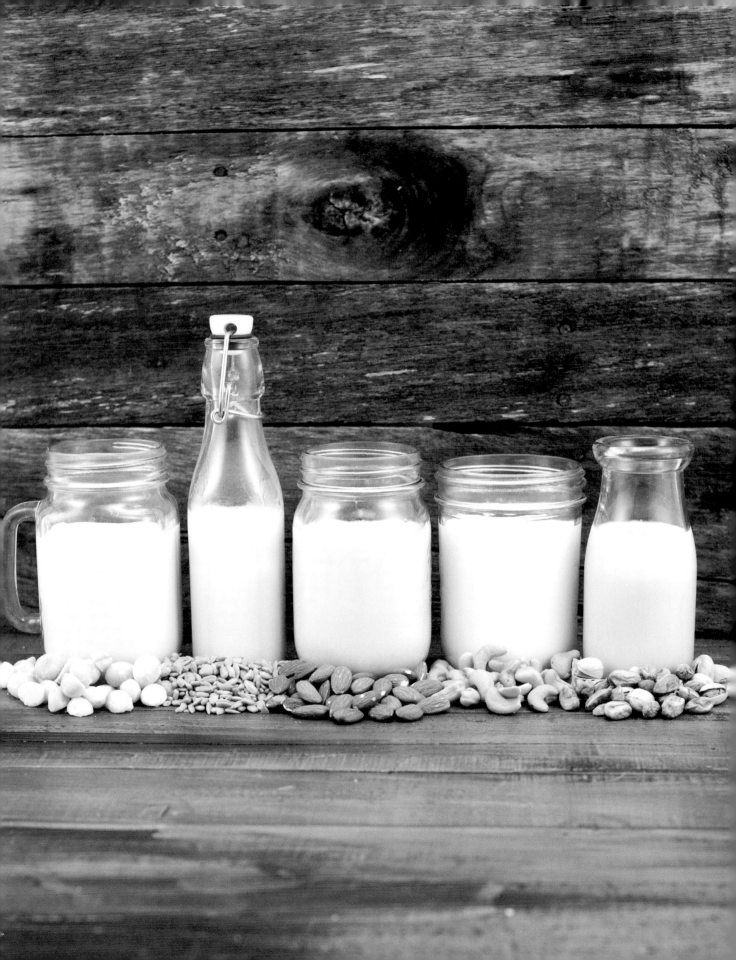

GHEE

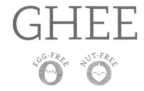

Ghee is one of the first fats I reach for in cooking and baking. It is everything I love about butter but without all the negatives that can come with dairy, and it has a very high smoke point, which means it is great for cooking at high temperatures. Many people who are sensitive to dairy find they can tolerate ghee because the cooking process removes almost all of the lactose and casein (that's the stuff that makes many folks' stomachs hurt when they eat dairy). And most important of all, it tastes great. So let's get your ghee on!

Cook Time: 50 minutes   Yield: 2 cups

1 pound high-quality unsalted butter (grass-fed preferred)

1. Melt the butter in a saucepan over medium heat, stirring occasionally. This will take around 10 minutes.

2. Once all of the butter has melted, reduce the heat to low and simmer without stirring for 30 to 40 minutes. After about 20 minutes, you will see a layer has formed on the top of the ghee. This is the milk proteins separating. Carefully skim the proteins from the top of the ghee with a small spoon and discard. Skim again after another 10 minutes. The ghee is done once it has a very light toffee scent and the milk solids at the bottom of the pan start to turn a light brown (watch them as you do not want them to burn).

3. Remove the pan from the heat and set aside to cool for 5 minutes, then strain the ghee through a fine-mesh strainer or coffee filter into resealable, heatproof containers. Allow to cool completely, then store in the refrigerator for up to 2 months or in the freezer for up to 6 months.

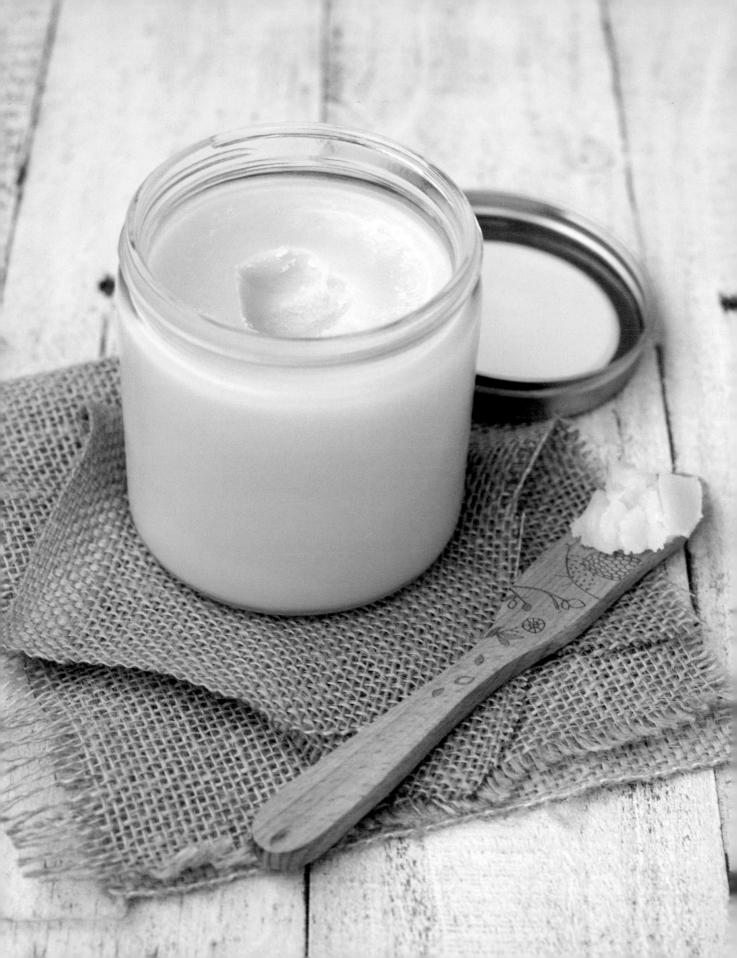

LARD

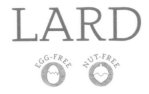

Lard is one of my favorite fats to use in savory dishes, second only to ghee, and it's fairly easy to make at home. While you can order the pork fat to make lard online, finding it locally can be easier than you'd think. When starting out on a Paleo diet, it's a good idea to become friends with your local butcher or the folks at the meat counter. Things like chicken and beef bones for stock (page 310) and quality fat for making lard may not always be out on display for everyone to buy, but you'd be surprised at what is hidden behind the counter. Even if you are limited to one grocery store in your area, chances are the people at the meat counter will be able to get you what you need, or know where you can get it.

Prep Time: 10 minutes   **Cook Time:** 2 hours 30 minutes   **Yield:** 6 cups

4 pounds pure pork fat (leaf fat if possible), cut into 1-inch chunks

1 cup water

1. Working in batches, place the fat chunks in a food processor or blender and pulse a few times, until ¼-inch pieces are formed.

2. In a large Dutch oven or heavy-bottomed pot over low heat, combine the water and pork fat. Allow the fat to very slowly melt for 1 hour, then carefully strain the liquid through a fine-mesh strainer into a resealable, heatproof container. Return the pan to the stove and allow the remaining solid fat to melt for another hour, then strain again into the same container. Return the pan to the stove one more time and melt the remaining solid fat for another 30 minutes, or until cracklings at the bottom are browned but not crispy or burnt. Strain the remaining melted fat into the container, seal, and allow to cool completely. Store for up to 3 months in the refrigerator.

KITCHEN TIP

After all of the lard has been rendered, you can return the pan to the stove, turn the heat up to medium-high, and fry the cracklings until they are crispy. Use a slotted spoon to transfer them to a paper towel-lined plate to drain, then munch away!

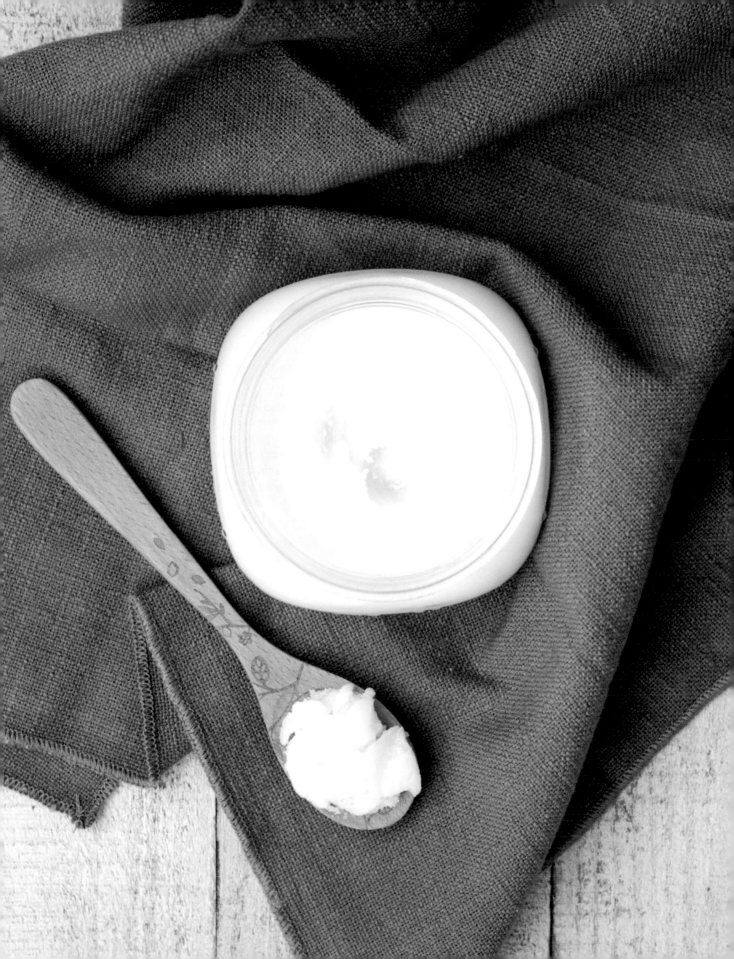

TALLOW

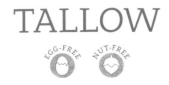

Tallow, like ghee and lard, is one of my favorite fats to use in savory cooking. Tallow is available at some natural food stores, from your local butcher, and online. You can also make it at home yourself. The key to rendering tallow is to cook the fat on very low heat and ensure it does not burn, which makes it perfect for a slow cooker. Make sure that you buy pure fat—if there's any protein mixed in with the fat, the tallow can go rancid fairly quickly.

Prep Time: 10 minutes   **Cook Time:** 6 to 7 hours   **Yield:** 3 to 4 cups

2 pounds pure beef fat

1. Keep the fat cold in the refrigerator until right before you're ready to use it, so it doesn't melt. Cut the fat into chunks, making sure to remove any pieces of meat and other detritus, so you have just the fat. Chop into ¼-inch pieces or, if you have a strong food processor or blender, pulse the chunks in batches until ground into very small pieces.

2. Place the ground fat in a slow cooker, cover, and cook on low for 6 to 7 hours, until completely rendered, stirring every hour or two. As the fat begins to render, small pieces may rise to the top.

3. The tallow is done when the bottom is a clear liquid. There will be pieces floating at the top, and that's okay. Place a double layer of cheesecloth over the mouth of a large mason jar or sealable container and strain the tallow through it to remove any impurities. Allow the tallow to cool and solidify at room temperature, then place the lid on tightly. Store for up to 3 months in the refrigerator.

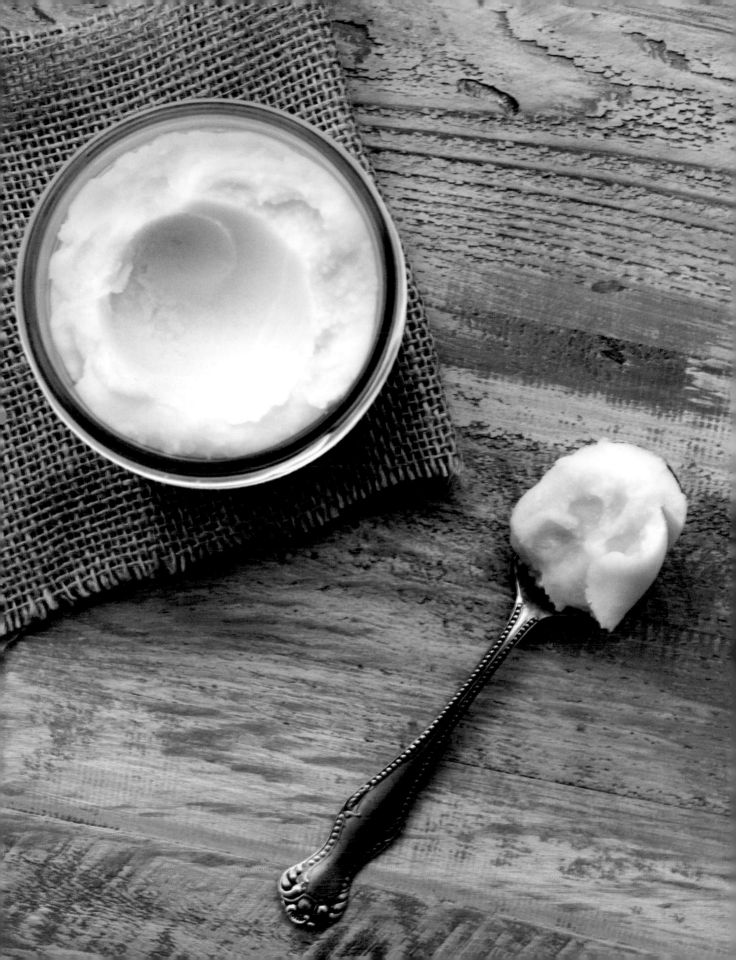

SPAGHETTI SQUASH NOODLES

I was on the last day of writing this cookbook when I realized that I wanted to include a quick recipe for making spaghetti squash noodles. I started to get the noodles ready for a photo, but when I ran a fork down the length of the squash, all I got was mush. I tried again and again but kept getting the same results. I figured I just purchased a bad squash and decided to try again the next day. It wasn't until I was lying in bed later that night that it suddenly dawned on me: I had picked out, purchased, brought home, sliced, cooked, cooled, and attempted to shred noodles from a BUTTERNUT squash, not a spaghetti squash. They are not the same shape, color, size, or smell, and I have been cooking both for about twenty years. Sleep is important, people.

Just FYI, the squash that is yellow both inside and outside, cylindrical in shape, and labeled as a spaghetti squash at the store is the one you want.

Prep Time: 5 minutes   Cook Time: 45 minutes   Yield: 2 to 4 servings

1 (3-pound) spaghetti squash, halved lengthwise and seeded

⅓ cup water

1 tablespoon extra-virgin olive oil or melted ghee (page 320)

¼ cup chopped fresh parsley, for garnish (optional)

Pesto (page 280) or other sauce, for serving

1. Preheat the oven to 400°F.

2. Place the squash cut side down in a roasting pan and pour the water around it. Bake for 35 to 45 minutes, until the squash is tender.

3. Remove the pan from the oven and place a large bowl next to the squash. Gently run a fork in the same direction as the noodle strands (top to bottom) and transfer the noodles to the bowl. Once all of the noodles are removed, you can discard the squash rind, or use it as a serving bowl.

4. To serve, toss the noodles with the olive oil and top with chopped fresh parsley, if desired, or your favorite sauce, such as pesto.

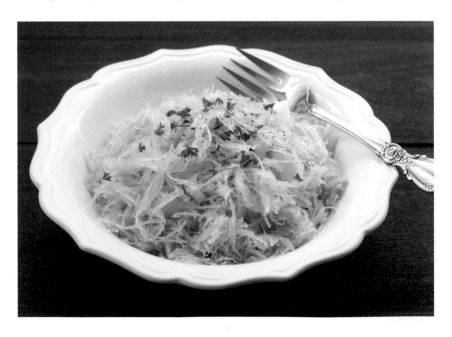

SWEET
POTATO
NOODLES

 EGG-FREE NUT-FREE KID-FAVORITES 40 MINUTES OR LESS

The first time I made my mother sweet potato noodles, she declared them one of the best things she had ever tasted. She proceeded to ask me for at least a week what sort of wizardry I had used to create these magical noodles. I never did tell her my secret or how easy they are to make. But it is very possible that she is reading this and the cat is out of the bag. In which case, love you Mom, happy noodling!

Prep Time: 10 minutes   **Cook Time:** 10 minutes   **Yield:** 4 servings

1 pound red- or white-skinned sweet potatoes, peeled

1 tablespoon ghee (page 320), lard (page 322), or tallow (page 324)

¼ teaspoon fine sea salt

¼ teaspoon ground black pepper

1 teaspoon chopped fresh parsley, for garnish (optional)

1. Slice the ends off the potatoes. Use a spiral slicer or a julienne slicer to turn the potatoes into noodles.

2. Melt the ghee in a large skillet over medium heat. Add the sweet potato noodles, salt, and pepper and cook for 7 to 10 minutes, until just tender, tossing occasionally. Taste and add more salt and pepper if desired. Garnish with chopped parsley, if desired, and serve.

TRY THIS!
Turn cooked sweet potato noodles into a fun dessert by tossing them with a few dashes of cinnamon and nutmeg and a drizzle of raw honey.

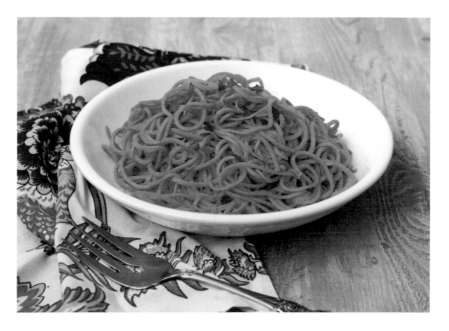

ZUCCHINI
NOODLES

If you've been following a Paleo diet for a while now, you've probably already made zucchini noodles. But if you're new to the world of Paleo, you'll find that these noodles make a great substitute for wheat-based noodles. Because zucchini is about 95 percent water, you need to salt them before cooking to help release excess liquid; otherwise that liquid will be released during cooking and you will wind up with a soggy mess. You can also use yellow summer squash instead of zucchini, and you'll need to salt those as well.

Prep Time: 10 minutes, plus up to 45 minutes to salt the zucchini   **Cook Time:** 5 minutes   **Yield:** 4 servings

6 to 8 large zucchinis (about 3 pounds), peeled

1 teaspoon fine sea salt

2 tablespoons ghee (page 320), lard (page 322), or tallow (page 324)

Ground black pepper

1. Use a julienne slicer or spiral slicer to make noodles of the peeled zucchinis. Place the noodles in a colander or strainer over a large bowl or pan. Sprinkle with the salt and toss, then allow to sit for at least 20 minutes and up to 45 minutes, until most of the moisture has been released, occasionally tossing the noodles to help the liquid drain. Wrap a few paper towels or a clean kitchen towel around the noodles and gently squeeze to remove as much additional moisture as possible. If the noodles are very long, cut them in half to make them easier to work with.

2. Melt the ghee in a large skillet over medium heat. Add the noodles and sauté for 3 minutes, or until just softened. Season with salt and pepper to taste.

KITCHEN TIP
If you're not making the noodles right away, roll them in paper towels or a kitchen towel and let them sit in the refrigerator for up to 24 hours before cooking. This also helps draw out even more moisture, which makes for noodles with an even better texture.

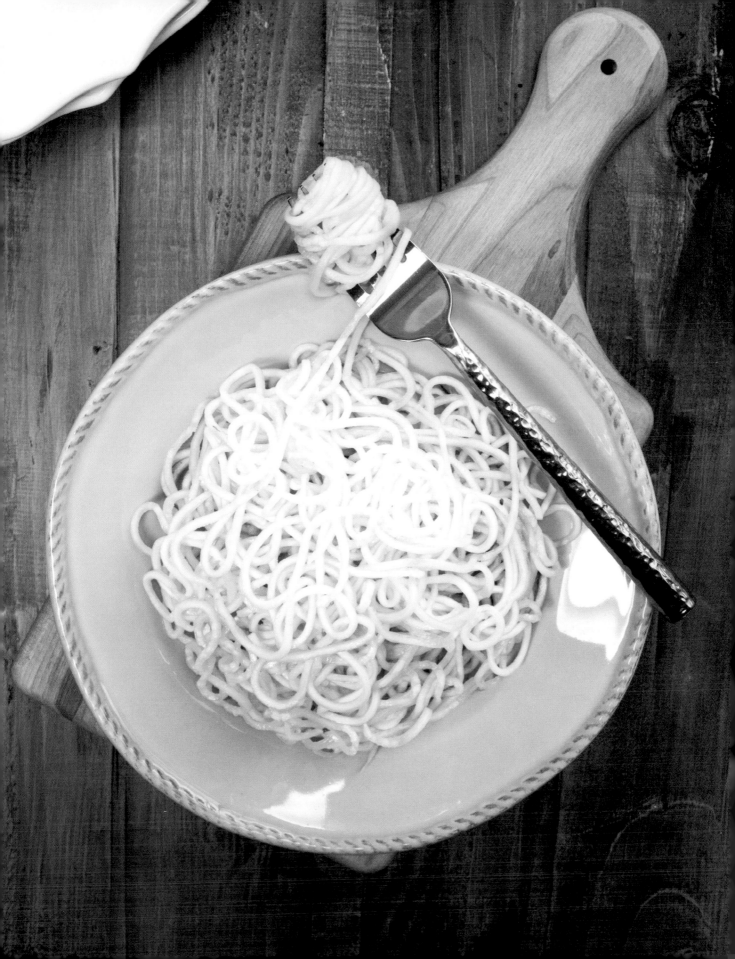

SEASONING BLENDS *and* RUBS

EGG-FREE · NUT-FREE · 40 MINUTES OR LESS

These seasoning blends will give you a good idea of which spices generally work well together, so you can use them as guidelines when creating your own recipes. But since everyone's taste is slightly different, you can check if you'll like the seasoning blend you're making by mixing a tiny bit of each ingredient together and placing a bit of the blend on the tip of your tongue. If you don't like it, taste each spice individually and figure out if there is one in particular that you don't care for. You can omit that spice entirely or use more of one of the other spices instead.

To make these seasoning blends, mix all the spices together in a small bowl and then store in an airtight container in a dark, dry place for up to a year. You can use these mixes to season meat, fish, poultry, and vegetables. Sprinkle them on your food as minimally or generously as your taste buds allow. As a general rule, if using a seasoning blend as a rub, use 2 tablespoons for every 1 pound of boneless or 2 pounds of bone-in meat, poultry, or fish. If using as a seasoning to enhance food, start off with ¼ to ½ teaspoon for each pound of meat or 2 cups of sauce.

Yield: ½ cup

ALL-PURPOSE SEASONING

2 tablespoons fine sea salt

1 tablespoon garlic powder

1 tablespoon onion powder

1 tablespoon dried parsley

2 teaspoons ground black pepper

1½ teaspoons dried basil

1½ teaspoons dried thyme

1½ teaspoons dried oregano

1½ teaspoons rubbed sage

1 teaspoon coriander

ITALIAN

2 tablespoons dried oregano

2 tablespoons dried thyme

1 tablespoon dried rosemary

1 tablespoon dried basil

1 tablespoon rubbed sage

2 teaspoons garlic powder

1 teaspoon fine sea salt

MEDITERRANEAN

2 tablespoons garlic powder

1½ tablespoons dried basil

1½ tablespoons dried oregano

2 teaspoons fine sea salt

2 teaspoons ground black pepper

2 teaspoons dried parsley

1½ teaspoons dried rosemary

1½ teaspoons dried thyme

1 teaspoon ground nutmeg

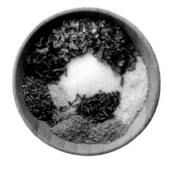

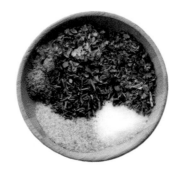

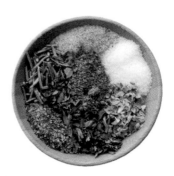

MEXICAN

2 tablespoons ground cumin

2 tablespoons paprika

1 tablespoon chili powder

1 tablespoon garlic powder

1 tablespoon onion powder

1½ teaspoons dried oregano

1½ teaspoons fine sea salt

MIDDLE EASTERN

1½ tablespoons ground black pepper

1½ tablespoons coriander

1½ tablespoons ground cumin

1½ tablespoons ground paprika

2 teaspoons ground allspice

1½ teaspoons cardamom

1½ teaspoons ground cloves

½ teaspoon ground cinnamon

½ teaspoon ground nutmeg

INDIAN

2 tablespoons ground cumin

1½ tablespoons ground coriander

1½ tablespoons turmeric

1 tablespoon ground cardamom

2 teaspoons ground black pepper

2 teaspoons ground cinnamon

1 teaspoon dry yellow mustard

1 teaspoon ground cloves

1 teaspoon ground nutmeg

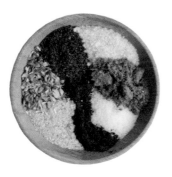

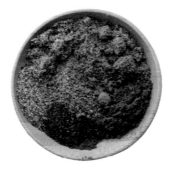

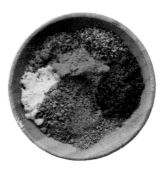

CAJUN

1½ tablespoons fine sea salt

1½ tablespoons garlic powder

1 tablespoon paprika

1 tablespoon onion powder

2½ teaspoons dried oregano

2½ teaspoons dried thyme

2 teaspoons ground black pepper

2 teaspoons cayenne pepper

THAI

1 tablespoon dried basil

1 tablespoon garlic powder

1 tablespoon onion powder

1 tablespoon coriander

1 tablespoon paprika

1 tablespoon ground ginger

1½ teaspoons cayenne pepper

1½ teaspoons ground cumin

1½ teaspoons ground black pepper

1½ teaspoons fine sea salt

JAMAICAN JERK

1½ tablespoons onion powder

1½ tablespoons garlic powder

1½ tablespoons dried thyme

2 teaspoons fine sea salt

2 teaspoons dried parsley

2 teaspoons paprika

1 teaspoon allspice

1 teaspoon ground black pepper

1 teaspoon cayenne pepper

1 teaspoon ground cumin

½ teaspoon ground cinnamon

½ teaspoon crushed red pepper

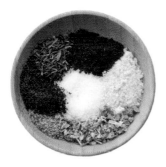

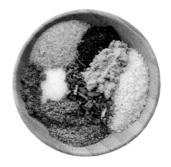

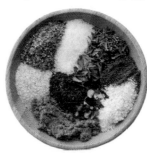

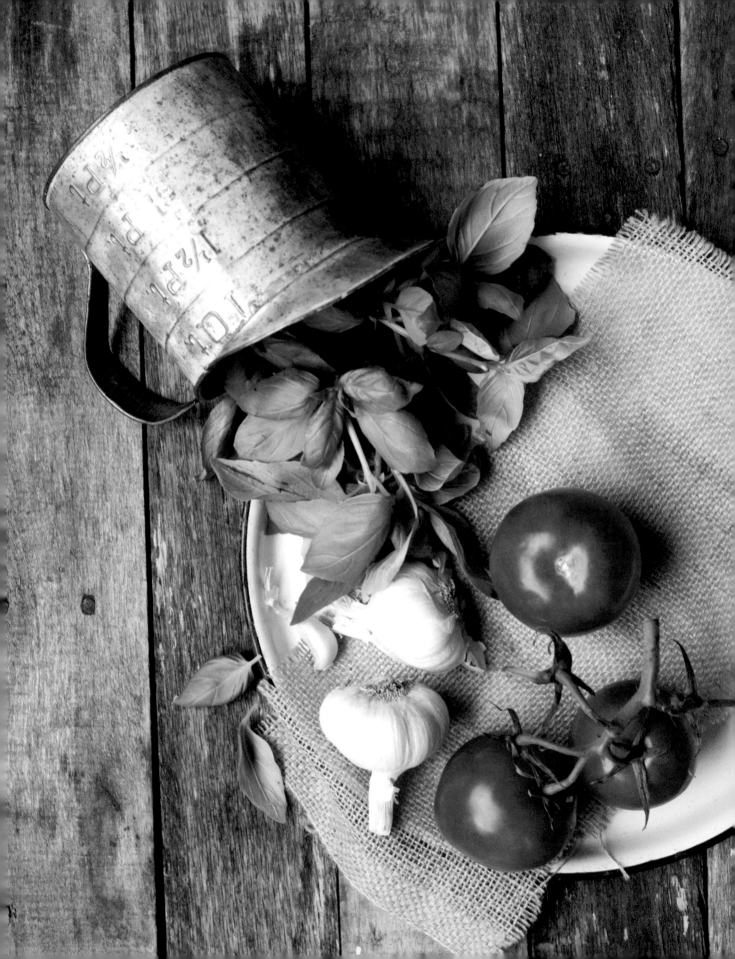

resources

Products

Because the ingredients in some products and their availability change so frequently, I keep a continuously updated list on my website of the brands, products, and resources I recommend.

For a list of my favorites, visit:

www.PaleoCupboard.com/resources

Recommended Reading

These are some of the books I recommend to help give you a better understanding of the science and nutritional aspects behind the Paleo diet. Each has a slightly different perspective, which can help give you a well-rounded view of what may or may not work best for you.

The Paleo Solution by Robb Wolf

It Starts with Food by Dallas Hartwig and Melissa Hartwig

Eat the Yolks by Liz Wolfe

Grain Brain by David Perlmutter

If you find that you are still having negative reactions to some of the foods on a Paleo diet, or you already know you suffer from inflammation or an autoimmune disorder, you may find the following books particularly helpful:

The Autoimmune Solution by Amy Myers

The Paleo Approach by Sarah Ballantyne

Informational Websites

Local Food Sources: Directories for local farmers, farmers markets, and resources for finding local produce and pasture-raised meats, poultry, and eggs

www.localharvest.org

www.eatwild.com

www.eatwellguide.org

Monterey Bay Aquarium's Seafood Watch Program: Up-to-date recommendations for seafood that's fished or farmed in ways that have less impact on the environment

www.seafoodwatch.org

Natural Resources Defense Council: Mercury Contamination in Fish: Guide to mercury levels in different kinds of fish

www.nrdc.org/health/effects/mercury/guide.asp

Dirty Dozen and Clean Fifteen: Lists of conventionally grown fruits and vegetables that test lowest and highest for pesticide residue

www.ewg.org/foodnews/summary.php

Food Safety Guidelines: Recommendations on how long to store different foods in the refrigerator, freezer, or cupboard, as well as the most recent recommended cooking times

www.foodsafety.gov/keep/charts/index.html

Nutrition Calculators: Online tools for finding nutritional information, such as calories, fat, protein, carbs, and more, for ingredients and recipes

nutritiondata.self.com/mynd/myrecipes

recipes.sparkpeople.com/recipe-calculator.asp

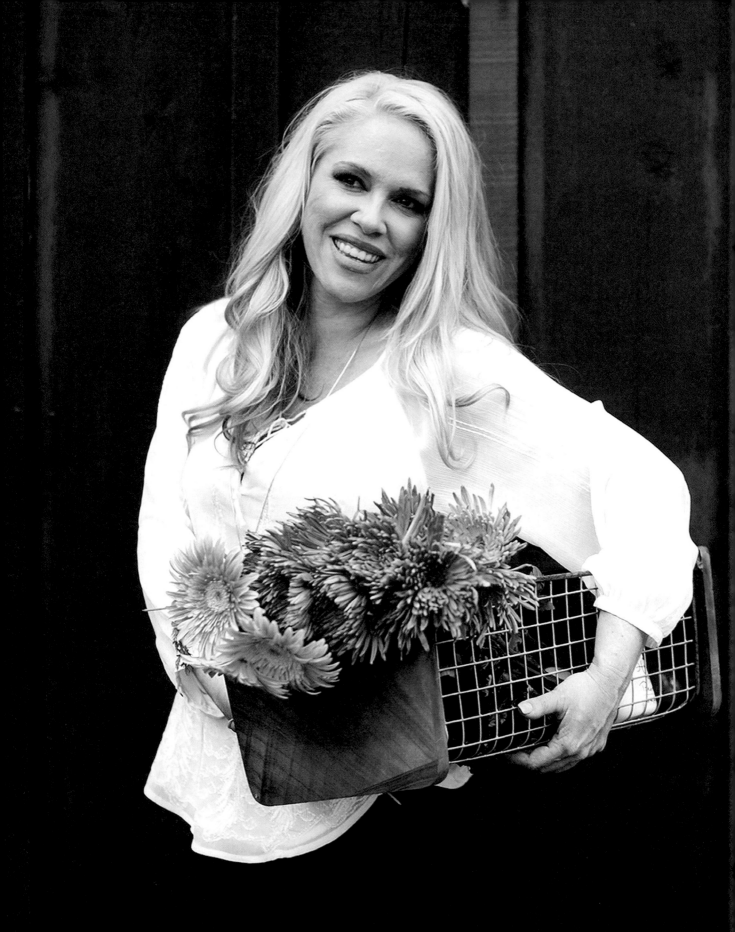

acknowledgments

To my laptop

Thank you for not suddenly deleting my entire manuscript, despite my many nightmares that had me convinced that you would do so. I enjoyed the many late nights we spent together.

To my followers

Thank you for the support and joy you give me on a daily basis. I am honored to be able to share my experiences, stories, and love of food and cooking with you. Your emails, comments, and words of encouragement mean the world to me. Thank you so much for letting me be a part of your journey.

To the Victory Belt team

Thank you for giving me this incredible opportunity to share my ideas and recipes with others. You had me the moment you told me I could "do things my way," and you have supported my vision all the way through to the end. Thank you for believing in me.

To my friends

Thank you for keeping me sane through this process, and for convincing me to take a risk and write a cookbook. There were many days I silently wanted to throw in the "tea towel," and it was your constant support that carried me forward. I am so lucky to have such amazing people in my life. Thank you for sticking by me, for being my sounding boards, and for laughing at my bad jokes.

To my mom

Thank you for everything you do for me. If it wasn't for your support I wouldn't be able to accomplish everything I can every single day. No matter how headstrong I am and how much I dig in my heels, you continue to motivate me to be the best person I can be. Thank you for reminding me to pause, enjoy life, and live in the moment.

To my small but mighty family

Thank you for being so understanding while I turned our lives upside-down for a few months. I know it wasn't fun having me spend all of my free time playing mad scientist in the kitchen, but you still patiently supported me and helped me every step of the way. Thank you for being my food choppers, taste testers, dish washers, hug givers, and my biggest fans.

To my grandmother

Thank you for teaching me that I can do anything I set my mind to. You taught me that cooking is about so much more than just eating, and that nourishing family and friends is a true act of love. I miss you every single day, and while you might only be with me in spirit, you inspire everything I do. This book is for you.

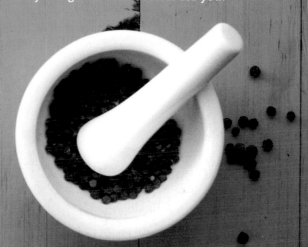

recipes by category

40 Minutes or Less

- Almond Flour (page 316)
- Aloha Chicken Dippers (page 106)
- Apple and Sage Sausage Patties (page 54)
- Apple Cider (page 288)
- Apple Mojito (page 290)
- Asian Sesame Chicken Salad (page 216)
- Avocado Basil Cream Sauce (page 270)
- Balsamic Rosemary Mushrooms (page 182)
- BLT Scallops with Herb Mayo (page 156)
- Blueberry Muffins (page 56)
- Breakfast Pizza (page 58)
- Broccoli and Mushroom Frittata (page 60)
- Broccoli Raisin Salad (page 217)
- Brussels Sprouts and Bacon Salad (page 218)
- Brussels Sprouts with Capers and Pancetta (page 184)
- Calamari Fritti with Tomato Basil Dipping Sauce (page 160)
- Chicken Salad on Apple Slices (page 114)
- Chile Rellenos with Ranchero Sauce (page 100)
- Chimichurri (page 273)
- Cilantro Lime Shrimp with Avocado Puree (page 164)
- Coconut Cream Tarts (page 250)
- Coconut Flour (page 313)
- Creamsicle Smoothie (page 302)
- Creamy Coleslaw (page 188)
- Creamy Mushroom Soup (page 226)
- Creamy Thai Pasta with Beef Strips (page 86)
- Crispy Sweet Potato Wedges (page 190)
- Eggplant Dip (page 271)
- Eggs Baked in Tomato Sauce (page 66)
- Fried Cauliflower Rice (page 202)

- Grab-and-Go Omelets (page 68)
- Guacamole (page 274)
- Honey Chipotle Meatballs (page 88)
- Honeydew Mint Agua Fresca (page 296)
- Hot Dulce de Leche (page 294)
- Hummus (page 276)
- Ketchup (page 275)
- Lemon and Thyme Chicken Thighs (page 120)
- Lemon Poppyseed Waffles (page 72)
- Mashed Sweet Potatoes (page 189)
- Mayonnaise (page 278)
- Melon Granita (page 258)
- Mexican Cauliflower Rice (page 204)
- Mexican Shrimp Bisque (page 232)
- Mongolian Beef (page 90)
- Mussels in Thai Curry Sauce (page 170)
- Pan-Roasted Carrots with Gremolata (page 192)
- Pasta (page 194)
- Pesto (page 280)
- Pico de Gallo (page 282)
- Piña Colada Smoothie (page 304)
- Pizza Stuffed Mushrooms (page 142)
- Pork Schnitzel (page 152)
- Roasted Asparagus with Lemon Sauce (page 196)
- Roasted Squash and Pesto (page 198)
- Seafood Fra Diavolo (page 174)
- Seasoned Cauliflower Rice (page 200)
- Seasoning Blends and Rubs (page 330)
- Sesame Ginger Broccolini (page 206)
- Smoked Salmon Deviled Eggs (page 176)
- Sour Cream (page 281)
- Soy Sauce Substitute (page 283)
- Spaghetti Squash Noodles (page 326)

- Spicy Beef and Pepper Stir-Fry (page 98)
- Spinach and Bacon Salad (page 220)
- Strawberry Avocado Smoothie (page 306)
- Sweet and Sour Pork (page 146)
- Sweet Potato Hash with Spicy Hollandaise (page 76)
- Sweet Potato Noodles (page 327)
- Tartar Sauce (page 284)
- Tex-Mex-Style Pork Chops (page 148)
- Thai Coconut Soup (page 238)
- Thai Iced Tea (page 300)
- Tomato Avocado Stack with Crispy Prosciutto (page 222)
- Tortillas (page 210)
- Watermelon Cake (page 266)
- Whipped Coconut Cream (page 261)
- Zucchini Noodles (page 328)
- Zuppa Toscana (page 242)

Egg-Free

Nut-Free

- Aloha Chicken Dippers (page 106)
- Apple and Sage Sausage Patties (page 54)
- Apple Cider (page 288)
- Apple Mojito (page 290)
- Avocado Basil Cream Sauce (page 270)
- Balsamic Rosemary Mushrooms (page 182)
- Bangers and Mash (page 134)
- Barbacoa (page 80)
- BBQ Sauce (page 272)
- Beef Osso Buco (page 82)
- BLT Scallops with Herb Mayo (page 156)
- Broccoli and Mushroom Frittata (page 60)
- Broccoli Raisin Salad (page 217)
- Cajun Chicken Pasta (page 108)
- Chicken Curry (page 110)
- Chicken or Beef Stock (page 310)
- Chile Rellenos with Ranchero Sauce (page 100)
- Chimichurri (page 273)
- Chipotle Shrimp Tacos (page 162)
- Chocolate Soufflé with Strawberry Sauce (page 248)
- Cilantro Lime Shrimp with Avocado Puree (page 164)
- Cioppino (page 224)
- Coconut Cream (page 315)
- Coconut Flour (page 313)
- Coconut Milk (page 314)
- Coconut Milk Yogurt (page 62)
- Comforting Beef Stew (page 230)
- Creamsicle Smoothie (page 302)
- Creamy Chocolate Mousse (page 252)
- Creamy Coleslaw (page 188)
- Crème Brûlée (page 254)
- Crispy Sweet Potato Wedges (page 190)
- Deviled Scotch Eggs (page 64)
- Eggplant Dip (page 271)
- Eggs Baked in Tomato Sauce (page 66)
- Fish Stock (page 312)
- Fried Cauliflower Rice (page 202)

- Ghee (page 320)
- Grab-and-Go Omelets (page 68)
- Grilled Seafood Skewers (page 168)
- Guacamole (page 274)
- Honey Chipotle Meatballs (page 88)
- Honeydew Mint Agua Fresca (page 296)
- Hot Dulce de Leche (page 294)
- Hummus (page 276)
- Jerk Chicken (page 116)
- Ketchup (page 275)
- Lard (page 322)
- Lemon and Thyme Chicken Thighs (page 120)
- Lemonade (page 298)
- Mayonnaise (page 278)
- Mediterranean Fish (page 178)
- Melon Granita (page 258)
- Mexican Cauliflower Rice (page 204)
- Mexican Shrimp Bisque (page 232)
- Mongolian Beef (page 90)
- Moroccan Chicken (page 122)
- Mussels in Thai Curry Sauce (page 170)
- Orange and Ginger Glazed Salmon (page 172)
- Orange Chicken (page 118)
- Pan-Roasted Carrots with Gremolata (page 192)
- Pico de Gallo (page 282)
- Piña Colada Smoothie (page 304)
- Piri Piri Chicken (page 124)
- Pork Chile Verde (page 136)
- Pork Ragout (page 138)
- Pork Vindaloo (page 140)
- Provençal Chicken (page 126)
- Roasted Asparagus with Lemon Sauce (page 196)
- Salted Caramel Sauce (page 260)
- Seafood Fra Diavolo (page 174)
- Seasoned Cauliflower Rice (page 200)
- Seasoning Blends and Rubs (page 330)
- Sesame Chicken Wings (page 128)
- Sesame Ginger Broccolini (page 206)

- Simple Slow Cooker Chicken (page 130)
- Slow Cooker Applesauce (page 207)
- Slow Cooker Pork Ribs (page 144)
- Smoked Salmon Deviled Eggs (page 176)
- Sour Cream (page 281)
- Soy Sauce Substitute (page 283)
- Spaghetti Squash Noodles (page 326)
- Spiced Carrot and Ginger Soup (page 234)
- Spicy Beef and Pepper Stir-Fry (page 98)
- Spicy Smashed Sweet Potatoes (page 208)
- Spinach and Bacon Salad (page 220)
- Strawberry Avocado Smoothie (page 306)
- Summer Vegetable Casserole (page 212)
- Sweet and Sour Pork (page 146)
- Sweet Potato Hash with Spicy Hollandaise (page 76)
- Sweet Potato Noodles (page 327)
- Taco Soup (page 236)
- Tallow (page 324)
- Tartar Sauce (page 284)
- Tex-Mex-Style Pork Chops (page 148)
- Thai Coconut Soup (page 238)
- Thai Iced Tea (page 300)
- Tomato Avocado Stack with Crispy Prosciutto (page 222)
- Tomato Basil Soup with Crispy Shallots (page 240)
- Tuscan Pork Roast (page 150)
- Watermelon Cake (page 266)
- Whipped Coconut Cream (page 261)
- Zucchini Noodles (page 328)

Kid Favorites

- Almond Milk (page 318)
- Aloha Chicken Dippers (page 106)
- Apple and Sage Sausage Patties (page 54)
- Apple Cider (page 288)
- Asian Sesame Chicken Salad (page 216)
- Balsamic Rosemary Mushrooms (page 182)
- Bangers and Mash (page 134)
- BBQ Sauce (page 272)
- Blackberry Peach Upside-Down Cake (page 246)
- Blueberry Muffins (page 56)
- Breakfast Pizza (page 58)
- Broccoli Raisin Salad (page 217)
- Cajun Chicken Pasta (page 108)
- Chicken Piccata (page 112)
- Chicken Salad on Apple Slices (page 114)
- Chocolate Soufflé with Strawberry Sauce (page 248)
- Cider Baked Apples (page 262)
- Coconut Cream Tarts (page 250)
- Coconut Milk (page 314)
- Coconut Milk Yogurt (page 62)
- Colcannon (page 186)
- Comforting Beef Stew (page 230)
- Cottage Pie (page 84)
- Creamsicle Smoothie (page 302)
- Creamy Chocolate Mousse (page 252)

- Creamy Coleslaw (page 188)
- Creamy Mushroom Soup (page 226)
- Crème Brûlée (page 254)
- Crispy Sweet Potato Wedges (page 190)
- Fish & Chips (page 166)
- Fried Cauliflower Rice (page 202)
- Grab-and-Go Omelets (page 68)
- Granola (page 70)
- Horchata (page 292)
- Hot Dulce de Leche (page 294)
- Ketchup (page 275)
- Lemon and Thyme Chicken Thighs (page 120)
- Lemon Bars (page 256)
- Lemon Poppyseed Waffles (page 72)
- Lemonade (page 298)
- Mashed Sweet Potatoes (page 189)
- Mayonnaise (page 278)
- Melon Granita (page 258)
- Mexican Cauliflower Rice (page 204)
- Mongolian Beef (page 90)
- Orange Chicken (page 118)
- Pasta (page 194)
- Pasta Bolognese (page 92)
- Piña Colada Smoothie (page 304)
- Pizza Stuffed Mushrooms (page 142)
- Popcorn Chicken-Fried Steak and Gravy (page 94)
- Pork Ragout (page 138)
- Pork Schnitzel (page 152)

- Provençal Chicken (page 126)
- Roasted Squash and Pesto (page 198)
- Salted Caramel Sauce (page 260)
- Seasoned Cauliflower Rice (page 200)
- Sesame Chicken Wings (page 128)
- Simple Slow Cooker Chicken (page 130)
- Slow Cooker Applesauce (page 207)
- Slow Cooker Pork Ribs (page 144)
- Sour Cream (page 281)
- Spaghetti Squash Noodles (page 326)
- Strawberry Avocado Smoothie (page 306)
- Summer Vegetable Casserole (page 212)
- Swedish Meatballs (page 102)
- Sweet and Sour Pork (page 146)
- Sweet Crêpes (page 74)
- Sweet Potato Noodles (page 327)
- Sweet Potato Pie (page 264)
- Taco Soup (page 236)
- Tex-Mex-Style Pork Chops (page 148)
- Tortillas (page 210)
- Tuscan Pork Roast (page 150)
- Watermelon Cake (page 266)
- Whipped Coconut Cream (page 261)
- Zucchini Noodles (page 328)
- Zuppa Toscana (page 242)

recipe index

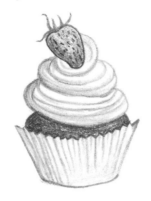

Breakfast

54

Apple and Sage Sausage Patties

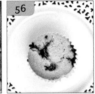
56

Blueberry Muffins

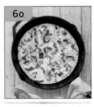
58

Breakfast Pizza

60

Broccoli and Mushroom Frittata

62

Coconut Milk Yogurt

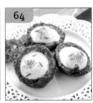
64

Deviled Scotch Eggs

66

Eggs Baked in Tomato Sauce

68

Grab-and-Go Omelets

70

Granola

72

Lemon Poppy-seed Waffles

74

Sweet Crêpes

76

Sweet Potato Hash with Spicy Hollandaise

Beef

80

Barbacoa

82

Beef Osso Buco

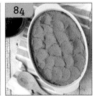
84

Cottage Pie

86

Creamy Thai Pasta with Beef Strips

88

Honey Chipotle Meatballs

90

Mongolian Beef

92

Pasta Bolognese

94

Popcorn Chicken-Fried Steak and Gravy

96

Satay with Dipping Sauce

98

Spicy Beef and Pepper Stir-Fry

100

Chile Rellenos with Ranchero Sauce

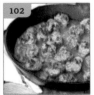
102

Swedish Meatballs

Chicken

 106
Aloha Chicken Dippers

 108
Cajun Chicken Pasta

 110
Chicken Curry

 112
Chicken Piccata

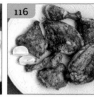 114
Chicken Salad on Apple Slices

 116
Jerk Chicken

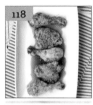 118
Orange Chicken

 120
Lemon and Thyme Chicken Thighs

 122
Moroccan Chicken

 124
Piri Piri Chicken

 126
Provençal Chicken

 128
Sesame Chicken Wings

 130
Simple Slow Cooker Chicken

Pork

 134
Bangers and Mash

 136
Pork Chile Verde

 138
Pork Ragout

 140
Pork Vindaloo

 142
Pizza Stuffed Mushrooms

 144
Slow Cooker Pork Ribs

 146
Sweet and Sour Pork

 148
Tex-Mex-Style Pork Chops

 150
Tuscan Pork Roast

 152
Pork Schnitzel

Seafood

 156
BLT Scallops with Herb Mayo

 158
Cajun Shrimp and Grits

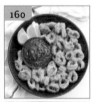 160
Calamari Fritti with Tomato Basil Dipping Sauce

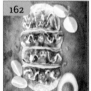 162
Chipotle Shrimp Tacos

 164
Cilantro Lime Shrimp with Avocado Puree

 166
Fish & Chips

 168
Grilled Seafood Skewers

 170
Mussels in Thai Curry Sauce

 172
Orange and Ginger Glazed Salmon

 174
Seafood Fra Diavolo

 176
Smoked Salmon Deviled Eggs

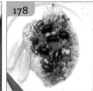 178
Mediterranean Fish

Side Dishes

 182
Balsamic Rosemary Mushrooms

 184
Brussels Sprouts with Capers and Pancetta

 186
Colcannon

 188
Creamy Coleslaw

 189
Mashed Sweet Potatoes

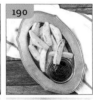 190
Crispy Sweet Potato Wedges

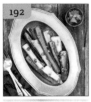 192
Pan-Roasted Carrots with Gremolata

 194
Pasta

 196
Roasted Asparagus with Lemon Sauce

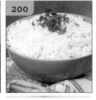 198
Roasted Squash and Pesto

 200
Seasoned Cauliflower Rice

 202
Fried Cauliflower Rice

204
Mexican Cauliflower Rice

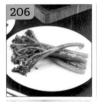 206
Sesame Ginger Broccolini

 207
Slow Cooker Applesauce

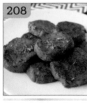 208
Spicy Smashed Sweet Potatoes

 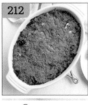 210
Tortillas

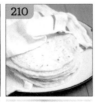 212
Summer Vegetable Casserole

Soups, Stews, and Salads

 216
Asian Sesame Chicken Salad

 217
Broccoli Raisin Salad

 218
Brussels Sprouts and Bacon Salad

 220
Spinach and Bacon Salad

 222
Tomato Avocado Stack with Crispy Prosciutto

 224
Cioppino

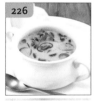 226
Creamy Mushroom Soup

 228
Gumbo

 230
Comforting Beef Stew

 232
Mexican Shrimp Bisque

 234
Spiced Carrot and Ginger Soup

 236
Taco Soup

 238
Thai Coconut Soup

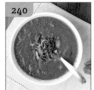 240
Tomato Basil Soup with Crispy Shallots

 242
Zuppa Toscana

Desserts

246
Blackberry Peach Upside-Down Cake

248
Chocolate Soufflé with Strawberry Sauce

250
Coconut Cream Tarts

252
Creamy Chocolate Mousse

254
Crème Brûlée

256
Lemon Bars

258
Melon Granita

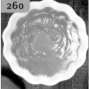
260
Salted Caramel Sauce

261
Whipped Coconut Cream

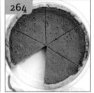
262
Cider Baked Apples

264
Sweet Potato Pie

266
Watermelon Cake

Dips and Sauces

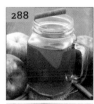
270
Avocado Basil Cream Sauce

271
Eggplant Dip

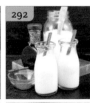
272
BBQ Sauce

273
Chimichurri

274
Guacamole

275
Ketchup

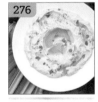
276
Hummus

278
Mayonnaise

280
Pesto

281
Sour Cream

282
Pico de Gallo

283
Soy Sauce Substitute

284
Tartar Sauce

Drinks

288
Apple Cider

290
Apple Mojito

292
Horchata

294
Hot Dulce de Leche

296
Honeydew Mint Agua Fresca

298
Lemonade

300
Thai Iced Tea

302
Creamsicle Smoothie

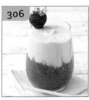
304
Piña Colada Smoothie

306
Strawberry Avocado Smoothie

Basics

310

313

314

316

318

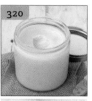
320

Chicken or Beef Stock

Coconut Flour

Coconut Milk

Almond Flour

Almond Milk

Ghee

322

324

326

327

328

330

Lard

Tallow

Spaghetti Squash Noodles

Sweet Potato Noodles

Zucchini Noodles

Seasoning Blends and Rubs

index